FREE Study Skills Videos/DVD Offer

Dear Customer,

Thank you for your purchase from Mometrix! We consider it an honor and a privilege that you have purchased our product and we want to ensure your satisfaction.

As part of our ongoing effort to meet the needs of test takers, we have developed a set of Study Skills Videos that we would like to give you for FREE. These videos cover our *best practices* for getting ready for your exam, from how to use our study materials to how to best prepare for the day of the test.

All that we ask is that you email us with feedback that would describe your experience so far with our product. Good, bad, or indifferent, we want to know what you think!

To get your FREE Study Skills Videos, you can use the **QR code** below, or send us an **email** at studyvideos@mometrix.com with *FREE VIDEOS* in the subject line and the following information in the body of the email:

- The name of the product you purchased.
- Your product rating on a scale of 1-5, with 5 being the highest rating.
- Your feedback. It can be long, short, or anything in between. We just want to know your impressions and experience so far with our product. (Good feedback might include how our study material met your needs and ways we might be able to make it even better. You could highlight features that you found helpful or features that you think we should add.)

If you have any questions or concerns, please don't hesitate to contact me directly.

Thanks again!

Sincerely,

Jay Willis
Vice President
jay.willis@mometrix.com
1-800-673-8175

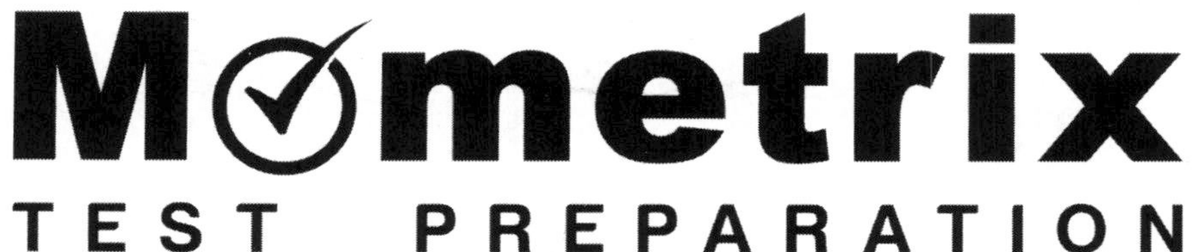

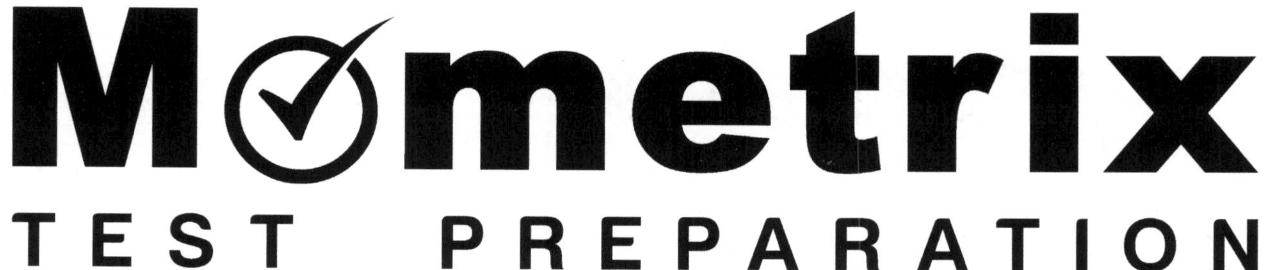

MLT

Exam Secrets Study Guide

MLT Test Review for the Medical Laboratory Technician Examination

Written and edited by Mometrix Test Prep

Printed in the United States of America

This paper meets the requirements of ANSI/NISO Z39.48-1992 (Permanence of Paper).

Mometrix offers volume discount pricing to institutions. For more information or a price quote, please contact our sales department at sales@mometrix.com or 888-248-1219.

Paperback
ISBN 13: 978-1-61072-019-9
ISBN 10: 1-61072-019-9

Ebook
ISBN 13: 978-1-62120-591-3
ISBN 10: 1-62120-591-6

DEAR FUTURE EXAM SUCCESS STORY

First of all, **THANK YOU** for purchasing Mometrix study materials!

Second, congratulations! You are one of the few determined test-takers who are committed to doing whatever it takes to excel on your exam. **You have come to the right place.** We developed these study materials with one goal in mind: to deliver you the information you need in a format that's concise and easy to use.

In addition to optimizing your guide for the content of the test, we've outlined our recommended steps for breaking down the preparation process into small, attainable goals so you can make sure you stay on track.

We've also analyzed the entire test-taking process, identifying the most common pitfalls and showing how you can overcome them and be ready for any curveball the test throws you.

Standardized testing is one of the biggest obstacles on your road to success, which only increases the importance of doing well in the high-pressure, high-stakes environment of test day. Your results on this test could have a significant impact on your future, and this guide provides the information and practical advice to help you achieve your full potential on test day.

Your success is our success

We would love to hear from you! If you would like to share the story of your exam success or if you have any questions or comments in regard to our products, please contact us at **800-673-8175** or **support@mometrix.com**.

Thanks again for your business and we wish you continued success!

Sincerely,
The Mometrix Test Preparation Team

Need more help? Check out our flashcards at:
http://mometrixflashcards.com/MLT

Written and edited by the Mometrix Exam Secrets Test Prep Team
Printed in the United States of America

TABLE OF CONTENTS

Introduction

Thank you for purchasing this resource! You have made the choice to prepare yourself for a test that could have a huge impact on your future, and this guide is designed to help you be fully ready for test day. Obviously, it's important to have a solid understanding of the test material, but you also need to be prepared for the unique environment and stressors of the test, so that you can perform to the best of your abilities.

For this purpose, the first section that appears in this guide is the **Secret Keys**. We've devoted countless hours to meticulously researching what works and what doesn't, and we've boiled down our findings to the five most impactful steps you can take to improve your performance on the test. We start at the beginning with study planning and move through the preparation process, all the way to the testing strategies that will help you get the most out of what you know when you're finally sitting in front of the test.

We recommend that you start preparing for your test as far in advance as possible. However, if you've bought this guide as a last-minute study resource and only have a few days before your test, we recommend that you skip over the first two Secret Keys since they address a long-term study plan.

If you struggle with **test anxiety**, we strongly encourage you to check out our recommendations for how you can overcome it. Test anxiety is a formidable foe, but it can be beaten, and we want to make sure you have the tools you need to defeat it.

Secret Key #1 – Plan Big, Study Small

There's a lot riding on your performance. If you want to ace this test, you're going to need to keep your skills sharp and the material fresh in your mind. You need a plan that lets you review everything you need to know while still fitting in your schedule. We'll break this strategy down into three categories.

Information Organization

Start with the information you already have: the official test outline. From this, you can make a complete list of all the concepts you need to cover before the test. Organize these concepts into groups that can be studied together, and create a list of any related vocabulary you need to learn so you can brush up on any difficult terms. You'll want to keep this vocabulary list handy once you actually start studying since you may need to add to it along the way.

Time Management

Once you have your set of study concepts, decide how to spread them out over the time you have left before the test. Break your study plan into small, clear goals so you have a manageable task for each day and know exactly what you're doing. Then just focus on one small step at a time. When you manage your time this way, you don't need to spend hours at a time studying. Studying a small block of content for a short period each day helps you retain information better and avoid stressing over how much you have left to do. You can relax knowing that you have a plan to cover everything in time. In order for this strategy to be effective though, you have to start studying early and stick to your schedule. Avoid the exhaustion and futility that comes from last-minute cramming!

Study Environment

The environment you study in has a big impact on your learning. Studying in a coffee shop, while probably more enjoyable, is not likely to be as fruitful as studying in a quiet room. It's important to keep distractions to a minimum. You're only planning to study for a short block of time, so make the most of it. Don't pause to check your phone or get up to find a snack. It's also important to **avoid multitasking**. Research has consistently shown that multitasking will make your studying dramatically less effective. Your study area should also be comfortable and well-lit so you don't have the distraction of straining your eyes or sitting on an uncomfortable chair.

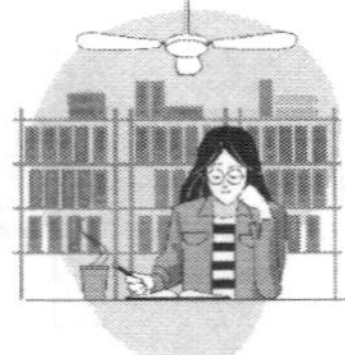

The time of day you study is also important. You want to be rested and alert. Don't wait until just before bedtime. Study when you'll be most likely to comprehend and remember. Even better, if you know what time of day your test will be, set that time aside for study. That way your brain will be used to working on that subject at that specific time and you'll have a better chance of recalling information.

Finally, it can be helpful to team up with others who are studying for the same test. Your actual studying should be done in as isolated an environment as possible, but the work of organizing the information and setting up the study plan can be divided up. In between study sessions, you can discuss with your teammates the concepts that you're all studying and quiz each other on the details. Just be sure that your teammates are as serious about the test as you are. If you find that your study time is being replaced with social time, you might need to find a new team.

Secret Key #2 – Make Your Studying Count

You're devoting a lot of time and effort to preparing for this test, so you want to be absolutely certain it will pay off. This means doing more than just reading the content and hoping you can remember it on test day. It's important to make every minute of study count. There are two main areas you can focus on to make your studying count.

Retention

It doesn't matter how much time you study if you can't remember the material. You need to make sure you are retaining the concepts. To check your retention of the information you're learning, try recalling it at later times with minimal prompting. Try carrying around flashcards and glance at one or two from time to time or ask a friend who's also studying for the test to quiz you.

To enhance your retention, look for ways to put the information into practice so that you can apply it rather than simply recalling it. If you're using the information in practical ways, it will be much easier to remember. Similarly, it helps to solidify a concept in your mind if you're not only reading it to yourself but also explaining it to someone else. Ask a friend to let you teach them about a concept you're a little shaky on (or speak aloud to an imaginary audience if necessary). As you try to summarize, define, give examples, and answer your friend's questions, you'll understand the concepts better and they will stay with you longer. Finally, step back for a big picture view and ask yourself how each piece of information fits with the whole subject. When you link the different concepts together and see them working together as a whole, it's easier to remember the individual components.

Finally, practice showing your work on any multi-step problems, even if you're just studying. Writing out each step you take to solve a problem will help solidify the process in your mind, and you'll be more likely to remember it during the test.

Modality

Modality simply refers to the means or method by which you study. Choosing a study modality that fits your own individual learning style is crucial. No two people learn best in exactly the same way, so it's important to know your strengths and use them to your advantage.

For example, if you learn best by visualization, focus on visualizing a concept in your mind and draw an image or a diagram. Try color-coding your notes, illustrating them, or creating symbols that will trigger your mind to recall a learned concept. If you learn best by hearing or discussing information, find a study partner who learns the same way or read aloud to yourself. Think about how to put the information in your own words. Imagine that you are giving a lecture on the topic and record yourself so you can listen to it later.

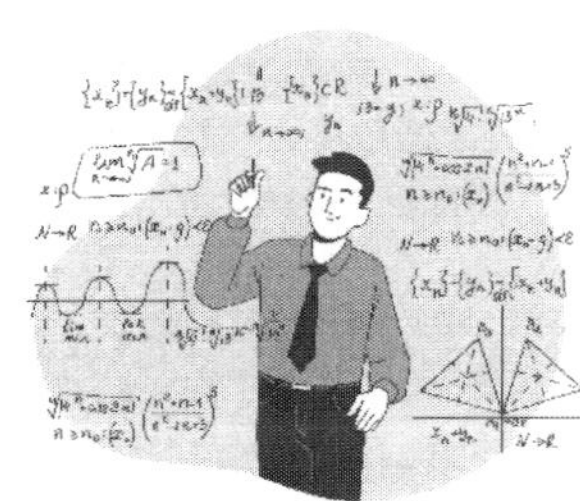

For any learning style, flashcards can be helpful. Organize the information so you can take advantage of spare moments to review. Underline key words or phrases. Use different colors for different categories. Mnemonic devices (such as creating a short list in which every item starts with the same letter) can also help with retention. Find what works best for you and use it to store the information in your mind most effectively and easily.

Secret Key #3 – Practice the Right Way

Your success on test day depends not only on how many hours you put into preparing, but also on whether you prepared the right way. It's good to check along the way to see if your studying is paying off. One of the most effective ways to do this is by taking practice tests to evaluate your progress. Practice tests are useful because they show exactly where you need to improve. Every time you take a practice test, pay special attention to these three groups of questions:

- The questions you got wrong
- The questions you had to guess on, even if you guessed right
- The questions you found difficult or slow to work through

This will show you exactly what your weak areas are, and where you need to devote more study time. Ask yourself why each of these questions gave you trouble. Was it because you didn't understand the material? Was it because you didn't remember the vocabulary? Do you need more repetitions on this type of question to build speed and confidence? Dig into those questions and figure out how you can strengthen your weak areas as you go back to review the material.

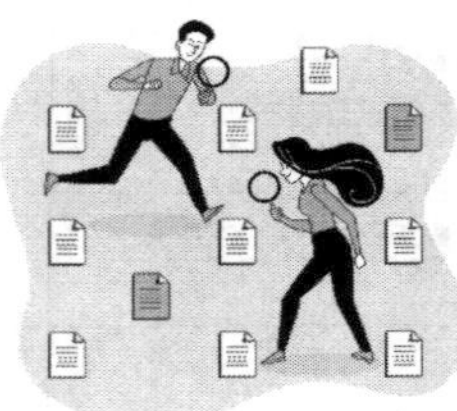

Additionally, many practice tests have a section explaining the answer choices. It can be tempting to read the explanation and think that you now have a good understanding of the concept. However, an explanation likely only covers part of the question's broader context. Even if the explanation makes perfect sense, **go back and investigate** every concept related to the question until you're positive you have a thorough understanding.

As you go along, keep in mind that the practice test is just that: practice. Memorizing these questions and answers will not be very helpful on the actual test because it is unlikely to have any of the same exact questions. If you only know the right answers to the sample questions, you won't be prepared for the real thing. **Study the concepts** until you understand them fully, and then you'll be able to answer any question that shows up on the test.

It's important to wait on the practice tests until you're ready. If you take a test on your first day of study, you may be overwhelmed by the amount of material covered and how much you need to learn. Work up to it gradually.

On test day, you'll need to be prepared for answering questions, managing your time, and using the test-taking strategies you've learned. It's a lot to balance, like a mental marathon that will have a big impact on your future. Like training for a marathon, you'll need to start slowly and work your way up. When test day arrives, you'll be ready.

Start with the strategies you've read in the first two Secret Keys—plan your course and study in the way that works best for you. If you have time, consider using multiple study resources to get different approaches to the same concepts. It can be helpful to see difficult concepts from more than one angle. Then find a good source for practice tests. Many times, the test website will suggest potential study resources or provide sample tests.

Practice Test Strategy

If you're able to find at least three practice tests, we recommend this strategy:

Untimed and Open-Book Practice

Take the first test with no time constraints and with your notes and study guide handy. Take your time and focus on applying the strategies you've learned.

Timed and Open-Book Practice

Take the second practice test open-book as well, but set a timer and practice pacing yourself to finish in time.

Timed and Closed-Book Practice

Take any other practice tests as if it were test day. Set a timer and put away your study materials. Sit at a table or desk in a quiet room, imagine yourself at the testing center, and answer questions as quickly and accurately as possible.

Keep repeating timed and closed-book tests on a regular basis until you run out of practice tests or it's time for the actual test. Your mind will be ready for the schedule and stress of test day, and you'll be able to focus on recalling the material you've learned.

Secret Key #4 – Pace Yourself

Once you're fully prepared for the material on the test, your biggest challenge on test day will be managing your time. Just knowing that the clock is ticking can make you panic even if you have plenty of time left. Work on pacing yourself so you can build confidence against the time constraints of the exam. Pacing is a difficult skill to master, especially in a high-pressure environment, so **practice is vital**.

Set time expectations for your pace based on how much time is available. For example, if a section has 60 questions and the time limit is 30 minutes, you know you have to average 30 seconds or less per question in order to answer them all. Although 30 seconds is the hard limit, set 25 seconds per question as your goal, so you reserve extra time to spend on harder questions. When you budget extra time for the harder questions, you no longer have any reason to stress when those questions take longer to answer.

Don't let this time expectation distract you from working through the test at a calm, steady pace, but keep it in mind so you don't spend too much time on any one question. Recognize that taking extra time on one question you don't understand may keep you from answering two that you do understand later in the test. If your time limit for a question is up and you're still not sure of the answer, mark it and move on, and come back to it later if the time and the test format allow. If the testing format doesn't allow you to return to earlier questions, just make an educated guess; then put it out of your mind and move on.

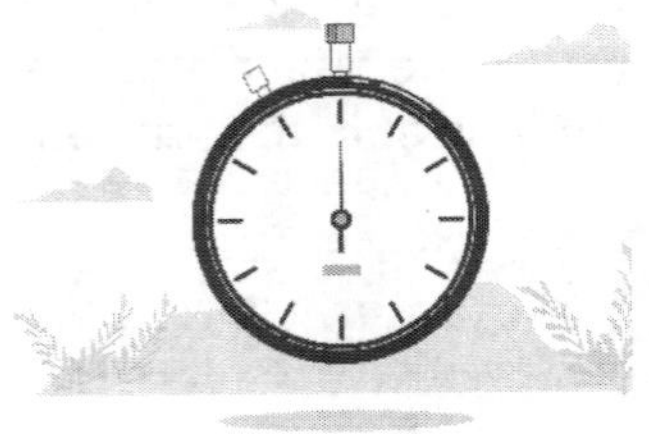

On the easier questions, be careful not to rush. It may seem wise to hurry through them so you have more time for the challenging ones, but it's not worth missing one if you know the concept and just didn't take the time to read the question fully. Work efficiently but make sure you understand the question and have looked at all of the answer choices, since more than one may seem right at first.

Even if you're paying attention to the time, you may find yourself a little behind at some point. You should speed up to get back on track, but do so wisely. Don't panic; just take a few seconds less on each question until you're caught up. Don't guess without thinking, but do look through the answer choices and eliminate any you know are wrong. If you can get down to two choices, it is often worthwhile to guess from those. Once you've chosen an answer, move on and don't dwell on any that you skipped or had to hurry through. If a question was taking too long, chances are it was one of the harder ones, so you weren't as likely to get it right anyway.

On the other hand, if you find yourself getting ahead of schedule, it may be beneficial to slow down a little. The more quickly you work, the more likely you are to make a careless mistake that will affect your score. You've budgeted time for each question, so don't be afraid to spend that time. Practice an efficient but careful pace to get the most out of the time you have.

Secret Key #5 – Have a Plan for Guessing

When you're taking the test, you may find yourself stuck on a question. Some of the answer choices seem better than others, but you don't see the one answer choice that is obviously correct. What do you do?

The scenario described above is very common, yet most test takers have not effectively prepared for it. Developing and practicing a plan for guessing may be one of the single most effective uses of your time as you get ready for the exam.

In developing your plan for guessing, there are three questions to address:

- When should you start the guessing process?
- How should you narrow down the choices?
- Which answer should you choose?

When to Start the Guessing Process

Unless your plan for guessing is to select C every time (which, despite its merits, is not what we recommend), you need to leave yourself enough time to apply your answer elimination strategies. Since you have a limited amount of time for each question, that means that if you're going to give yourself the best shot at guessing correctly, you have to decide quickly whether or not you will guess.

Of course, the best-case scenario is that you don't have to guess at all, so first, see if you can answer the question based on your knowledge of the subject and basic reasoning skills. Focus on the key words in the question and try to jog your memory of related topics. Give yourself a chance to bring the knowledge to mind, but once you realize that you don't have (or you can't access) the knowledge you need to answer the question, it's time to start the guessing process.

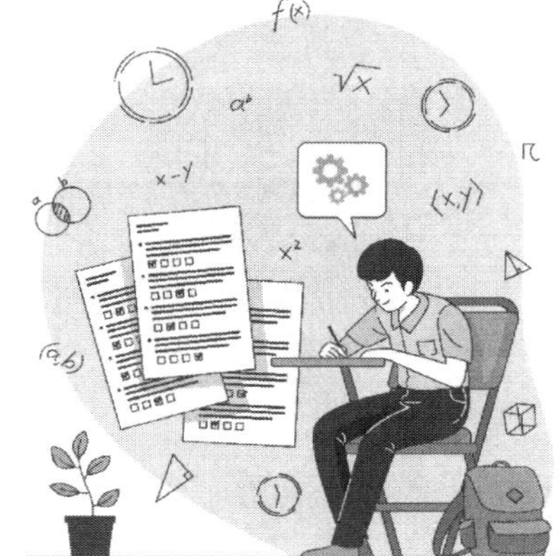

It's almost always better to start the guessing process too early than too late. It only takes a few seconds to remember something and answer the question from knowledge. Carefully eliminating wrong answer choices takes longer. Plus, going through the process of eliminating answer choices can actually help jog your memory.

Summary: Start the guessing process as soon as you decide that you can't answer the question based on your knowledge.

How to Narrow Down the Choices

The next chapter in this book (**Test-Taking Strategies**) includes a wide range of strategies for how to approach questions and how to look for answer choices to eliminate. You will definitely want to read those carefully, practice them, and figure out which ones work best for you. Here though, we're going to address a mindset rather than a particular strategy.

Your odds of guessing an answer correctly depend on how many options you are choosing from.

Number of options left	5	4	3	2	1
Odds of guessing correctly	20%	25%	33%	50%	100%

You can see from this chart just how valuable it is to be able to eliminate incorrect answers and make an educated guess, but there are two things that many test takers do that cause them to miss out on the benefits of guessing:

- Accidentally eliminating the correct answer
- Selecting an answer based on an impression

We'll look at the first one here, and the second one in the next section.

To avoid accidentally eliminating the correct answer, we recommend a thought exercise called **the $5 challenge**. In this challenge, you only eliminate an answer choice from contention if you are willing to bet $5 on it being wrong. Why $5? Five dollars is a small but not insignificant amount of money. It's an amount you could afford to lose but wouldn't want to throw away. And while losing $5 once might not hurt too much, doing it twenty times will set you back $100. In the same way, each small decision you make—eliminating a choice here, guessing on a question there—won't by itself impact your score very much, but when you put them all together, they can make a big difference. By holding each answer choice elimination decision to a higher standard, you can reduce the risk of accidentally eliminating the correct answer.

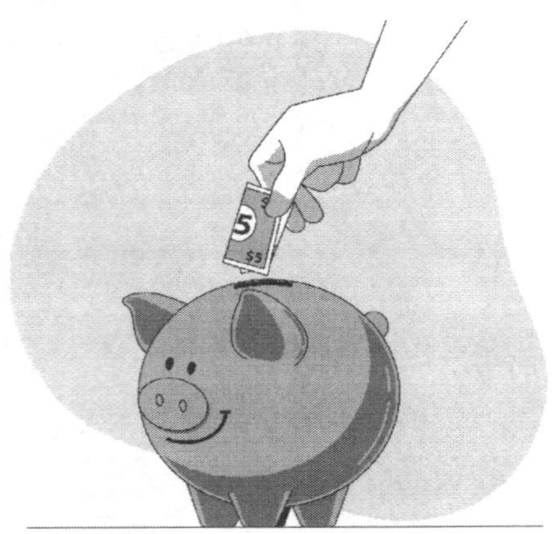

The $5 challenge can also be applied in a positive sense: If you are willing to bet $5 that an answer choice *is* correct, go ahead and mark it as correct.

Summary: Only eliminate an answer choice if you are willing to bet $5 that it is wrong.

Which Answer to Choose

You're taking the test. You've run into a hard question and decided you'll have to guess. You've eliminated all the answer choices you're willing to bet $5 on. Now you have to pick an answer. Why do we even need to talk about this? Why can't you just pick whichever one you feel like when the time comes?

The answer to these questions is that if you don't come into the test with a plan, you'll rely on your impression to select an answer choice, and if you do that, you risk falling into a trap. The test writers know that everyone who takes their test will be guessing on some of the questions, so they intentionally write wrong answer choices to seem plausible. You still have to pick an answer though, and if the wrong answer choices are designed to look right, how can you ever be sure that you're not falling for their trap? The best solution we've found to this dilemma is to take the decision out of your hands entirely. Here is the process we recommend:

Once you've eliminated any choices that you are confident (willing to bet $5) are wrong, select the first remaining choice as your answer.

Whether you choose to select the first remaining choice, the second, or the last, the important thing is that you use some preselected standard. Using this approach guarantees that you will not be enticed into selecting an answer choice that looks right, because you are not basing your decision on how the answer choices look.

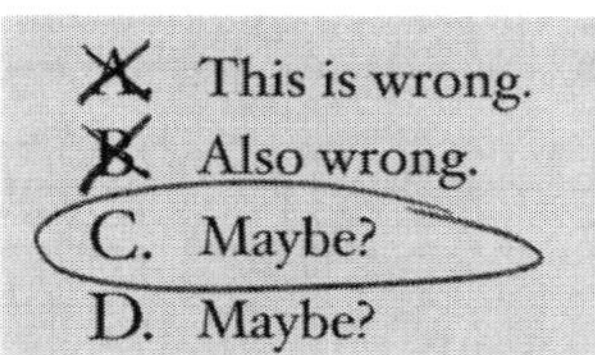

This is not meant to make you question your knowledge. Instead, it is to help you recognize the difference between your knowledge and your impressions. There's a huge difference between thinking an answer is right because of what you know, and thinking an answer is right because it looks or sounds like it should be right.

Summary: To ensure that your selection is appropriately random, make a predetermined selection from among all answer choices you have not eliminated.

Test-Taking Strategies

This section contains a list of test-taking strategies that you may find helpful as you work through the test. By taking what you know and applying logical thought, you can maximize your chances of answering any question correctly!

It is very important to realize that every question is different and every person is different: no single strategy will work on every question, and no single strategy will work for every person. That's why we've included all of them here, so you can try them out and determine which ones work best for different types of questions and which ones work best for you.

Question Strategies

✓ Read Carefully

Read the question and the answer choices carefully. Don't miss the question because you misread the terms. You have plenty of time to read each question thoroughly and make sure you understand what is being asked. Yet a happy medium must be attained, so don't waste too much time. You must read carefully and efficiently.

✓ Contextual Clues

Look for contextual clues. If the question includes a word you are not familiar with, look at the immediate context for some indication of what the word might mean. Contextual clues can often give you all the information you need to decipher the meaning of an unfamiliar word. Even if you can't determine the meaning, you may be able to narrow down the possibilities enough to make a solid guess at the answer to the question.

✓ Prefixes

If you're having trouble with a word in the question or answer choices, try dissecting it. Take advantage of every clue that the word might include. Prefixes can be a huge help. Usually, they allow you to determine a basic meaning. *Pre-* means before, *post-* means after, *pro-* is positive, *de-* is negative. From prefixes, you can get an idea of the general meaning of the word and try to put it into context.

✓ Hedge Words

Watch out for critical hedge words, such as *likely, may, can, sometimes, often, almost, mostly, usually, generally, rarely,* and *sometimes.* Question writers insert these hedge phrases to cover every possibility. Often an answer choice will be wrong simply because it leaves no room for exception. Be on guard for answer choices that have definitive words such as *exactly* and *always.*

✓ Switchback Words

Stay alert for *switchbacks.* These are the words and phrases frequently used to alert you to shifts in thought. The most common switchback words are *but, although,* and *however.* Others include *nevertheless, on the other hand, even though, while, in spite of, despite,* and *regardless of.* Switchback words are important to catch because they can change the direction of the question or an answer choice.

⊘ Face Value

When in doubt, use common sense. Accept the situation in the problem at face value. Don't read too much into it. These problems will not require you to make wild assumptions. If you have to go beyond creativity and warp time or space in order to have an answer choice fit the question, then you should move on and consider the other answer choices. These are normal problems rooted in reality. The applicable relationship or explanation may not be readily apparent, but it is there for you to figure out. Use your common sense to interpret anything that isn't clear.

Answer Choice Strategies

⊘ Answer Selection

The most thorough way to pick an answer choice is to identify and eliminate wrong answers until only one is left, then confirm it is the correct answer. Sometimes an answer choice may immediately seem right, but be careful. The test writers will usually put more than one reasonable answer choice on each question, so take a second to read all of them and make sure that the other choices are not equally obvious. As long as you have time left, it is better to read every answer choice than to pick the first one that looks right without checking the others.

⊘ Answer Choice Families

An answer choice family consists of two (in rare cases, three) answer choices that are very similar in construction and cannot all be true at the same time. If you see two answer choices that are direct opposites or parallels, one of them is usually the correct answer. For instance, if one answer choice says that quantity *x* increases and another either says that quantity *x* decreases (opposite) or says that quantity *y* increases (parallel), then those answer choices would fall into the same family. An answer choice that doesn't match the construction of the answer choice family is more likely to be incorrect. Most questions will not have answer choice families, but when they do appear, you should be prepared to recognize them.

⊘ Eliminate Answers

Eliminate answer choices as soon as you realize they are wrong, but make sure you consider all possibilities. If you are eliminating answer choices and realize that the last one you are left with is also wrong, don't panic. Start over and consider each choice again. There may be something you missed the first time that you will realize on the second pass.

⊘ Avoid Fact Traps

Don't be distracted by an answer choice that is factually true but doesn't answer the question. You are looking for the choice that answers the question. Stay focused on what the question is asking for so you don't accidentally pick an answer that is true but incorrect. Always go back to the question and make sure the answer choice you've selected actually answers the question and is not merely a true statement.

⊘ Extreme Statements

In general, you should avoid answers that put forth extreme actions as standard practice or proclaim controversial ideas as established fact. An answer choice that states the "process should be used in certain situations, if..." is much more likely to be correct than one that states the "process should be discontinued completely." The first is a calm rational statement and doesn't even make a definitive, uncompromising stance, using a hedge word *if* to provide wiggle room, whereas the second choice is far more extreme.

✅ Benchmark

As you read through the answer choices and you come across one that seems to answer the question well, mentally select that answer choice. This is not your final answer, but it's the one that will help you evaluate the other answer choices. The one that you selected is your benchmark or standard for judging each of the other answer choices. Every other answer choice must be compared to your benchmark. That choice is correct until proven otherwise by another answer choice beating it. If you find a better answer, then that one becomes your new benchmark. Once you've decided that no other choice answers the question as well as your benchmark, you have your final answer.

✅ Predict the Answer

Before you even start looking at the answer choices, it is often best to try to predict the answer. When you come up with the answer on your own, it is easier to avoid distractions and traps because you will know exactly what to look for. The right answer choice is unlikely to be word-for-word what you came up with, but it should be a close match. Even if you are confident that you have the right answer, you should still take the time to read each option before moving on.

General Strategies

✅ Tough Questions

If you are stumped on a problem or it appears too hard or too difficult, don't waste time. Move on! Remember though, if you can quickly check for obviously incorrect answer choices, your chances of guessing correctly are greatly improved. Before you completely give up, at least try to knock out a couple of possible answers. Eliminate what you can and then guess at the remaining answer choices before moving on.

✅ Check Your Work

Since you will probably not know every term listed and the answer to every question, it is important that you get credit for the ones that you do know. Don't miss any questions through careless mistakes. If at all possible, try to take a second to look back over your answer selection and make sure you've selected the correct answer choice and haven't made a costly careless mistake (such as marking an answer choice that you didn't mean to mark). This quick double check should more than pay for itself in caught mistakes for the time it costs.

✅ Pace Yourself

It's easy to be overwhelmed when you're looking at a page full of questions; your mind is confused and full of random thoughts, and the clock is ticking down faster than you would like. Calm down and maintain the pace that you have set for yourself. Especially as you get down to the last few minutes of the test, don't let the small numbers on the clock make you panic. As long as you are on track by monitoring your pace, you are guaranteed to have time for each question.

✅ Don't Rush

It is very easy to make errors when you are in a hurry. Maintaining a fast pace in answering questions is pointless if it makes you miss questions that you would have gotten right otherwise. Test writers like to include distracting information and wrong answers that seem right. Taking a little extra time to avoid careless mistakes can make all the difference in your test score. Find a pace that allows you to be confident in the answers that you select.

⊘ Keep Moving

Panicking will not help you pass the test, so do your best to stay calm and keep moving. Taking deep breaths and going through the answer elimination steps you practiced can help to break through a stress barrier and keep your pace.

Final Notes

The combination of a solid foundation of content knowledge and the confidence that comes from practicing your plan for applying that knowledge is the key to maximizing your performance on test day. As your foundation of content knowledge is built up and strengthened, you'll find that the strategies included in this chapter become more and more effective in helping you quickly sift through the distractions and traps of the test to isolate the correct answer.

Now that you're preparing to move forward into the test content chapters of this book, be sure to keep your goal in mind. As you read, think about how you will be able to apply this information on the test. If you've already seen sample questions for the test and you have an idea of the question format and style, try to come up with questions of your own that you can answer based on what you're reading. This will give you valuable practice applying your knowledge in the same ways you can expect to on test day.

Good luck and good studying!

Blood Banking

Blood Products

Blood Donor Requirements, Blood Collection Methods, and Directed or Autologous Donations

Collection methods include whole blood collection and apheresis. Collection is an aseptic technique that requires a closed collection system. The volume of donation and testing samples taken cannot exceed 10.5 mL of whole blood per kilogram of patient body weight. **Directed** donations are made for a specific patient, and **autologous** donations are for oneself, typically before surgery. **Apheresis** collections follow the same criteria and preparation as whole blood donations, but a machine removes the elements needed and returns the remainder back to the body.

Blood donor criteria:

- Must be **healthy;** i.e., must feel well and chronic conditions must be controlled
- **Age**: ≥ 16 years
- **Oral temperature**: ≤37.5 °C or ≤99.5 °F
- **Blood pressure**: must be within normal limits, as defined by the individual institutions
- **Hgb/Hct**: ≥12.5 g/dL/≥38%
- **Weight:** minimum 110 lb/50 kg

Common deferrals:

- **1 year:** possible human immunodeficiency virus (HIV), hepatitis, or malaria exposure; recipient of blood products; tattoos; mucous membrane or skin penetration exposure to blood; or >72 hours spent in a correctional facility
- **3 years:** asymptomatic visitor/immigrant from malarial endemic area or previously diagnosed with malaria
- **Indefinite/Permanent:** viral hepatitis (after age 11); positive HBsAg or hepatitis B virus nucleic acid testing result; repeatedly reactive anti-HBc or anti-human T cell leukemia-lymphoma virus (HTLV); past infection of hepatitis C virus (HCV), HTLV, HIV, or *Trypanosoma cruzi*; or a family history/risk of Creutzfeldt-Jakob disease.

Determining Whether Whole Blood Donation is Possible

Example Scenario	Decision	Reason
A 33-year-old woman with a hematocrit of 38	Allowed	Hematocrit is above minimum acceptable level of 36
A 48-year-old man who received a blood transfusion 5 months ago	Not allowed	Recent blood transfusion creates possibility of hepatitis transmission; hepatitis B has an incubation period of six months

Example Scenario	Decision	Reason
A 21-year-old woman who received a tattoo 14 months ago	Allowed	Individuals are not allowed to donate blood within 12 months of receiving a tattoo
A 35-year-old man who went on a trip to Nigeria 3 months ago	Not allowed	Individuals who do not take a prophylactic for malaria before visiting Africa may donate within six months of their return; individuals who do take a prophylactic must wait three years from their return

Adverse Reactions

On occasion, an individual will experience an adverse reaction when donating blood. Fainting, nausea, rapid breathing, and dizziness are all common side effects of donation. When these or more severe side effects, like convulsions or heart trouble, occur, the tech should immediately remove the tourniquet and blood collection bag. Cold compresses and smelling salts may be appropriate. In especially severe cases, one should make sure that the individual's airway is open and that his or her pulse rate is normal.

Label Requirements of Donated Blood Products

Donated blood products must have a label with the following information: contents; amount of blood collected; volume of blood collected; expiration date; unique number for that particular donated unit; ABO and D type of the blood component; donor classification; prescription requirements; warning regarding infectious agents; FDA license number; information regarding the Circular of Information; type and amount of anticoagulant; and recommended storage temperature.

Routine Processing and Testing of Donor Blood

Each unit of **blood** or **blood component** is required to be **labeled** with the following:

- Name of the product (red blood cells [RBCs], whole blood, etc.)
- Type and amount of anticoagulant
- Unit volume
- Storage temperature
- Name and address of the collecting facility and the Food and Drug Administration (FDA) registration or license number
- Expiration date
- Unique donor ID number
- Volunteer, autologous, or paid donor must be denoted
- The following phrases must be present on all blood component labels:
    - Properly identify intended recipient
    - ℞ only
    - See the circular of information for indications, contraindications, cautions, and methods of infusion.

Routine screening tests performed on donor samples:

- ABO, Rh, antibody screen
- Syphilis
- HIV
- Cytomegalovirus (CMV)
- Hepatitis B and C — HBsAg, anti-HCV, anti-HBc

- Human T cell lymphotropic virus 1 and 2 (HTLV-I/II) antibody
- West Nile virus
- Trypanosoma cruzi antibodies.

Temperature Requirements, Additives, and Anticoagulants

Anticoagulants and preservatives added to **RBCs** are typically a combination of citrate and dextrose (citrate phosphate dextrose [**CPD**] or citrate phosphate double dextrose [**CP2D**] solutions). **Citrate** acts as an anticoagulant by binding to calcium in the blood and effectively preventing the coagulation cascade from being activated. **Dextrose** provides an energy source to RBCs for viability. An inorganic phosphate buffer (**A-1**) may also be added to prolong RBC viability by increasing the production of adenosine triphosphate (**ATP**). Blood products containing CPD or CP2D may be stored at 1–6 °C for 21 days, and those containing CPDA-1 may be stored at 1–6 °C for 35 days.

Saline adenine glucose (**SAG**) solutions can be added to RBCs to extend the primary anticoagulant storage (**AS**) stability to 42 days at 1–6 °C. Common SAG uses include:

- AS-1 (SAG plus mannitol) with CPD
- AS-3 (SAG plus sodium phosphate, sodium citrate, and citric acid) with CP2D
- AS-5 (ADSOL).

Blood components are available for transfusion until 11:59 pm (2359) on the date of expiration posted on the unit's label. After expiration, components that are not eligible for rejuvenation must be removed from stock and disposed of into biohazard waste bins.

Transporting Blood Components and Visual Properties of Stored Products

RBCs: 1–6 °C — insulated cooler with cold packs to sustain optimal temperature; cannot have direct contact with cool pack; towels or bubble wrap may be used as a barrier between them.

Platelets 20–24 °C (room temperature) — container insulted from exposure to external temperatures.

Frozen components (fresh frozen plasma [FFP] or cryoprecipitated antihemophilic factor [AHF], more commonly known as cryoprecipitate, or cryo): must be kept frozen using an insulated cooler with dry ice.

During storage, it is imperative that all blood products remain in a closed system to avoid loss of quality and to avoid potential bacterial contamination. Storage at proper temperatures will also aid in reducing contamination risks. Upon visual inspection, RBCs should be a deep-red color, with no cloudiness or clots observed. Platelets, FFP, and cryo should not have any clots or particulate matter observed during the storage process.

Blood Components

Packed Red Blood Cells (PRBCs)

Packed red blood cells (**PRBCs**) are prepared by collecting whole blood and separating the RBCs from the plasma by sedimentation or centrifugation. PRBCs are kept at 1–6 °C until issued for transfusion and cannot be returned to the lab if the seal is disturbed or if the unit temperature exceeds 10 °C. This product achieves the same oxygen-carrying capacity as transfusing whole blood, with less volume of product.

- **Storage/Stability:** 1–6 °C for 21 days with CPD or CP2d, 35 days with CPDA-1
- **Indications**: Low O_2-carrying capacity — anemias, ongoing or massive bleed
- **Expected outcome**: One unit of PRBCs will raise hemoglobin by 1 g or hematocrit by 3%

Cryoprecipitated Antihemophilic Factor (AHF)

Cryoprecipitated antihemophilic factor (AHF), more commonly known as cryoprecipitate, or **cryo**, is a cold-insoluble portion of plasma formed when FFP is brought to 1–6 °C, separated from the thawed FFP, and refrozen within 1 hour. Units of cryo must contain ≥150 mg of fibrinogen and ≥80 IU/bag of factor VIII. Clotting factors also found in cryo include von Willebrand factor (vWF), ristocetin cofactor activity, fibronectin, and factor XIII.

- **Storage/Stability**: 1 year after collection at −18 °C, 6 hours at room temperature after being thawed
- **Indications:** Fibrinogen loss due to disseminated intravascular coagulation (DIC) or massive bleeding, dysfibrinogenemia with bleeding
- **Expected outcome**: Clotting in efforts to achieve hemostasis

Plasma

Plasma separated from cells through centrifugation and frozen within 8 hours of collection is known as fresh frozen plasma (**FFP**). FFP is used to introduce clotting factors to the body when it is deficient. This product must be ABO compatible to the recipient to avoid transfusion reactions to residual RBC antibodies.

- **Storage/Stability**: 1 year after collection at −18 °C, 7 years at ≤−18 °C, 24 hours at 1–6 °C once thawed at 30–37 °C
- **Indications:** Coagulation deficiencies, factor XI deficiencies, congenital deficiencies, warfarin toxicity, massive transfusions
- **Expected outcome**: Clotting in efforts to achieve hemostasis

Platelets

Platelets can be collected via whole blood samples or apheresis. Whole blood-derived platelets are collected by a low-speed spin to separate and remove RBCs, followed by a second centrifugation at more rotations per minute to separate platelets and white cells. Plasma forms a supernatant, which is separated, and the remaining elements (platelets, white blood cells [WBCs], and some plasma) are kept for platelet transfusion. Apheresis platelets are separated at collection with an instrument that separates the blood components and returns the remainder to the donor.

- **Storage/Stability**: 5 days at room temperature (20–24 °C) with constant, gentle agitation
- **Indications:** Severe thrombocytopenia or platelet dysfunction, prophylactic use for low platelet count and moderate/high risk of bleeding, massive transfusions resulting in thrombocytopenia
- **Expected outcome** (the average adult):
  - One unit of platelets increases the platelet count by 5,000–10,000/μL
  - One unit of apheresis platelets increases the platelet count by 20,000–60,000/μL

Leukocyte-Reduced Components

Leukocyte-reduced components are prepared by filtration and require a $< 5 \times 10^6$ white blood cell (**WBC**) concentration per unit of product. The purpose for transfusing leukocyte-reduced products is to prevent **human leukocyte antigen (HLA)** alloimmunization, CMV transmission, and febrile nonhemolytic reactions in recipients. Common factors that increase the probability of such reactions include the presence of cytokines released from WBCs, prior alloimmunization to HLA, or other leukocyte antigens.

- **Storage/Stability**: Consistent with recommended storage conditions for each individual product (RBCs, platelets, etc.)
- **Indications**: Recipient with repeated febrile nonhemolytic reactions to blood products
- **Expected outcome**: Transfusion of blood products without adverse reactions

Apheresis Products and Fractionation Products

Apheresis products are collected with a process that separates out a specific component and returns the remaining blood components back to the donor's body. The advantage of collecting products with this method is there are fewer inadvertent WBCs present in donations, reducing the risk of adverse recipient reaction to WBC antigens during transfusion.

Fractionation of blood products occurs across multiple steps. Whole blood is slowly spun to separate RBCs from platelet-rich plasma. From this plasma, one unit of donor platelets and one unit of FFP can be collected. FFP can be further separated into individual clotting factor concentrates, or cryo, by flash freezing and collecting the plasma protein precipitates. Fractionating blood products allows for more direct transfusions, focused on a specific product, effectively introducing less volume to a recipient's system and limiting unnecessary transfusions.

Plasmapheresis, Plateletpheresis, and Leukapheresis

- **Plasmapheresis**: Form of apheresis in which plasma alone is removed from the blood of the donor; remaining blood products are returned to the donor, who may undergo this process once every eight weeks
- **Plateletpheresis**: Only platelets are removed from donor blood; performed with an electronic apheresis instrument; donors may undergo this process once every 48 hours
- **Leukapheresis**: White blood cells alone are removed from donor blood; performed with electronic apheresis instrument; donors may undergo this process no more than twice a week or 24 times in one year

Whole Blood, Washed RBCs, and Frozen/Deglycerolized RBCs

Units of **whole blood** are not typically transfused due to the availability of various individual blood components. Transfusions of whole blood are most often used in cases of severe shock and hypovolemia with ≥25% loss of blood volume. RBCs will increase O_2 levels, and plasma will replace lost volume in recipients.

Washed RBCs are prepared by removing plasma from the product with successive saline washes. Removing residual plasma from RBCs will remove complement and diminish the presence of IgA on the cells. Washed RBCs are transfused in patients with anti-IgA to reduce the risk of anaphylactic shock from IgA in plasma. Neonatal transfusions also use washed RBCs from maternal blood to remove anti-HPA-1a for safe transfusion.

Frozen/deglycerolized RBCs are treated with a 40% glycerol cryoprotective agent that allows RBCs to be stored at extremely low (≤65 °C) temperatures for up to 10 years. Cells must be thawed at 37 °C, and the glycerol agent must be removed prior to transfusion. This preparation is typically performed on autologous donations or rare units, in which there is a lack of high-incidence antigens.

REJUVENATED RBCS AND IRRADIATED COMPONENTS

Autologous or rare RBC units may be **rejuvenated** to extend their date of expiration. A solution is added to a unit of PRBCs to restore metabolites that have been depleted over time, such as 2,3 DPG and ATP. Cells must be washed prior to transfusion to remove inosine, which may be toxic. Rejuvenation may be done at any point in a unit's shelf life and up to 3 days past its expiration to extend the RBC unit's shelf life an additional 24 hours when stored at 1–6 °C.

Blood components are **irradiated** to inactivate donor T lymphocytes and prevent graft-versus-host disease (GVHD). If not inactivated, donor T lymphocytes may recognize recipient cells as foreign and destroy them. Recipients at risk of GVHD include those receiving blood components from a family member, a fetus in utero, and patients who are immunocompromised by either inherited disease or induced by drug therapy. Irradiated components expire at the original outdate or 28 days after radiation occurs, whichever is first.

STANDARDS FOR BLOOD COMPONENTS

Standards that blood components must meet to be eligible for transfusion are as follows:

Component	Standard
RBCs	Minimum of 80% hematocrit
Leukocyte-reduced RBCs	$< 5 \times 10^6$ leukocytes per unit
Apheresis RBCs	> 60 g hemoglobin per unit
Apheresis RBCs leukocyte-reduced	> 51 g of hemoglobin per unit
Frozen RBCs	≥ 80% original RBC concentration glycerol removed before transfusion
FFP	Frozen within 8 hours of collection
Cryo	≥ 80 IU per unit and 150 mg fibrinogen per unit
Single donor and pooled platelets	$\geq 5.5 \times 10^{10}$ platelets per unit and pH ≥ 6.2
Leukocyte-reduced platelets	$\geq 5.5 \times 10^{10}$ platelets per unit $< 8.3 \times 10^5$ leukocytes per unit (single donor) $< 5 \times 10^6$ leukocytes per unit (pooled)
Apheresis leukocyte-reduced platelets	$\geq 3.0 \times 10^{11}$ platelets per unit pH ≥ 6.2 $< 5 \times 10^6$ leukocytes per unit
Apheresis granulocytes	$\geq 1.1 \times 10^{10}$ granulocytes per unit

Blood Group Systems

MOLECULAR STRUCTURE OF AN ANTIBODY

Every antibody has four molecular chains, two light chains and two heavy chains. The light chains contain a variable region in which the antibody bonding site is found. Some antibodies produce agglutination because of their reactions with the antigens on red blood cells. The heavy chains, on the other hand, determine the antibody's immunoglobulin type

Antibody Enhancer

An antibody enhancer is the chemical that stimulates the formation of antigen-antibody complexes. For instance, the proteolytic enzymes papain, ficin, and bromelain are frequently used as antibody enhancers, because they increase red blood cell agglutination. Bovine albumin, on the other hand, encourages sensitized red blood cells to form agglutination lattices. Low ionic strength solution, known by the abbreviation LISS, is often used to stimulate the formation of antigen-antibody complexes. Finally, polyethylene glycol additive, or PEG, concentrates antibodies.

Human Leukocyte Antigens

Human leukocyte antigens (HLA) exist on both tissue cells and white blood cells, and are encoded by genes in the Major Histocompatibility Complex (MHC). This complex is found on the number six chromosome. For transfusions to be successful, human leukocyte antigens must be the same between donor and recipient for all stem cell, tissue, organ, and bone marrow donations. Otherwise, graft versus host disease is likely. Chills and fevers are the most common immune response to the presence of human leukocyte antigens.

Antigen-Antibody Interactions

The interactions between antigens and antibodies may result in the formation of a complex. An antigen will bond to the variable region on the light molecular chain of a corresponding antibody. These interactions may be stronger or weaker depending on the compatibility of the antigens and the antibody. In vitro, the reactions between an antigen and an antibody cause agglutination or hemolysis; in vivo, they may result in an immune response. The following forces conspire to hold together antigen-antibody complexes: hydrophobic bonding, hydrogen bonding, electrostatic charge, and Van der Waal's force.

Grades of Agglutination Reactions

Red blood cells can manifest six grades of agglutination reaction:

0	Lowest grade; no agglutinative red blood cells are present
+w	Red blood cell button divides into almost invisible or invisible clumps
1 +	Red blood cell button divides into a number of small and medium-sized clumps
2 +	Red blood cell button divides into numerous medium-sized clumps
3 +	Red blood cell button divides into large clumps
4 +	Red blood cell button does not break into clumps; free red blood cells cannot be seen in the background

ABO Blood System

The ABO blood system differentiates based on the amount of A antigens and B antigens on the outside of red blood cells. Individuals who have red blood cells with both A and B antigens on the surface are said to have AB blood. This indicates that such individuals do not have antibodies (IgM) against these antigens in their blood serum. In like fashion, individuals who only have the B antigens on the surface are said to have B blood. Individuals will only have IgM antibodies against the A antigen. Similarly, individuals with type O blood will have red blood cells with neither A nor B antigens on the surface, but blood serum will contain antibodies against both A and B antigens.

Determining Successful Blood Transfusions

Donor	Recipient	Result
A	AB	Successful transfusion, no agglutination
AB	A	Unsuccessful transfusion, agglutination
O	B	Successful transfusion, no agglutination; type O are universal donors
A	O	Unsuccessful transfusion, agglutination
O	AB	Successful transfusion, no agglutination; type AB are universal recipients

Determining Compatibility in Major Crossmatch Test

Donor	Recipient	Reasoning
O+	A-	Incompatible: Recipients blood may contain anti-D antibodies; donors blood contains D antigens
A+	AB+	Compatible: Recipients blood contains neither anti-A nor anti-B antibodies in serum, so donors blood is acceptable
A-	O-	Incompatible: Recipients blood contains both anti-A and anti-B antibodies in serum, so A antigens in the blood of donor will agglutinate
AB-	B-	Incompatible: Recipients blood contains anti-A antibodies in serum, which will agglutinate when mixed with A antigens

Determining Possible Blood Genotypes and Probability of Blood Types for the Offspring

Mother	Father	Offspring	Probability
AB	AO	AA, AO AB BO	A: 50% AB: 25% B: 25%
BO	BO	BB, BO OO	B: 75% O: 25%
OO	AO	AO OO	A: 50% O: 50%
AO	BO	AB AO BO OO	AB: 25% A: 25% B: 25% O: 25%

H Antigen

The H antigen is part of the A and B antigens, functioning as an acceptor molecule for sugars. Blood type A is the H antigen with N-acetylgalactosamine affixed. Blood type B is H antigen with D-galactose affixed. Blood type B is also H antigen with no sugar affixed. Only 0.01% of the world's population has the h antigen rather than the H antigen, known as the Bombay blood group (phenotype hh). These individuals are universal donors because they lack A, B, and H antigens, but can only be transfused with Bombay blood group blood.

Antibody Class Abbreviations

- Kell: abbreviation K; antibody class IgG
- Kidd: Jk; IgG
- Duffy: Fy; IgG
- Lutheran: Lu; IgG and IgM
- Lewis: Le; IgM
- P: P; IgM
- MNS: MNS; IgG and IgM
- Ii: I; IgM

Antigens Related to Blood Group Systems

- Kell: K (kell), k (Cellano), Kpa, Kpb, Kpc, Jsa, Jsb, K11 (Cote), Wka, and Ku; the most common antigens are K12, K13, K16, K18, K19, K20, and K22
- Duffy: Fy^a, Fy^b, Fy3, Fy4, Fy5, and Fy6
- Kidd: Jka, Jkb, and Jk3
- MNS: M, N, S, s, and U; both of the M and N antigens are associated with glycophorin A; the S, s, and U antigens are associated with glycophorin B

Duffy Blood Group System

The Duffy blood group system is a group of antigens (proteins) found on the outsides of erythrocytes (red blood cells). They are distinguished based on their reactions with anti-Fy^a serum. Blood can be said to be Duffy positive, meaning that the Duffy antigen is present on the red blood cells. Blood can also be said to be Duffy negative, meaning that there is no Duffy antigen present. There are three common Duffy phenotypes, and they are Fy(a+b+), Fy(a+b-), and Fy(a-b+). Almost all white people are Duffy positive, and almost all black people of African descent are Duffy negative. Because the Duffy antigen is a receptor for the parasites that can cause malaria, being Duffy negative (not having the Duffy antigen) can help provide resistance against contracting malaria. Furthermore, if a person who is Duffy negative receives blood that is Duffy positive in a blood transfusion, an allergic reaction can occur.

Distinctive Aspects of Blood Groups

- Resistance to malaria infection: Duffy blood group; phenotype Fy(a-b-) is most resistant
- Hemolytic disease of the newborn: Related to Rh, ABO, Kell, MNS, and Duffy blood group systems
- Infection with Mycoplasma pneumoniae: Related to Ii blood group system
- Chronic granulomatous disease: Related to Kell blood group system, especially phenotype K-k-Kp(a-b-)
- Paroxysmal cold hemoglobinuria: Related to P blood group system, especially the Donath-Landsteiner antibody

Determining If RhIg Dose is Needed

Situation	Decision
Rh positive mother, Rh negative baby	The mother is not a candidate for Rhlg because she is Rh positive.
Rh negative mother, Rh negative baby	The mother is not a candidate for Rhlg because even though she is Rh negative, she gave birth to a Rh negative baby.

Situation	Decision
Rh negative mother, D^u negative mother, Rh positive baby	The mother is a candidate for RhIg because she is Rh negative (D^u negative), and she gave birth to a Rh positive baby.
Rh negative mother, D^u negative mother, triplets (one is Rh positive, and two are Rh negative)	The mother is a candidate for RhIg because she is Rh negative, and at least one of her triplets is a Rh positive baby.

Kleihauer-Betke Test

The Kleihauer-Betke test is an acid elution test used to determine the severity or presence of fetal-maternal hemorrhage postpartum. This is accomplished by determining the quantity of fetal red blood cells or hemoglobin present in the mother's blood stream after delivery. This test is performed when a Rh-negative mother has given birth. In this particular test, at a pH of 3.2, a sample of maternal blood is stained with erythrosine B-hematoxylin. Once the stain is applied, the adult hemoglobin (which is soluble in the acid solution) will turn pale. Sometimes the adult hemoglobin is said to become ghost-like. The fetal hemoglobin, on the other end, is not soluble in the acid solution, and remains bright pink. Depending on the amount of fetal hemoglobin present in the maternal blood sample, the appropriate dosage of Rh immune globulin (RhIg) can be administered to the mother to help prevent the formation of Rh antibodies in the mother's blood.

Blood Group Immunology

Immune Response

The immune system's first response to a foreign antigen is the **primary response**. In the primary immune response, there are no circulating antibodies immediately detectable. IgM antibodies are present between 10 and 14 days after immunogenic antigen stimulation. The body's response to a second exposure to the same antigen is known as the **secondary response**. During the secondary immune response, lymphocytes induce an immediate antibody response and detectable amounts of IgM antibody are rapidly present in serum or plasma, followed by detectable IgG antibodies.

T lymphocytes mature in the thymus from CD34+ progenitor cells and participate in cell-mediated immune responses. T cells differentiate into subpopulations with specific functions that include cytotoxicity and the secretion of cytokines. Making up the majority of lymphocytes circulating in peripheral blood, T cells participate in allograft rejection, graft-versus-host reactions, and delayed hypersensitivity. **B lymphocytes** mature from hematopoietic stem cells in the fetal liver and adult bone marrow and contribute to humoral immunity and the adaptive immune system. B cells differentiate into active plasma cells that form and secrete immunoglobulins, and inactive memory B cells that participate in secondary immune responses.

Macrophages participate in the induction of immune responses through antigen presentation and phagocytosis. Embedded in tissues, macrophages are attracted and adhere to foreign organisms by chemotaxis. Macrophages then engulf the foreign material and destroy it with digestive enzymes found in the cells' granules.

Immunoglobulins

Immunoglobulins are antibodies produced by B lymphocytes in response to exposure of foreign material in the body. These immunogenic gamma globulin (Ig) serum antibodies are composed of protein and carbohydrates. All glycoprotein antibody classes share the same basic monomer structure consisting of four polypeptide chains in a Y shape. Pairs of identical heavy and light chains are connected to each other at a hinged region by disulfide bonds to form polypeptide chains. Although only two types of light chains, kappa (κ) and lambda (λ), are common to all immunoglobulin classes, there are a variety of heavy chain chemical structures that differentiate Ig classes from one another. Immunoglobulins contain three constant regions on each heavy chain and one on each light chain that remain the same in every antibody. They also contain one variable region located at the terminal end of each heavy and light chain, with differing amino acid compositions relative to each class of antibody. Immunoglobulins are classified by their molecular weight, structure, and biological activity into the following five classes: IgA, IgD, IgE, IgG, and IgM.

Physical and Biological Properties of Immunoglobulins

IgA molecules are between 160,000 and 500,000 daltons in size, contain alpha (α) heavy chains, and comprise 13% of total circulating antibodies. The two subclasses of IgA molecules are IgA1 and IgA2. **IgA1** is primarily found in serum and is a monomer structure, whereas **IgA2** is structured as a dimer that is most often a secretory immunoglobulin present in tears, saliva, and nasal mucosa. The primary function of IgA molecules is to defend against local infections at mucosal surfaces.

IgD molecules are 180,000 daltons in size, contain delta (δ) heavy chains, and make up 1% of circulating antibodies. IgD molecules are monomers that are present on the surface of B cell lymphocytes that signal the cells to begin activation.

IgE molecules are monomers that are 196,000 daltons in size and contain epsilon (ε) heavy chains. These antibodies circulate in serum in trace amounts and act to release histamines from mast cells in response to an allergy.

IgG molecules are 150,000 daltons in size, contain gamma (γ) heavy chains, and make up 80% of the concentration of total circulating antibodies in serum. IgG antibodies are the only class that is able to cross the placenta from mother to fetus. Four subclasses of IgG antibodies exist, each with a functional difference due to their difference in location and number of disulfide bonds at the constant region of their heavy chains: IgG1, IgG2. IgG3, and IgG4. The variation in IgG subclasses allows for a variety of avenues for antigen binding, immune complex formations, complement activation, and triggering effector cells.

IgM molecules are the largest immunoglobulin at 900,000 daltons in size, contain mu (μ) heavy chains, and have a pentamer structure. IgM accounts for 6% of circulating antibodies in serum and are the best immunoglobulin for fixing with complement due to their multiple binding sites. Participating in the early phases of immune responses, an increased concentration of IgM antibodies indicates a current or acute infection in the body.

Antigen–Antibody Interactions

In an immunocompetent host, organisms and other sources with antigenic properties will induce a response from antibodies. Foreign antigens are recognized by lymphocytes and stimulate the plasma cell production of antibodies that are specific to the epitopes, or antigenic determinants of a foreign antigen. After antibody production, the variable portion of its polypeptide chain, known as the paratope, recognizes the antigen-specific epitopes. The antibody paratope is created with a high affinity for its specific antigen's epitope that will cause the antigen and antibody to bind together in a lock-and-key manner. The type of weak, noncovalent bond formed between the antigen and antibody is determined by the site on the antibody where the bond takes place. The following bonds and interactions are typical of antigen–antibody complexes: electrostatic bonds, hydrogen bonds, van der Waals forces, and hydrophobic interactions. The immune complex formed by antigen–antibody interactions is transported to cellular systems, most commonly macrophages, to be destroyed or deactivated.

ANTIGEN–ANTIBODY INTERACTION TESTING

The presence or absence of an antigen–antibody complex can be visually observed due to agglutination and precipitation. Agglutination and precipitation rely on the aggregation of test antigens with the corresponding antibodies present in a sample. If the antibody is present, the test antigen will bind to the antigen-binding fragment site of two antibodies and create a lattice formation resulting in the visible end product. **Precipitation** testing methods use soluble test antigens that will aggregate with an antibody to cause a precipitate to settle out of a solution. **Agglutination** methods are based on the use of particulate antigens forming a bridge between antibodies, resulting in clumping. Agglutination occurs in two stages, sensitization and lattice formation. **Sensitization** represents the physical attachment of antibodies to antigens and is dependent on certain physical conditions such as pH, temperature, and incubation period. It is imperative to know the properties of specific antibodies because each one reacts best at different pH levels, temperatures, and with or without periods of incubation. Once the sensitization phase is complete, cross-links between sensitized antibodies will result in aggregation during the final phase of lattice formation.

Clumping due to precipitation or agglutination indicates the presence of the suspected antibody in patient serum, aiding in the diagnosis or establishment of exposure to a particular antigen-bearing entity. The absence of a precipitant or agglutinin determines the lack of a specific antibody in serum.

PRECIPITATION TESTING METHODS TO IDENTIFY AND DETERMINE ANTIGEN–ANTIBODY INTERACTION

Precipitation methods for antigen–antibody reactions include the following:

- **Single** or **radial immunodiffusion** is used to determine the concentration of antigen present in a serum sample. Antibodies are imbedded in the agar of a plate with circular wells, where patient serum and known standards are added. The plate is incubated, and diffusion occurs, forming rings of precipitate around the wells. The diameter of each ring is measured and compared on a plotted standard curve, where the concentration of antigen present in the sample is able to be determined.
- **Double immunodiffusion** or **ouchterlony** methods are used to determine a relationship between an antigen and an antibody. A known antibody is added to the wells of an agar plate, with patient sera and known standards added to its surrounding wells. The plate is incubated and diffusion occurs, resulting in a visible band of precipitation. The location of precipitant bands from patient wells is compared to standard wells to determine antigen–antibody identification.
- **Immunoelectrophoresis** uses gel diffusion and electrophoresis to determine the heavy and light chains in immunoglobulins. The trough of the agar is filled with known antibody that is diffused across the gel by electrophoresis with patient serum proteins. At the zone of equivalence, a precipitation arc appears, and the size of the arc is determined by the concentration of antigen present.
- **Immunofixation** combines protein electrophoresis and immunoprecipitation to classify monoclonal gammopathies by determining the heavy and light chains involved. Patient serum is added to six positions on the agarose plate that are electrophoresed to separate proteins. Monospecific antisera are added to five of the lanes, leaving the sixth lane as a reference. If antigen is present in patient sera, bands of antigen–antibody complexes precipitate, wash, and stain, to become easily visible and able to compare to reference immunoglobulin bands.

Agglutination Testing Methods to Identify and Determine Antigen–Antibody Interaction

Agglutination-based methods for antigen–antibody reactions include the following:

- **Direct agglutination** detects antibodies against cellular antigens. A known antigen in the form of an insoluble particulate is added to the patient sample. If antibodies for the antigen are present, an antigen–antibody complex will form and visual clumping is observed. If the antibody is not present, there will be no agglutination in the test field.
- **Passive hemagglutination** uses a soluble antigen to detect an RBC antibody. A patient samples suspected of containing an RBC antibody is serial diluted, and a suspension of reagent RBCs is added to the sample. Cross-links will form between RBCs and visual agglutination will be observed if the antibody is present in the sample. If no antibody is present, the RBC suspension will fail to agglutinate.
- **Passive latex agglutination** uses latex beads coated in soluble reagent antigen to act as a passive carrier. The latex beads are combined with the patient sample to establish the presence or absence of the specific antibody to the reagent antigen. Visible aggregates of the latex beads will form when the antibody binds to antigens on the surface of the beads. If there is no antibody present in a sample, no binding will occur and the latex beads will not agglutinate.

Classical and Alternative Pathways for Complement Activation

Complement is a group of serum proteins that become activated in response to a foreign substance in the body, producing inflammation and **chemotaxis**, or movement, of phagocytic cells to the site of infection. The process of coating target cells for the enhancement complement attachment to phagocytic cells is known as **opsonization**. Activation of complement is achieved through different avenues based on the biologic interaction between a foreign substance and the immune system.

The **classical complement pathway** is activated by the formation of an IgG or IgM antigen–antibody immune complex on the surface of foreign material and begins with the esterase inhibitor, **C1;** the binding protein, **C4;** and a serine protease, **C2**. Complement's **alternative pathway** requires lipopolysaccharides or polysaccharides on that surface of microbes for activation of **C3**.

The classical and alternative pathways converge at the convertase protein, C3, which cleaves into C3a and C3b. **C3a** stimulates inflammation and the release of histamines from complement bound material of the classical pathway. **C3b** binds to microbial cell walls in the alternative pathway, attracting macrophages for the ingestion of the microbe. Following the cleavage of C3, the convertase **C5** is formed, further inducing inflammation and cell lysis with the membrane attach complex.

Physiology and Pathophysiology

Physiology of Blood

Blood Volume Regulation

The average adult has approximately **5 liters** of blood circulating throughout their body. This total volume is comprised of blood flowing through the chambers of the heart, veins, venules, arteries, and capillaries at any given time. Maintaining the appropriate blood volume is necessary for normal functioning of the body to ensure constant perfusion to tissues, for nutrient delivery and waste removal, and to avoid hyper- or hypovolemic shock. The **kidneys** are responsible for regulating blood volume by filtering water and solutes out of the blood and then reabsorbing filtrates and water necessary for maintaining proper blood volume. In response to a change in blood volume, the **cardiovascular system** will adjust arterial pressure to ensure adequate perfusion to tissues. The **bone marrow** is responsible for creating the cells, which make up the solid portion of the blood volume. The **nervous system** stimulates the portions of the body that are necessary for maintaining proper blood circulation and volume.

Oxygenation and Circulation of Blood

Blood from the superior and inferior venae cavae enters the right atrium of the heart. From there, it flows through the right tricuspid and into the right ventricle, where right ventricular contraction opens the pulmonary semilunar valve. Blood flows through the pulmonary valve and into the pulmonary trunk. It is then distributed to the lungs by the left and right pulmonary arteries to lose carbon dioxide (CO_2) and gain O_2. Blood then flows from the lungs to the left atrium via the pulmonary veins and then through the mitral valve to the left ventricle. Left ventricular contraction opens the aortic semilunar valve, where oxygenated blood from the aorta is distributed to all parts of the body via the arteries and capillaries. Necessary fluids and nutrients are dispersed to interstitial tissues, and waste products are then picked up by the blood. The veins carry the O_2-poor and waste-containing blood back to the heart to begin the process again.

Composition and Functions of Blood

The blood is composed of 55% liquid and 45% cellular elements. The liquid and cellular composition of blood and its functions are as follows:

- **Plasma**: the liquid portion, composed of several substances with differing functions
  - **Water**: absorbed from the intestines to maintain adequate blood volume
  - **Proteins**: maintain osmotic pressure
    - **Albumin**: maintains blood volume and pressure
    - **Globulins**: aid in substance transport and fighting infection
    - **Fibrinogen**: aids in coagulation
  - Gases:
    - **O_2**: necessary for cellular respiration
    - **CO_2**: end product of cellular metabolism
  - **Nutrients**: lipids, glucose, and amino acids absorbed from the intestines and used as food for cells
  - **Nitrogenous waste**: uric acid and urea produced in the liver and excreted by the kidneys
  - Hormones and vitamins: aid in metabolism
- **RBCs**: transport O_2 and aid in the transport of carbon dioxide (CO_2)
- **WBCs**: fight infections
  - **Neutrophils**: phagocytize pathogens
  - **Lymphocytes**: provide humoral and cell-mediated immunity
  - **Eosinophils**: engulf and destroy allergens and antigen–antibody complexes
  - **Monocytes**: act as macrophages to engulf and destroy pathogens and debris created by cellular breakdown
  - **Basophils**: inflammation response mediator; releases histamine and heparin to promote blood flow to injured tissue
- **Platelets**: aid in clotting and hemostasis.

Effects of Abnormal Blood Composition Physiology

Blood is composed of cells and substances from various systems of the body. A variety of clinical signs and symptoms may be caused by abnormalities in the blood composition. Dehydration causes the plasma volume to decrease and the hematocrit level to increase. The decrease in fluid volume will also elevate serum sodium levels and serum osmolality, while decreasing the volume of urine output. A lack of O_2 in the blood does not allow for proper cellular respiration to take place, and tissues will become damaged if O_2 levels remain low. Low hemoglobin caused by the lysing of RBCs or a large amount of blood loss can be responsible for a lack of O_2 being delivered to important tissues and organs. The buildup of waste materials in the blood due to the failure or impairment of another organ system can cause toxic consequences if waste materials are not cleared from a patient's system. A decreased amount of circulating WBCs in blood can cause a system to become immunocompromised and more susceptible to life-threatening infections. Low WBC counts can be caused by chemotherapy treatments or other immunosuppressive drugs. Increased bleeding can occur due to a lack of clotting caused by a decrease in platelet numbers and function. Abnormalities of blood composition are often related to a failure or disturbance in another portion of the body and can be corrected with the appropriate medical interventions.

Survival and Metabolization of RBCs, WBCs, and Platelets in Circulation

RBCs have a life span of **120 days** after they have been released from the bone marrow and into peripheral circulation. Degraded RBCs are removed from circulation by phagocytic cells located in the blood vessels of the liver, spleen, bone marrow, and lining of lymph node channels. Iron and protein from the hemoglobin molecule are stored and transported back to the bone marrow to be used in the formation of new RBCs. Ironless heme molecules become waste products on RBC metabolism. The waste products are converted to bilirubin and urobilinogen and excreted in the stool and urine.

After being released from the bone marrow, **WBCs** circulate in peripheral blood for approximately **10 hours** before they accumulate into the walls of blood vessels and tissues where they survive for **4–5 days**. As phagocytic white cells begin to degrade due to their digestive granules, macrophages will surround and consume them. Portions of WBCs may be removed, whereas waste products will be metabolized in the liver and excreted by the intestinal and urinary tracts and the lungs and through saliva.

Platelets survive in the peripheral blood for **5–10 days** once that are released into circulation. Old and degraded platelets are removed from circulation, destroyed, and digested by macrophages that reside in the spleen and liver.

Hemostasis and Coagulation

Role of Platelets in Coagulation

Some 30% of platelets are stored in the spleen, and 70% are present in the circulating peripheral blood. Normal platelets function to maintain the endothelial lining of blood vessels by activating the coagulation response, aiding in coagulation mechanisms, and decreasing or halting blood loss during an injury to the endothelium. Adhesion of platelets to the injured endothelium takes place with glycoprotein Ib on platelets binding to exposed collagen and secreting ADP, factor V, and fibrinogen to stimulate other platelets. ADP-stimulated platelets change shapes from disks, to spheres, to pseudopods, and they assemble in links to best adhere and aggregate at the injury site. Fibrinogen binds together links of platelets in the first phase of aggregation, and, with strong stimuli, an irreversible platelet plug is formed. Platelets secreting arachidonic acid, and ultimately producing thromboxane A2, will allow the platelet plug to stay localized to an injury and prevent excess clotting throughout the body.

FUNCTIONS OF COAGULATION FACTORS

Coagulation factors, along with plasma proteins, tissues, and calcium, work with one another on the surface of platelets to form fibrin clots. A cascade must be followed through these factors and mechanisms properly for adequate clot formation. Listed below are the coagulation factors and their functions in the coagulation cascade:

Factor	Name	Function
I	Fibrinogen	Forms clots
II	Prothrombin	Activates I, I, VII, VIII, XI, XIII, protein C, and platelets
III	Tissue factor	Cofactor of VIIa
IV	Ionized calcium	Needed for factors to bind to phospholipids
V	Labile factor	Cofactor of X; forms the prothrombinase complex
VII	Stable factor	Activates IX and X
VIII:C	AHF	Cofactor of IX; forms tenase complex
VIII:vWF	von Willebrand factor (vWF)	Cofactor; accelerates enzymatic reactions
IX	Plasma thromboplastin component	Activates X; forms a tenase complex with VIII
X	Stuart–Prower factor	Activates II; forms a prothrombinase complex with V
XI	Plasma thromboplastin antecedent	Activates IX
XII	Hageman factor	Activates XI, VII, PK, and plasminogen
XIII	Fibrin-stabilizing factor	Crosslinks fibrin
PK	Prekallikrein	Activates XII and PK; cleaves HMWK
HMWK	High-molecular-weight kininogen	Supports activation of XII, XI, and PK

COAGULATION FACTOR DISORDERS

Coagulation factor disorders cause a deficiency or dysfunction of coagulation factors that leads to a disruption in the coagulation process. These disorders and their causes are listed below:

- Hereditary:
    - Hemophilia A and hemophilia B are X-chromosome, sex-linked recessive disorders that almost exclusively affect males as spontaneous bleeding into joints. **Hemophilia A** is caused by a deficiency of **factor VIII:C,** and **Hemophilia B** occurs from a **factor IX** deficiency. Treatment is achieved by transfusing commercial factor VIII and factor IX concentrates, respectively.
    - **Hemophilia C** is an incomplete autosomal recessive disorder that causes a **factor XI** deficiency, with symptoms presenting in a wide range of severity and treated with plasma infusions.
    - **Von Willebrand disease** is caused by a primary defect of **factor VIII:vWF** and a deficiency of **factor VIII**. This autosomal-dominant disease causes defects in platelet adhesion and affects males and females equally. To maintain hemostasis, von Willebrand disease is treated with cryo transfusions and mild cases are treated with desmopressin (DDAVP).
    - **Factor XIII deficiency** is an extremely rare, autosomal-recessive disorder that causes significant bleeding and poor wound healing and is treated with factor XIII concentrate.

- Acquired:
  - **Inhibitors** such as **lupus anticoagulant antibodies** and **factor VIII inhibitors** are IgG antibodies directed against a factor or phospholipids causing clotting issues.
  - **Vitamin K deficiency** due to poor diet or broad-spectrum antibiotic use causes a functional deficiency of factors II, VII, IX, and X. Clotting is disrupted by proteins in vitamin K's absence being present but not functional.

Thrombocytopenia and Thrombocytosis

Thrombocytopenia is defined as a platelet count of $\leq 100 \times 10^9/L$. A patient's platelet count may be low due to the decreased production of platelets, certain diseases and deficiencies, sequestration, or the destruction of platelets. Decreased platelet production can be caused by decreased or absent megakaryocytes in bone marrow, which is common in patients with leukemia or aplastic anemia and in those taking chemotherapy drugs. Decreased platelet production can also be alcohol induced, HIV associated, or due to vitamin B_{12} and folate deficiencies. An enlarged spleen related to cirrhosis, congestive splenomegaly, or sarcoidosis may sequester platelets, removing them from circulation. Antiphospholipid antibody syndrome, connective tissue disorders, and lymphoproliferative disorders can cause immunologic destruction of platelets, resulting in thrombocytopenia. Nonimmunologic destruction of platelets due to systemic infection or pregnancy can also result in a low platelet count.

A platelet count of $\geq 450 \times 10^9/L$ is classified as **thrombocytosis**. Essential thrombocytosis is due to a myeloproliferative disorder, caused by a clonal abnormality of a hematopoietic stem cell. Overproduction of platelets may also be caused by other disorders such as an acute infection, chronic inflammatory disorder, iron deficiency, or cancer. This is considered reactive thrombocytosis.

Hereditary and Acquired Dysfunctions of Platelets

Hereditary dysfunction of platelets can cause an inability for platelets to properly aggregate or adhere**.** **Glanzmann disease** is an autosomal recessive disorder causing a defect in the glycoprotein IIb/IIIa receptor. Due to this activation dysfunction, platelets cannot aggregate properly. Bernard-Soulier syndrome and von Willebrand disease cause dysfunction in the adhesion process of platelet function. **Bernard-Soulier syndrome** is an autosomal recessive disorder causing a defect in the glycoprotein Ib/IX complex that binds with endothelial von Willebrand factor (vWF). A defect or deficiency in the vWF that is needed for proper adhesion is known as **von Willebrand disease.**

Acquired platelet dysfunction can be caused by long-term use of nonsteroidal anti-inflammatory drugs (NSAIDs), systemic disorders, or cardiopulmonary bypass. Aspirin is a common NSAID that can induce dysfunction of platelet activation and aggregation by preventing the production of thromboxane A2. The mechanism in which cardiopulmonary bypass works to oxygenate blood and return it to the body can cause platelet dysfunction. During the process of cardiopulmonary bypass, fibrinolysis can be activated on the platelets' surface causing the loss of glycoprotein Ib/IX necessary for binding to vWF. The decrease in bound vWF reduces the platelets' ability to adhere to the location of a bleed.

Hemolytic Disease of the Fetus and Newborn (HDFN)

Hemolytic disease of the fetus and newborn (**HDFN**) occurs when a baby's RBCs are positive for an antigen that a mother's RBCs are negative for. Most often, HDFN develops due to ABO or Rh incompatibilities, but it can also occur with potentially any RBC-group incompatibility (anti-c, anti-K, anti-E are common). If the baby's blood enters the mother's circulation during pregnancy or childbirth, the mother's immune system will recognize the foreign antigen and subsequently produce IgG antibodies against it. After sensitization of the mother's RBCs occurs, the IgG antibody can cross the placenta and enter the fetus' circulation. Antibodies react with antigens on the baby's RBCs, coat them, and destroy the RBCs, causing anemia and hyperbilirubinemia.

Ultrasound, including color Doppler, and amniocentesis tests for bilirubin and fetal maturity can detect HDFN and its severity in utero. HDFN can also be detected after birth with samples from the mother and/or baby. Tests performed on samples from the mother can include the rosette test or detection of fetal hemoglobin (HbF) via acid elution, chromatography, or flow cytometry.

Samples from the baby may be tested with the following methods: cord blood ABO/Rh, DAT, hemoglobin, peripheral smear, reticulocyte count, and bilirubin levels.

Treatment and Prevention for HDFN

Treating HDFN can be done in the antepartum or postpartum period depending on the severity of the disease. In mild cases, neonates can be treated with **phototherapy** to clear excess bilirubin from their system. More severe cases may be treated with RBC **exchange transfusions**, with a significant portion of the newborn's blood (most commonly O negative) being transfused with donor RBCs compatible for the mother's blood. **Intrauterine or umbilical vein transfusions** are also an option when delivering the baby is too great of a risk. This will correct severe HDFN and aid in the delivery of a healthy baby.

Prevention of HDFN begins with maternal screening early in pregnancy to establish ABO/Rh type and the presence of antibodies present in her blood. Rh-negative women will be administered **Rh immunoglobulin** at 28 weeks antepartum and within 72 hours after giving birth. Rh immunoglobulin allows for passive immunization of the mother's RBC antibodies and keeps them from attacking incompatible fetal RBCs. Women positive for antibodies due to previous pregnancy or transfusions will have a titer of that antibody monitored throughout pregnancy to detect an active immune response. If the antibody titer increases, the potential for HDFN arises and must be monitored for its severity.

Anemias

Congenital and Acquired Anemias

Congenital anemias are due to an internal dysfunction or deficiency, whereas **acquired anemias** are the result of an external injury or cause. Congenital anemias are caused by dysfunction of the RBC membrane, hemoglobin abnormalities, or enzyme deficiencies that have been genetically inherited by the patient. There are numerous external causes that can contribute to acquired anemia including nutritional deficiencies, DIC, artificial heart valves, alloimmunization, and more.

Detection of congenital and acquired anemias is dependent on the cause of the anemia because they manifest in different ways. Correlation among a patient's signs and symptoms, RBC indices, chemistry tests, and hemoglobin electrophoresis studies allows for the determination of the cause of the anemia.

The treatment of congenital and acquired anemias differs depending on their cause, but the most common treatment for both is blood transfusions. Acquired anemias due to nutritional deficiencies may be treated with supplements of the deficient element, whereas congenital causes for anemia may only be able to be managed with transfusion.

Warm, Cold, and Drug-Induced Immune Hemolytic Anemias

Immune hemolytic anemias develop from the production and binding of antibodies to a patient's own RBC antigens resulting in increased RBC destruction. **Warm immune hemolytic anemia** is induced by **IgG** antibodies coating RBCs, causing them to be prematurely and rapidly lysed in the spleen. **Cold immune hemolytic anemia** is a response to **IgM**-coated RBCs that become fixed with complement and are rapidly destroyed in the liver. These anemias can be induced by certain drugs, other systemic autoimmune diseases, or malignancy, or they may potentially be idiopathic with an unknown etiology.

Detection of immune hemolytic anemias begins with low hemoglobin and hematocrit values. Upon further investigation, **increased reticulocyte counts, spherocytes**, and **polychromatic RBCs** will be observed. **High** RBC distribution widths and mean corpuscular volume indices are a result of the increase in production and the release of immature RBCs into circulation. Diagnosis of immune hemolytic anemias comes from a collective observation of the previously noted signs and symptoms along with a **positive DAT**.

Treatment of this disease includes steroids or other immunosuppressive drugs, removal or resolution of the underlying condition, and blood transfusions to increase the patient's hemoglobin and hematocrit.

Solid Organs and Hematopoietic Progenitor Cells for Transplantation

Solid organ transplantation occurs in patients with failing organs due to chronic conditions that do not respond to alternative forms of treatment. Recipients are administered immunosuppressive drugs prior to transplantation to decrease the risk of the donor organ being rejected. Solid organs require ABO blood group and HLA compatibility for transplantation and the best opportunity for long-term survival of the organ. Most solid organs for transplant come from deceased donors; however, living donors are an option for organs such as a kidney or liver. The geographic distance between the donor and recipient of solid organs also plays an important role in a successful transplant because these tissues are delicate and their survival is time sensitive.

Hematopoietic progenitor cells are stem cells that are obtained from bone marrow, umbilical cord blood, or apheresis peripheral blood. Hematopoietic progenitor cell transplants are used to replenish bone marrow after chemotherapy or radiation treatments or to replace abnormal bone marrow cells with properly functioning cells. Abnormal bone marrow activity can result from congenital immune deficiencies, RBC disorders, anemias, or bone marrow malignancies. Allogenic stem cells for transplant do not need to be ABO compatible but should be HLA-identical to the recipient to decrease the risk of GVHD.

Serologic and Molecular Testing

Routine Tests

Routine Blood Grouping Tests

Blood grouping tests are completed for **ABO** and **Rh** typing of patient and donor blood. ABO typing is determined through forward- and reverse-typing methods, whereas Rh is determined only through forward typing. The reactions and outcomes are as follows:

Anti-A	Anti-B	A_1 Cell	B Cell	ABO Type
+	–	–	+	A
–	+	+	–	B
+	+	–	–	AB
–	–	+	+	O

Anti-D	Rh
+	Pos
–	Neg

Serological testing is also available for the detection of other common clinically significant antigens present on RBCs. A positive antigen test result confirms that the corresponding antibody is not present in patient or donor RBCs, whereas a negative result cannot confirm or deny antibody presence. Following manufacturer procedures, each antiserum may be tested at a variety of temperatures, with enhancement material added; check the cells to verify negative results. Common antisera available include anti-c, anti-C, anti-e, anti-E, anti-K, anti-Jka, anti-Jkb, anti-M, and anti-Fya.

Antibody Detection and Crossmatch Testing

Antibody screen and panel cells are used in testing patient serum to detect and identify the presence of clinically significant antibodies in a patient's blood circulation. Screen and panel cells are commercially produced group O blood cells with specific antigens present on each of the cells. By testing with different enhancement techniques and at a variety of temperatures, positive reactions to these cells aid in the detection and identification of unexpected antibodies in blood recipient samples that may cause transfusion-related reactions if unnoticed.

Crossmatch testing is performed with recipient serum and donor RBCs to determine if the transfusion of donor cells will be compatible with the recipient's blood in vivo. Immediate-spin crossmatches consist of combining patient serum with donor RBCs in a test tube, centrifuging the sample, and grading the reaction on the RBC button that forms in the bottom of the tube. A negative reaction occurs when the RBC button completely breaks apart with slight agitation of the test tube, resulting in a compatible crossmatch. Positive reactions will result in agglutinated RBCs in patient serum, indicating that donor cells are incompatible for transfusion. In instances in which antibodies are present in patient samples, crossmatches are extended to 37 °C and antihuman globulin (AHG) phases to ensure compatibility with donor RBCs.

Clinical Significance of Antibody Identification in Blood Bank Samples

Antibody identification is pertinent in assuring donor cells are compatible and safe for transfusion into recipients. Unexpected antibodies detected with 2–3 commercial screening cells will be further tested with a panel of 10–20 different commercial cells. These cells are mixed with patient serum and are tested at a variety of temperatures with different enhancement media because circulating antibodies react best under different conditions. Further testing may be necessary to identify the specific antibodies present, such as antigen testing or elution and adsorption.

Clinically significant antibodies are those that can cause a reaction within the recipient if their system is exposed to RBCs with the corresponding antigen. Reactions can vary from a fever and hives to hemolytic reactions with life-threatening consequences. Proper identification of these antibodies is necessary to ensure safe transfusion practices and to help patients rather than harm them.

Direct Antiglobulin Testing (DAT)

Direct antiglobulin testing (**DAT**) is performed to determine the presence of IgG antibody or complement-coated RBCs, which indicate several hemolytic anemias. The DAT procedure is comprised of adding antihuman globulin (**AHG**) reagent to patient cells that have been washed in saline three to four times. Cells that have been coated with IgG and/or complement in vivo will react with the antiglobulin and agglutinate (+ DAT). Cells that do not agglutinate (– DAT) must have

IgG and complement-coated checks cells added to prove that AHG was added to the sample and was not neutralized by insufficient washing of patient RBCs. Samples collected in ethylenediaminetetraacetic acid (EDTA)-coated tubes are best for DAT because EDTA chelates Ca^{2+}, preventing complement activation by plasma antibodies and false positives.

Indirect Antiglobulin Test

The indirect antiglobulin test (IAT) measures the sensitization of red blood cells in vitro. The test is performed as follows: patient's blood serum is mixed with red blood cells and incubated at body temperature. Once the IgG antibodies in the serum have had a chance to attach to the red blood cells, the mixture is washed and antihuman globulin is added. Any agglutination indicates IgG antibodies. A false negative may occur when the washing is not done properly or when antihuman globulin is not added to the solution. A false positive may occur when red blood cells are agglutinated before being washed.

Donath-Landsteiner (D-L) Test

The Donath-Landsteiner test indicates whether paroxysmal cold hemoglobinuria is present. When this condition is present, individuals will contain hemoglobin cold temperatures. The roots of this disorder are in the anti-P antibody of the P blood group system. This antibody connects to the surfaces of red blood cells in temperatures below 37 °C and at warmer temperatures causes hemolysis. The Donath-Lansteiner test is performed as follows: a test tube of serum and red blood cells is placed at 4 °C, while a control to his place at 37 °C. The test tube of serum and blood is gradually warmed to 37 °C, at which point the tubes are centrifuged. If after centrifuging neither displays an indication of hemolysis, the test is negative. When the tube containing serum and red blood cells shows evidence of hemolysis, but the control tube does not, the test is positive. If both tubes show evidence of hemolysis, the test is rendered invalid.

Reagents

Antiglobulin Sera

Antisera reagents are a highly purified solution of an antibody used to detect the presence of antigens on human RBCs. Named after their antibody of detection, antisera reagents can be prepared from monoclonal hybridization or through deliberate animal inoculation of antigen, resulting in a purified antibody serum. **Monoclonal hybridization** fuses one clone of human neoplastic antibody-producing cells with splenic lymphocytes from rodents that have been sensitized. Both methods of antisera production allow for standardized and purified antibody concentrations to a specific antigen.

Antisera reagent standards that must be met include the following:

- Antibody specific with proper concentration of antibody to detect antigen
- Meets a certain strength of reaction with corresponding RBCs
- Sterile, clear
- Container with a dropper, labeled with an expiration date
- Stored at 4 °C when not in use
- Manufacturer directions are to be followed; quality assurance procedures must be established and documented.

Blood Grouping Sera and Reagent RBCs

In **forward** or **direct blood typing**, blood grouping sera are mixed with patient RBCs and the presence of absence of a reaction is used to determine the blood type. Reactions that indicate the presence of an antigen are agglutination and hemolysis. **Agglutination** is clumping of RBCs, occurring when antigen in patient cells combines with antibodies in reagent antiserum. This reaction occurs at various strengths and is graded (0 to 4+) depending on its strength. **Hemolysis** occurs when antisera antibodies and patient RBC antigens react with one another's RBCs releasing hemoglobin and producing a clear, cherry-red solution with or without agglutination present.

Reagent RBCs coated in A1- and B-cell antigens and suspended in saline are used to perform **reverse blood type** testing on patient serum. Reactions for reverse type testing are based on the presence or absence of agglutination. No agglutination indicates no serum antibody to the specific reagent antigen, and an agglutinant reaction of varying strengths (0 to 4+) indicates that a serum antibody to the reagent antigen is present.

Special Tests and Reagents

Enzymes

Patient RBCs can be pretreated with enzymes to aid in identifying clinically significant antibodies. **Papain, bromelain, ficin,** and **trypsin** are the proteolytic enzymes used in treating the cells by removing the sialic acid layer of the RBC membrane, allowing more antigenic sites to become available for antibody binding. The use of enzymes aids in antibody identification because of their ability to enhance weakly reacting antibodies and one or multiple antibodies if they are present, while diminishing the reaction of other antibodies. Enzyme-treated cells are tested in an antibody panel, and the results are compared to the untreated patient results to identify an antibody or antibodies present.

- The following antibodies are **enhanced** by enzymes: Kidd, Rh, Lewis, I, P_1.
- The following antibodies are **destroyed** by enzymes: M, N, S, s, Duffy.

Enhancement Media and Lectins

Enhancement media are used to promote antibody binding for an increased ability to detect antigen–antibody interactions. Bovine serum **albumin** promotes antigen–antibody binding by dispersing ionic charges on the RBC surface and decreasing the zeta potential. **Low-ionic-strength saline** includes albumin and glycine to decrease the zeta potential near the RBC surface and increase antibody uptake. **Polyethylene glycol** enhances the interaction between RBCs and antibodies by excluding water molecules from the area surrounding the surface of the RBCs. Removing water molecules from the cell surface area allows RBCs to move closer together, concentrating the antibodies and increasing the antibody uptake.

Lectins are proteins derived from the seeds of plants with ABO blood group specificity that act similarly to IgM antibodies. The proteins are used as commercial antisera to distinguish ABO subgroups and aid in the workup of polyagglutination syndromes. Each lectin has a unique characteristic pattern and reaction against RBCs carrying a particular antigen; for example, *Dolichos biflorus* lectin differentiates A_1 RBCs from the A_2 subgroup by positively reacting with only A_1-coated RBCs.

Adsorptions and Elutions

The method of **adsorption** is used to bind antibodies to RBCs, removing them from plasma, allowing for the analysis and identification of antibodies that may have been masked. This testing method is also a tool for confirming an antigen's presence on RBCs or an antibody's presence in plasma. **Autoadsorption** methods are used to remove autoantibodies from patient plasma through the use of the patient's own RBCs. Most commonly, autoadsorption testing is completed to reveal and identify underlying alloantibodies by removing the interference of warm autoantibodies. **Alloadsorption** methods use reagent RBCs with specific antigens on their surface to remove certain alloantibodies from patient plasma, allowing analysis of underlying alloantibodies to be performed.

Elution methods are used to break the antigen–antibody bond on patient RBCs and release the antibody into a solution. The solution is centrifuged, and the supernatant containing free antibodies, deemed the **eluate**, is tested to determine the antibody specificity. ABO antibodies are often established using an elution method in which the sample is frozen, thawed, and heated, whereas alloantibodies and warm autoantibodies are commonly eluted using an acid solution such as acidic glycine. Elutions are used in complex antibody workups, warm autoantibody detection, HDFN, and during the investigation of transfusion reactions.

Titrations and Cell Separations

Titrations determine the concentration of an antibody in patient serum and the strength of an antigen's expression on RBC samples. The patient sample is serial diluted into tubes with the following dilution of serum to saline in each tube: 1, 2, 4, 8, 32, 64, 128, 256, and 512. Two drops of each dilution and one drop of reagent RBCs coated in antibody-specific antigens are combined in clean test tubes labeled with the corresponding dilution. Each test tube is centrifuged and examined macroscopically for agglutination. Antibody concentrations, or **titers,** are determined by the highest dilution of sample that has an observed reaction of 1+ agglutination.

Reticulocyte cell separation is performed on samples from recently transfused patients to distinguish the patient's native RBCs from donor RBCs in circulation. Reticulocytes are immature RBCs released from the bone marrow that are less dense than mature RBCs. This method uses the differing cell densities to differentiate patient and donor cells. Capillary tubes of the patient sample are centrifuged resulting in mature donor cells settling at the bottom of the tube and less dense immature patient cells remaining at the top. Patient reticulocytes separated off can then be tested for RBC antigens originating from the patient without contamination from donor cell antigens.

ELISA and Molecular Techniques

Enzyme-linked immunosorbent assay (ELISA) is used in testing donor blood samples for transfusion-transmitted diseases including HIV, hepatitis, and syphilis. ELISA methods rely on the formation of antigen–antibody immune complexes to determine the presence of potentially harmful substances in blood donor samples. The antibody to specific disease-causing antigens is imbedded in the ELISA area, the sample is added, and finally a chromogenic substrate is added to the test area. If the distinct antigen is present, the reagent antibody will bind with it on one side and an enzyme-labeled antibody will bind to the other creating an antibody–antigen–antibody "sandwich." The addition of chromogenic substrate will induce a color development of the immune complex to determine the presence of potentially harmful antigens in a sample.

Molecular techniques are used to more accurately identify RBC antigens in patients that are commonly transfused, in samples with weak or discrepant reactions, and for antigens that don't have a reliable antiserum. The **polymerase chain reaction (PCR)** is a common molecular method that amplifies a specific region of deoxyribonucleic acid (DNA) that contains the nucleotides that encode each individual antigen. DNA analysis of a sample will determine the presence or absence of the RBC antigen being tested for.

Thiol Reagents and Immunofluorescence

Thiol reagents dissolve the disulfide bonds made between cysteine amino acids of IgM antibodies and Kell antigens. **Dithiothreitol**, **2-mercaptoethanol (2-ME)**, and **ZZAP**, a mixture of papain and dithiothreitol, are the thiol reagents most commonly used. The use of thiol reagents allows for the

IgG antibodies to be distinguished from IgM by diminishing the activity of IgM antibodies while leaving IgG antibodies unaffected.

Immunofluorescence testing methods use the binding point of a specific antibody to determine the presence or absence of its corresponding antigen. The binding point, or epitope, of the reagent antibody is labeled with a fluorescent dye that will fluoresce if the specific antigen binds to the antibody, indicating its presence in the patient sample. Immunofluorescence techniques may be used for testing donor blood units for transfusion-related diseases.

Solid Phase and Column Agglutination Testing

Solid phase testing determines incompatibilities between plasma antibodies and target RBC antigens. Patient plasma is added to a microwell with a reagent antigen bound to the bottom of the well. Solid phase tests rely on the Fc portion of an antibody in patient plasma attaching to reagent antigens imbedded in the well. Immune complexes formed in a **positive reaction** cause RBCs to diffuse along the bottom of the microwell in a carpet-like appearance. Unbound reagent cells indicate a **negative reaction** by forming an RBC button on the bottom of the well. Solid phase testing can be used with automated systems for blood typing and antibody identification procedures.

Column agglutination, or **gel testing**, uses reagent RBCs and patient plasma added to the top of a viscous gel matrix in individual wells of a gel testing card. The card is incubated and centrifuged, and the reactions in each well are observed and interpreted. Patient samples that do not bind with reagent RBCs will completely settle to the bottom of the gel column for a **negative interpretation**. Agglutination and IgG binding of a **positive antigen–antibody reaction** inhibits RBCs from moving through the matrix, causing them to settle higher in the gel. Patterns of positive and negative antigen–antibody reactions between patient plasma and antigen-coated reagent cells are interpreted to determine blood types, antibody detection and identification, and crossmatch compatibility.

Chloroquine Diphosphate and EDTA Glycine Acid

Chloroquine diphosphate (CDP) and **EDTA glycine acid (EGA)** are reagents used to dissociate IgG antibodies from the surface of RBCs in samples with a positive direct antiglobulin test (DAT). The purpose of dissociating IgG from the RBC membrane is to be able to accurately phenotype patient RBCs. Whereas CDP is able to release IgG bound to RBCs without destroying the surface of the membrane, EGA reagents cause damage to certain antigens on the RBC surface. The main antigens that EGA destroys are from the Kell blood grouping system, making it impossible to phenotype for Kell antigens from an EGA-treated sample. CDP- and EGA-treated samples are commonly used in elutions and autoadsorptions in patients with warm autoimmune hemolytic anemia and in cases of HDFN.

Human Leukocyte Antigens and Cytotoxicity

Human leukocyte antigens (HLAs) are cell surface proteins that can sensitize donor and recipient cells and activate T lymphocytes causing a cytotoxic reaction in blood product recipients. A **cytotoxic reaction** occurs when an antibody combines with an HLA antigen on the surface of a cell, activating the complement system, which ultimately leads to the destruction of the cell. **Class I** HLA antigens are found on platelets, and **Class II** HLA antigens are present on the surface of WBCs. Leukocytes and platelets from donors and recipients can be tested to identify HLA sensitization, determine HLA typing, and find HLA-compatible donors for sensitized recipients.

Due to room-temperature storage conditions and O_2-permeable containers, each unit of platelets is tested for bacterial contamination before being deemed safe for transfusion. Twenty-four hours after collection, a sample of platelet product is obtained and a culture bottle is inoculated with the sample. Automated culture monitoring systems are used to detect metabolic changes that indicate bacterial growth. If the culture does not indicate bacterial growth after 24 hours of incubation, platelet products are released for use labeled "No growth to date."

QUALITY ASSURANCE

BLOOD LABELING REQUIREMENTS

The FDA requires that all blood products and materials used for transfusion be labeled with machine-readable **labeling language** to decrease incidence of errors related to the wrong patient or wrong product. The label must contain at least the unique facility ID, the donor's lot number, the product code, and the blood type of the donor. The two labeling languages in use include:

- **Codabar**: Labeling that includes an identifying barcode, a description of the contents (such as "RED BLOOD CELLS"), the volume, additives, storage requirements, and test results of FDA required tests (such as HIV and HBV.
- **ISB-128**: The international standard for identification and labeling as well as transfer of information about body products, including blood. ISB-128 provides a standard terminology, reference tables to apply the appropriate codes, data structures, delivery mechanisms, and standard layout for labels.

TRANSFUSION RECORD DOCUMENTATION AND TRANSFUSION ADMINISTRATION PROTOCOL

Transfusion record documentation must be maintained for at least 5 years and those required for tracing a blood product from donor to disposition maintained for at least 10 years following administration or 5 years after expiration date. Computerized records must be secure and software validated. Records must include all those associated with the donor, recipient, and blood product, including testing (all steps and results), storage, and disposition. The records must be easily accessible and allow for tracing of blood products. Donor records must be maintained and should include information about storage temperatures and visual blood inspections, and preparation of components. Recipient records should include blood type and information regarding antibodies history of transfusions, and adverse transfusion reactions. Records should also be maintained regarding therapeutic phlebotomy, policies and procedures, cytapheresis procedures, antibody identification, quality control, and shipping.

MAINTAINING PROPER RECORDS OF ALL QUALITY CONTROL AND BLOOD BANK PROCEDURES

Proper **record keeping and documentation** for quality control and blood bank procedures are maintained at 4 different levels:

- Blood bank **polices**: A statement of intent that should include the principles that will be utilized to guide decision-making and procedures and may outline the roles and responsibility of employees as well as financial basis for maintaining the program. An example: Employee practices that ensure blood safety.
- Blood bank **processes**: These should outline the way things happen, including the chain of command and basic methods of dealing with various functions of the blood bank, such as collecting, storing, and distributing blood products.

- Blood bank **procedures**: These are step-by-step explanations of how each blood bank procedure, such as collecting a blood sample or applying a label to a blood product, is carried out, including the equipment and supplies needed.
- Supporting documentation/Forms: These should include all forms of documentation that are required and samples to show the correct manner of completing and filling out forms required forms.

Proper Storage and Transportation of Blood and Blood Products for Transfusions

The FDA and AAB have established temperature standards for storage and transportation of blood and blood products:

Product	Storage	Transportation
Whole blood, red blood cells (including irradiated, deglycerolized, leukocyte reduced, washed, apheresis), and plasma (including any form after thawing and liquid).	1–6 °C	1–10 °C
Platelets (any form), apheresis granulocytes (including irradiated), anti-hemophilic factor (including cryoprecipitated, thawed cryoprecipitated, and plasma thawed cryoprecipitated).	20–24 °C with continuous agitation	20–24 °C
Antihemophilic factor (including plasma cryoprecipitated, pooled cryoprecipitated before freezing), plasma (including frozen within 24 hours of phlebotomy and cryoprecipitate reduced).	≤-18 °C	Frozen
Fresh frozen plasma	≤-18 °C or ≤-65 °C	≤-18 °C or ≤-65 °C

Visible Inspection of Units of Blood/Components

Contamination	Cryoprecipitate	Plasma	Platelets	RBCs
Bacteria	Bubbles, clots, fibrin strains, opaque	Bubbles, clots, fibrin strains, opaque	Bubbles, clots, fibrin strains, opaque, grey appearance	Dark purple to black
Bile	Bright yellow to brown	Bright yellow to brown	Bright yellow to brown	----
Color abnormality	Any abnormal color	Any abnormal color	Any abnormal color	Supernatant, grey/brown
Hemolysis	Pink to red	Pink to red	----	Bright red
Lipids	White appearance, opaque	White appearance, opaque	White appearance, opaque	Lighter red, opaque
Particulates	Clots, aggregates of cellular material	Clots, fibrin strands, white materials	Clots, fibrin strands, white materials	Clots, white materials
RBC contamination	Light pink to red	Light pink to red	Light pink	----

Blood Bank Regulations

OSHA and state regulations outline the requirements for **disposition of blood bags and patient samples**. Blood disposition must comply with OSHA's Bloodborne Pathogen's Standard (29 CFR 1910.1030), which covers blood (semi-liquid, liquid, dried) in containers, in other waste products, or on items, such as sharps. As a regulated waste, the blood must be placed in a container that is closable, leak-proof, labeled (proper color-coding), and closed before removal to avoid any spillage or loss of contents during transport to disposal site. **Temperatures:** Blood bank refrigerators are maintained at 2–4 °C with audible and visible alarm if the temperature falls to 6 °C. Freezers are maintained at -20 °C, with alerts when the temperature falls to -19 °C. Incubators usually provide for a range of temperatures (5–70 °C) with much incubation done at 37 °C. The alarm system for refrigerators, freezers, and incubators should be battery powered so it still functions if the electrical supply is cut.

Requirements for Blood Bank Operation

Requirements for blood bank operation include:

- Obtaining a blood bank license and renewing annually.
- Being available for inspection upon request.
- Participating in proficiency testing.
- Obtaining qualified director and adequate numbers of other qualified personnel.
- Supervising staff, identifying training needs, and implementing training.
- Having appropriate equipment for all functions.
- Using appropriate infection control practices and disposing contaminated materials appropriately.
- Carrying out a documented review for collection/preparation of all blood components.
- Maintaining a manual that outlines all policies and procedures.
- Maintaining correct and legible records that includes significant steps in procedures, test outcomes, ABO/Rh typing result, and donor records, and carrying out reporting responsibilities.
- Establishing criteria for blood collection, processing, storage, distribution, and testing.
- Labeling in compliance with Code of Federal Regulations.
- Storing blood/blood components appropriately and at correct temperature with temperature monitoring system in place.

Quality Control for All Reagents

Reagent solutions are used for most diagnostic tests, and results are often dependent on using the correct reagent (stock, working, or standard) at the correct concentration. Quality control procedures include ensuring:

- Accurate weighing and measuring when preparing reagent solutions.
- Carefully following of directions and/or using reagent kits when preparing reagent solutions.
- Choosing the correct reagent.
- Following recommended procedures when disposing of reagents.
- Using proper PPE when working with reagents.
- Neutralizing spilled acids/corrosive chemicals with sodium carbonate or sodium bicarbonate and alkali with dry sand.
- Labeling strong acids and alkali (corrosive compounds) and storing near the floor.

- Properly storing all reagents (acid in glass, flammable reagents in metal or glass, sodium/potassium hydroxide in plastic, hygroscopic chemicals in desiccator or air-tight container, photosensitive chemicals in dark, glass stoppered bottle).
- Monitoring volumes/concentration of chemicals that are explosive when dehydrated.
- Diluting stock only as needed.
- Labeling reagent solutions with date and other information according to directions.
- Labeling all poisonous, flammable, and otherwise hazardous materials.

Maintaining Quality of Patient Samples Collected for Blood Bank Testing

Preanalytical procedures must be followed to maintain the quality of patient samples collected and stored for blood banking purposes. Expired sample tubes cannot be used, and containers with the appropriate additive for blood bank testing must be collected. Identification of the correct patient is imperative prior to collecting a sample, as is correctly labeling the tube once the sample has been collected. Often, a separate, uniquely identifying wristband will be required for a patient receiving blood products. This wristband's identification number will be placed on all of the patient's blood bank samples and blood products assigned to them for an additional form of identification to ensure that the proper patient is receiving the correct products.

Bacterial Contamination

Occasionally, blood products in storage will suffer a bacterial contamination. The most common type of bacterial contaminant is *Yersinia enterocolitica*. Bacteria of this kind will grow while the product is being stored. Individuals who receive blood products that have been contaminated are likely to manifest symptoms similar to those of an adverse transfusion reaction: fever and chills, e.g. Clots, discoloration, or hemolysis in the blood unit indicates possible contamination.

Transportation Guidelines

Platelets should be transported at room temperature, and they should not be jostled. Red blood cells must be transported at a temperature at 1–10 °C; it is standard to place red blood cells in a Styrofoam box inside a cardboard box and on ice. Frozen blood components must be shipped on dry ice and wrapped well.

Maintaining Quality of Blood Bank Reagents

The following blood banking reagents are tested with quality control samples on each day of their use to ensure they are functioning properly:

- blood grouping reagents
- reverse typing cells
- antibody screen cells
- AHG reagent.

Decreased activity or complete inactivity of reagents with quality control material indicates deterioration of the reagents that can no longer be used for patient testing. AHG reagent quality is also verified for each sample yielding a negative result. IgG sensitized cells, known as check cells, are added to the negatively reacting sample and will agglutinate in the presence of properly functioning AHG. Check cells do not agglutinate in insufficiently washed samples where residual serum neutralizes the AHG.

Testing procedures implemented by reagent and equipment manufacturers' transfusion service facilities must be followed in a strict manner to ensure the accuracy and quality of blood bank processes. Quality assurance policies require comprehensive training of blood bank technologists as well as routine competency testing to ensure that procedures are properly being followed. Evaluation, validation, and the planning of new processes are also important quality assurance measures.

Transfusion Practice

Indications for Transfusion

Whole blood transfusions are only indicated in the events of a massive hemorrhage with greater than 30% blood loss or an exchange transfusion. **Packed RBC** transfusions are indicated in patients with a hemoglobin value of less than 7g/dL or a hemoglobin value of 7–9g/dL accompanied by symptoms that include shortness of breath, fatigue, dizziness, chest pain, and weakness. Cases of symptomatic anemia without an active hemorrhage, acute blood loss, sickle cell crisis, and cardiac failure are indicators for this component. **Platelet** transfusions are indicated in patients with platelet counts of less than 50,000/μL, patients with platelet dysfunction, or as a prophylactic prior to surgery in patients with an active bleed. A transfusion of **plasma** is indicated in patients with coagulation factor deficiencies, DIC, thrombotic thrombocytopenic purpura, and for emergent use in the reversal of a warfarin overdose. Hemophilia, von Willebrand disease, fibrinogen deficiency, and a massive bleed during surgery are common indicators for the transfusion of **cryoprecipitate**.

Avoiding Cold Antibodies with Prewarmed Technique

One of the ways that lab technicians try to avoid cold antibodies is by using what is known as the prewarmed technique. This technique is performed as follows: a drop of panel cells and auto control cells is put into a test tube, which is then warmed for 10 minutes at 37 °C. Simultaneously, a tube of serum from the patient is warmed for 10 minutes at 37 °C. The serum is then added to the warmed panel cells, and the mixture continues to incubate for 30 minutes. At this point, it is washed three times with saline that has been heated to 37 °C. Finally, antihuman globulin is added and the reactions of the materials can be interpreted.

Pre-Transfusion Steps and Transfusion Reaction Steps

Before a transfusion is begun, the lab technician should double-check the tag on the blood bag as well as the paperwork associated with the requisition. During a blood transfusion, the individual's vital signs should be checked every quarter hour. Vital signs that must be checked include body temperature, pulse, blood pressure, and respiration. If a transfusion reaction begins or is suspected, the transfusion should stop immediately. The patient's physician should then be notified.

Review Video: Blood Transfusions
Visit mometrix.com/academy and enter code: 759682

Component Therapy

Component therapy is the practice of transfusing individual blood component products instead of whole blood. This therapeutic method allows for the treatment of a specific deficiency in recipients, while preventing volume overload or a reaction to unnecessary products. Indications for transfusion are specific to each component and are determined in correlation with clinical signs and symptoms.

Immunologic Reactions Due to Transfusion

Immunologic transfusion reactions can present as an immediate or a delayed response depending on the cause of the reaction. Symptoms of a transfusion reaction vary by patient but commonly include fever, chills, low back pain, nausea, vomiting, or low blood pressure with a high heart rate indicating shock. Hemolytic, febrile, allergic, and transfusion-related acute lung injury reactions occur as an **immediate response** to an immunologic incompatibility of donor and recipient blood. Nonhemolytic febrile reactions are attributed to an immune response to donor granulocytes. Antibodies to leukocytes or the activation of complement results in noncardiac pulmonary edema. Anaphylaxis caused by IgA antibody interactions and urticaria arising from antibodies to plasma proteins are allergic immunologic effects. Transfusion-related acute lung injury is a life-threatening reaction of donor leukocyte antibodies against patient leukocytes. Immediate, or acute, hemolytic transfusion reactions are a result of ABO incompatibilities or specific antibodies to antigen in recipient blood. The antibody–antigen reaction activates the complement system and results in lysis of donor RBCs intravascular. **Delayed immunologic responses** to transfusion include alloimmunization, GVHD, and delayed hemolytic reactions. GVHD is the engraftment of functional donor lymphocytes that act against the recipient's immune system. Sensitization to and production of antibodies directed toward donor antigens can also cause a delayed reaction. Extravascular hemolytic reactions occur between 3 and 10 days after transfusion due to the reemergence of a previously developed alloantibody.

Nonimmunologic Reactions and Transfusion-Transmitted Diseases

Immediate nonimmunologic transfusion reactions marked by a fever and congestive heart failure (CHF) are caused by circulatory overload, hemolysis, and bacterial contamination. Transfusion-associated circulatory overload can be fatal, with a cough, tachypnea, and dyspnea developing within hours of a transfusion. Hemolysis of RBCs can occur in a nonimmunologic manner through the physical mechanism of infusion or due to mishandling of the product. Bacterial contamination is most common in platelet transfusions, but it is possible in all blood products. A fever and chills during or shortly after the completion of a transfusion can indicate sepsis due to bacterial contamination. **Delayed adverse nonimmunologic** reactions include iron overload from multiple transfusions and the acquisition of a transfusion-transmitted disease. **Transfusion-transmitted diseases** can develop over time if bacteria, a virus, or protozoa are present in the donor unit. Hepatitis, HIV, human T cell leukemia-lymphoma virus, CMV, syphilis, and parasites have the potential for transmission via transfusion. Deferral of blood donors with HIV, hepatitis, and other potential exposures and pretransfusion testing for highly transmittable diseases aid in the decrease of adverse events that could occur.

Extracorporeal Circulation and Apheresis Techniques

Extracorporeal circulation is the mechanism used to remove blood from a patient's circulatory system into a mechanical system for a treatment or process and return it back to the patient's circulation. Many therapeutic processes use an extracorporeal circuit to remove waste, administer medication, or oxygenate blood in a patient. **Hemodialysis** and **hemofiltration** are used for kidney failure. The process removes waste products that the kidneys cannot excrete on their own and returns the filtered blood back to the body. **Extracorporeal membrane oxygenation** replicates lung function when the lungs are inundated or are unable to properly oxygenate the body; it treats blood with an anticoagulant and filters it through an oxygenator before returning it to the body via a vein or artery. Allowing for a still heart to be operated on, **cardiopulmonary bypass** mechanisms assume the responsibility of pumping blood throughout the body during open heart surgeries. **Apheresis** techniques use an extracorporeal circuit to remove a specific component of blood and return the remaining components to the circulation. For the treatment of immune system disorders, **plasmapheresis** removes whole blood from circulation, separates the plasma by centrifugation, administers treatment to the plasma, and then returns the remaining components back to the patient. Individual blood components that are donated for transfusion purposes, such as platelets and plasma, are collected via apheresis techniques.

Blood Administration and Patient Blood Management

Patient blood management is an evidence-based approach used by healthcare professionals to avoid unnecessary blood product transfusions to reduce the number of products used and improve patients' overall outcome by limiting their exposure. Blood management tactics include considering all possible alternatives for care, before deciding that blood products are the best course of treatment.

The process of **blood administration** begins with the decision to transfuse by assessing a patient's diagnostic test results and their clinical presentation. Although test results may indicate the need for transfusion, a patient may not present with symptoms that warrant it. Prior to transfusion, patients must be educated and informed of pertinent transfusion-related information and are required to sign an "informed consent" or "informed refusal" form to agree to or refuse transfusion services. The patient must be positively identified at all times throughout the transfusion process, from sample collection to testing, product release, and product administration. Regular monitoring of the patient's vital signs 15–30 minutes after the start and hourly during a transfusion is important for detecting adverse reactions that may arise. If an adverse reaction is suspected, the transfusion must be stopped immediately with all tubing associated with the unit to be removed, and a transfusion workup is initiated.

Look-Back/Recall Procedures for Blood Products

Look-back procedures are triggered when a transfusion recipient becomes infected and all donors are traced or a donor is discovered to have an infection and all recipients are traced. For donors who convert to positive for HIV, recipients of any component within the previous 12 months must be notified by the hospital or physician. For donors who convert to positive for hepatitis C virus, the recipient or physician must be notified. The physician can make the decision about notifying the recipient. **Recall of blood products** occurs when additional information becomes available about the donor, but in many cases the products have already been transfused and the recipients must be located. The FDA issues recalls and specific directions for look-back, such as the look-back time period. Recall classifications include:

- Class I: Adverse health consequences or death likely.
- Class II: Temporary or reversible adverse health consequences may occur.
- Class III: Very little risk of adverse health consequences.

Urinalysis and Other Body Fluids

Urinalysis

Terms Associated with Urinalysis

Anuria: Almost no urine discharge, usually due to renal failure or other kidney damage

Oliguria: Sharp decrease in urine discharge; typically caused by diarrhea, vomiting, perspiration, or other forms of dehydration

Polyuria: Sharp increase in urine discharge, to a level over 3 L per day; often caused by ingestion of diuretics, caffeine, alcohol, or by diabetes insipidus or mellitus

Nocturia: Nocturnal increase in urine discharge; often caused by a reduction in bladder capacity due to increased ingestion of fluids, pregnancy, or enlargement of the prostate gland

Prerenal: Classification of kidney disorders caused by problems outside of (before) the kidney, such as inadequate blood flow.

Suprapubic: Above the pubic bone, often the place where suprapubic catheters are placed, especially in males requiring long-term catheterization.

Glycosuria: Presence of glucose in the urine.

Renal threshold: The concentration at which the kidneys begin to remove a substance from the blood and into the urine.

Ascites: Accumulation of serous fluid in the abdominal cavity.

Tamm-Horsfall protein: AKA uromodulin, the most common protein found in normal urine.

Myoglobin: Protein found in muscle tissue.

Amniocentesis: Transabdominal sampling of amniotic fluid from the amniotic sac for prenatal diagnoses of chromosomal disorders and infections.

Pass-through: Duration of time that a drug needs to pass-through the liver and/or kidney.

Osmolality: Concentration of a substance (blood/urine).

Xanthochromic: Yellow-colored, usually in reference to cerebrospinal fluid that has the appearance of urine.

Myoglobinuria: Condition in which urine contains myoglobin; often the result of muscle trauma, coma, or muscle destruction

Hematuria: Condition in which urine contains intact red blood cells; often caused by renal tumors, menstruation, or pregnancy

Hemoglobinuria: Condition in which urine contains hemoglobin; often caused by infections, transfusion reactions, hemolytic anemia, or burns

Ketonuria: Condition in which urine contains ketones; often the result of diabetes mellitus, dehydration, or chronic imbalance electrolytes

Bilirubinuria: Condition in which urine contains bilirubin; often caused by liver disease, hepatitis, or cirrhosis of the liver

Methods of Urine Collection

- Glucose tolerance test: Used to diagnose diabetes or to monitor a diabetic; urine collection every hour, for three hours
- Void: Also known as random sample; patient collects his or her own urine
- Midstream clean catch: Patient cleans pubic area and then collects sample in mid-urination
- 24-hour: All urine output is collected over a 24-hour period
- Suprapubic aspiration: A needle is placed into the bladder and urine is extracted
- Two-hour postprandial: Urine is collected two hours after a meal; often performed to measure levels of sugar

Renal Anatomy and Physiology and Formation of Urine

The **kidneys** are located on the right and left sides posterior to the peritoneal cavity and are responsible for the fluid and acid-base balance in the body. The cortex (body) is encased in a capsule. Inside the cortex are pyramids, papilla, major and minor calyces, and renal pelvis leading to the ureter that carries urine to the bladder. The nephron is the functional unit responsible for filtering the blood (about 1200 mL/min) and removing waste products. The nephron includes:

- Glomerulus (capillaries surrounded by Bowman's capsule): Fluids and solutes move from the blood across capillary membranes into Bowman's capsule but plasma proteins and blood cells stay in the blood because they are too large.
- Bowman's capsule: Glomerular filtrate (similar to plasma) moves into proximal convoluted tubule.
- Proximal convoluted tubule: Water and electrolytes reabsorbed.
- Loop of Henle: Solutes, including glucose, reabsorbed.
- Distal convoluted tubule: Sodium and water reabsorbed according to levels of antidiuretic hormone (ADH) (from pituitary gland) and aldosterone (from adrenal cortex).
- Collecting duct: Carries urine into calyces of kidney for excretion.

Urinalysis and Association with Disease States

Color	Pale yellow/ amber and darkens when urine is concentrated or other substances (such as blood or bile) or present.
Appearance	Clear but may be slightly cloudy.
Odor	Slight. Bacteria may give urine a foul smell, depending upon the organism. Some foods, such as asparagus, change odor.
Specific gravity	1.015–1.025. May increase if protein levels increase or if there is fever, vomiting, or dehydration.
pH	Usually ranges between 4.5 and 8, with average of 5 to 6.
Sediment	Red cell casts from acute infections, broad casts from kidney disorders, and white cell casts from pyelonephritis. Leukocytes >10/ml^3 are present with urinary tract infections.

Glucose, ketones, protein, blood, bilirubin, and nitrate	Negative. Urine glucose may increase with infection (with normal blood glucose). Frank blood may be caused by some parasites and diseases but also by drugs, smoking, excessive exercise, and menstrual fluids. Increased red blood cells may result from lower urinary tract infections.
Urobilinogen	0.1-1.0 units. *Increased* in liver disease.

Mathematical Equation for Creatinine Clearance

Average Sized Adult

The creatinine clearance for an average sized adult, in milliliters per minute (mL/min), can be calculated by the equation $\frac{U}{P} \times V$. In this equation, U represents the creatinine concentration in the urine, in milligrams per deciliter (mg/dL), P represents the creatinine concentration in the plasma, in milligrams per deciliter (mg/dL), and V represents the volume of urine per minute, with the volume expressed in milliliters. Use the conversion factor of 24 hours being equal to 1440 minutes to convert the volume of urine over a 24 hour period to the volume of urine per minute. One thing to keep in mind with calculating the creatinine clearance is that the body surface area and the kidney size of an individual can affect the creatinine clearance. In an average sized individual, these factors are not really taken into account.

Altering Creatinine Clearance for Infants

When calculating creatinine clearance for an infant, we need to take into account the body surface area of the infant. Therefore, use the equation $\frac{U}{P} \times V \times \frac{1.73}{A}$ to calculate the creatinine clearance of an infant (mL/min/standard surface area). In this equation, U represents the creatinine concentration in the urine in milligrams per deciliter (mg/dL), P represents the creatinine concentration in the plasma in milligrams per deciliter (mg/dL), and V represents the volume of urine per minute with the volume expressed in milliliters. Use the conversion factor of 24 hours being equal to 1440 minutes to convert the volume of urine over a 24-hour period to the volume of urine per minute. 1.73 represents the average body surface area in square meters (m^2) of an average sized adult. A is the body surface area in square meters (m^2) of the individual (the infant) in question.

Benedict's Test

Benedict's test is a laboratory test that is used to determine the presence of reducing substances in a urine sample. Some reducing substances that can be present in urine include glucose (which can be indicative of diabetes), other reducing sugars such as lactose and galactose, creatinine, uric acid, or ascorbic acid. The test can tell a technician or a doctor if reducing substances are present in the urine sample, but the test itself is nonspecific. In other words, the test cannot determine the specific reducing substance present. To perform the test, Benedict's reagent (a solution of copper sulfate, sodium carbonate, and sodium citrate) is added to a urine sample, and the mixture is heated. A red, yellow, or orange precipitate is indicative of the presence of a reducing substance in the urine. The precipitate is formed because the copper sulfate in the Benedict's reagent is reduced by any reducing substance contained in the urine.

Addis Count Procedure

The Addis count is a laboratory technique to calculate the number of formed elements in a urine sample. The formed elements include blood cells (white blood cells and red blood cells) and casts. In this test, a twelve-hour urine specimen is collected. Formalin is used as a preservative for the urine sample. After the twelve-hour period, a specified quantity of the urine specimen is put in a centrifuge. Part of any resuspended urine sediment is then placed into a Neubauer blood-counting chamber. The squares of the blood-counting chamber are then examined. Any formed elements, such as casts, white blood cells, or red blood cells, that are present are counted. The total number of formed elements in the entire urine sample is then calculated. This test can be used on the urine of patients that have kidney disease.

Urinalysis Procedures

pH	Insert indicator paper or reagent strip into urine, remove excess, wait time according to manufacturer's guidelines, and compare to color chart.
Glucose	Use reagent strip OR place 5 mL of Benedict solution in test tube and 8 drops of urine, and mix. Boil solution for 2 minutes with Bunsen burner or spirit lamp with tube at about 45° angle or place tube in boiling water for 5 minutes. Cool tube and check color for amount of glucose with blue equal to 1+ and orange/red, 4+.
Nitrate/ Nitrite	Enzymes produced by bacteria change nitrate into nitrite, which is measured as an indirect method to detect UTI. Urine must have been in bladder for at least 4 hours, so first morning sample is usually used. Dip reagent strip in the urine sample and read results at 30–60 seconds and match against color chart with positive findings indicated by change to light to dark pink.
Bilirubin	Protect urine specimen from light and examine when fresh. Dip reagent strip in urine and read test results at 30–60 seconds and match against color chart with colors ranging from buff (1+) to tan/purple (3+) for positive reaction OR use Ictotest®.
Urobilinogen	Test fresh specimen between 2 and 4 PM (peak levels), especially for liver function testing. Dip reagent strip in the urine sample, read results at 30–60 seconds, and match to color chart with positive color changes ranging from peach-colored (0.2 mg/dL) to bright pink (8 mg/dL).
Protein	Use reagent strip OR place 5 mL of urine in a test tube and add 2 drops of sulfosalicylic acid. Observe for formation of white precipitate and as negative or from + to ++++ (trace to large amount) depending on the amount of precipitate.
Ketones	Use Acetest® tablets OR dip ketone stick in urine, wait 15 seconds, and monitor color changes. Positive changes are light lavender (5 mg/dL) to purple (160 mg/dL).
Blood	Place 12 mL urine in conical tube, centrifuge 5 minutes (medium speed), pour off supernatant, shake tube, use pipette to remove 1 drop of sediment and place on slide for microscopic examination. RBCs appear colored (yellow/green).
Leukocyte esterase	Obtain clean catch urine sample in sterile container, dip reagent strip into urine and check color chart after 2 minutes. No color change is negative but shades of pink to purple indicate trace to large amounts.

HCG Hemagglutination Inhibition Test

The HCG hemagglutination test is used to determine pregnancy by examining a urine sample. Add a sample of urine to two drops of HCG antiserum. To this, add red blood cells that have been coated in HCG. If HCG is present in the urine sample, the HCG antiserum binds to the HCG present, therefore making it impossible for the HCG antiserum to react with the red blood cells coated in HCG. This leads to the red cells not agglutinating, and a donut shape consisting of red blood cells will form. This donut shape indicates HCG in the urine sample. However, if there is no HCG present in the urine sample, the HCG antiserum will bind with the HCG coated red blood cells. No donut pattern of red blood cells will form. Instead, there will be a diffuse pattern of red blood cells. This diffuse pattern indicates that no HCG is present in the urine sample. The patient is not pregnant, or is pregnant more than six months.

Confirmatory Urine Tests

Clinitest®	Confirms the presence of glucose in the urine. Drop alkaline copper reagent tables in a tube containing 5 drops of urine and 10 drops of distilled water, which will boil. Wait 15 seconds after boiling stops, gently shake tube, and check color against chart. Blue is negative and colors from green to orange indicate the presence of 1/4% (+) to 2% (++++) glucose.
Ictotest®	Confirms the presence of bilirubin in the urine. Place 10 drops of urine on a special absorbant mat, place a reagent table in the middle of the moistened are and then one drop of distilled water on the tablet. After 5 seconds, place another drop of distilled water on the table. Wait 60 seconds and observe the color about and under the tablet. Blue or purple color indicates the presence of bilirubin.
Acetest® (Acetone test)	Confirms the presence of ketones in the urine. Place tablet on clean dry white paper and place 1 drop of urine on top of tablet. Wait 30 seconds and check color against color chart. No change in color is negative and shades of lavender (light, medium, and dark) indicate small, moderate, and large amounts of ketones.
Sulfosalicylic acid (SSA)	Confirms the presence of protein in the urine. If urine is cloudy, centrifuge before test. Fill tube (10 × 75 mm) one-third full of urine and add one-third tube of 3% SSA solution. Cover with paraffin film/cap and mix by inverting. Check results by holding in front of lined/text test strip. If the lines/text are clear, the result is negative, slightly cloudy but lines/text visible, 1+; lines are visible but unable to read text, 2+; no lines/text visible, 3+; totally opaque/gelled, 4+.

Example Situations and Possible Causes

Observation	Possible Cause
Ketone bodies present in urine	The presence of ketone bodies in a urine or blood sample can be caused by diabetes mellitus or ketone producing diet. The ketone bodies are due to an excessive metabolism of fat because sugar cannot be utilized.
Human chorionic gonadotropin present in urine	The presence of human chorionic gonadotropin (HCG) in the urine is due to pregnancy or testicular tumor. Within a week or two after conception, human chorionic gonadotropin is excreted into the urine, and it can be detected by a variety of laboratory techniques, including a radioimmunoassay.
Urine sediment that vontains white blood cells	If white blood cells (usually neutrophils) are found in urine sediment that usually indicates the presence of a urinary tract or renal infection.
Urine that when shaken forms a yellow foam	Most samples of urine do not foam when shaken. However, if urine, when shaken, forms a yellow foam, that is due to an increased concentration of bilirubin in the urine.

Abnormal Urine Colorations

- Red: Most commonly caused by blood; additional causes may be red blood cells, hemoglobin, myoglobin caused by muscle trauma
- Dark yellow or amber: Dehydration, infection, fever, or liver problems like hepatitis
- Bright yellow or orange: Caused by increased bilirubin, or by medications such as pyridium, which is used to treat urinary tract infections
- Green: Caused by presence of biliverdin, which is introduced by the breakdown of hemoglobin
- Black or gray: Presence of melanin or homogentisic acid resulting from a metabolic disorder

Specific Gravity

Every urinalysis includes a measure of specific gravity, which indicates the degree to which the kidneys can reabsorb water and essential chemicals from the glomerular filtrate. Most kidney disorders impair this function immediately. Specific gravity tests also indicate whether hormone abnormalities or dehydration is present. A normal specific gravity will range from 1.001–1.035. If the specific gravity is greater than 1.010, it is called hypersthenuric urine. If the specific gravity is less than 1.010, it is called hyposthenuric urine. If the specific gravity is exactly 1.010, it is called isosthenuric urine.

Reagent Strips

Lab technicians use reagent strips to examine the chemical composition of a urine sample. The following chemicals can be assessed: bilirubin, glucose, nitrite, blood, protein, white blood cells, ketones, and urobilinogen. Also, reagent strips can determine the specific gravity and pH of urine. These strips work as follows: they are dipped into the urine sample and change colors depending on the composition of the urine. As long as basic restrictions regarding room temperature and procedure are followed, these reagent strips are highly accurate.

Urine pH

Lab technicians often use pH reagent strips to determine the pH of a urine sample. Such a strip will contain bromethol blue and methyl red, and these chemicals will cause the strip to change colors depending on the pH of the urine. If the pH is 5.0, the strip will turn orange. As the pH of the urine increases, the resulting color on the strip will go from orange to yellow to green to blue. At a pH of 9.0, the strip will turn blue. Individuals will typically not have a pH lower than 6.0 except for first thing in the morning, or if they eat a high protein diet or have diabetes mellitus. Typical pH level will not be higher than 7.0 except in cases of renal tubular acidosis, urinary tract infection, or metabolic or respiratory alkalosis.

Urine Components Associated with Reagent Strips

- Sodium nitroprusside or nitro ferricyanide: Used to test for the presence of ketones in a sample of urine
- Diazonium salt reaction: Used to test for the presence of bilirubin in a sample of urine
- Tetrabromophenol blue: Used to test for the presence of abnormal levels of proteins in a sample of urine
- Indoxyl carbonic acid ester: Used to test for the presence of white blood cells in a sample of urine

Urine Casts and Their Appearance Under a Microscope

- White blood cell casts: Any cast containing white blood cells; indicates infection or inflammation
- Red blood cell casts: Any casts that contain red blood cells, which will appear brown or yellow under a microscope; indicative of renal disease
- Hyaline casts: The most common kind of cast, typically the result of renal disease, heart failure, or glomerulonephritis; often seen after stress, excessive exercise, or dehydration

Urine Crystals and Their Appearance Under a Microscope

- Cystine: Colorless, hexagonal plates
- Tyrosine: Yellow or colorless thin needles
- Cholesterol: Clear, flat rectangular crystals
- Uric acid: Various; colorless or yellow, and shaped as cubes, diamonds, plates, or needles
- Bilirubin: Yellow to brown plates, granules, or needles
- Calcium oxalate: Various; dumbbell, octahedral, or envelope shapes
- Leucine: Yellow to brown spheres, often with striations

Alkaline Urine Crystals and Their Appearance Under a Microscope

- Triple phosphate: Triangular or hexagonal prisms, similar to a coffin shape
- Calcium phosphate: Crystals may be irregularly-shaped and large, or in granular sheets or plates
- Amorphous phosphate: Colorless granules
- Ammonium biurate: Brown or yellow, with striations; may contain irregular projections
- Calcium carbonate: Small and colorless, often dumbbell-shaped

Maple Syrup Urine Disease

Individuals with the genetic metabolic disorder known as maple syrup urine disease have a natural deficiency of branched-chain keto acid decarboxylase, resulting in a diminished metabolism of valine, leucine, and isoleucine. The condition gets its name from the aroma emanating from the urine, breath, and skin of infants with the condition. This condition is most common in the Amish and Mennonite communities, and can be identified with a Guthrie bacterial inhibition test. If it is not treated, it can lead to intellectual disability, hypoglycemia, convulsions, and even death.

Other Body Fluids

Cerebrospinal Fluid

Cerebrospinal fluid fulfills a number of functions in the human body. It removes waste products, supplies nutrients to the nervous system, and supports the brain and spinal column. The average human produces 20 mL of this substance every hour, and typically has between 140 and 170 mL at any given time. Normal cerebrospinal fluid is clear and colorless. If the fluid is cloudy, this may be due to meningitis or hemorrhage; if it is yellow, this may indicate an elevated level of bilirubin or protein.

Cerebrospinal fluid is collected as follows: a spinal tap, otherwise known as a lumbar puncture, is made either between the third and fourth or fourth and fifth lumbar vertebrae. Three tubes of fluid are removed: one for microbiological analysis; one for hematological analysis; and one for chemical and serological analysis.

Semen Analysis

These are the parameters for a semen analysis: General color and clarity of the semen should be a grayish-white and translucent. The pH should be between 7.3 and 7.8, and the viscosity of the semen (the resistance of the semen to flow) should get a rating of one on a scale of one to four. The volume of the entire ejaculate should be between two and five milliliters. Coagulation and liquefaction should occur within 30 minutes of collecting the sample. The motility of the sperm, or the percentage of sperm present that are moving, should be about 60% or higher. The percentage of sperm that are moving forward (forward progression) should be at least 50% or higher. The sperm count should be a minimum of 40 million sperm per total ejaculate. At least 30% of the sperm present should have a normal morphology, with no double or deformed tails or heads.

Before his semen may be collected for an infertility analysis, and a male must be abstinent for three days. Such a waiting period is not necessary before other laboratory tests. Semen is collected in a sterile container and cannot be obtained in the presence of condoms or spermicides. Semen is collected and stored at room temperature.

In a typical semen analysis, the following characteristics are considered:

- Viscosity: Rated from zero (very low) to four (very viscous)
- Volume: Normal range is between two and 5 mL
- Color: Milky is normal
- pH: Normal range is between 7.2 and 7
- Sperm count: Normal range is between 20 and 160 million sperm per milliliter
- Motility (degree to which sperm move forward): Normal range is between 50 and 60%, or three or four on a scale of zero to four
- Shape of sperm: Normal shape is one head and one straight tail

Types of Fecal Matter

- Watery: Indicates diarrhea
- Ribbon-like: Indicates bowel obstruction
- Black/tarry: Indicates bleeding in the gastrointestinal tract
- Frothy, bulky, or yellow colored: Indicates malabsorption syndrome, in which stool contains too much fat
- Containing mucus: Indicates colitis or inflammation of the intestinal wall

Synovial Fluid

Synovial fluid, also known as joint fluid, lubricates and cushions the joints and delivers nutrients to cartilage. Synovial fluid is thick and stringy, and should either be clear or light yellow. Infections, inflammations, and bleeding may affect the consistency and color of synovial fluid. Gout is indicated by crystals in the fluid. A typical analysis of synovial fluid includes an analysis of visual characteristics as well as a differential counts and Gram stain.

PKU

Phenylketonuria, otherwise known as PKU, is a metabolic disorder in which phenylalanine is not easily converted into tyrosine. This genetic disorder is often caused by a lack of the catalyzing enzyme hydroxylase. If this condition is not treated, it can result in intellectual disability. Infants born with PKU will have urine with a distinct odor. The smell is caused by an elevated level of ketones. Infants should be tested within their first day of life. There are a few different tests for PKU: ferric chloride strips and the Guthrie bacterial inhibition test are the most common methods.

Refractometers

Refractometers are used to measure fluid concentration by assessing light refraction through a prism. Refractometers vary in size and sophistication (simple handheld devices to more complex digital devices), so procedures may vary. Generally, the instrument is calibrated with water before the sample is tested. Testing:

- Turn on equipment.
- Clean prism with cotton ball and ethanol or according to manufacturer's guidelines.
- Place sample on prism or in sample well and secure prism.
- Look through the eyepiece, adjust as needed for manual equipment.
- Read results expressed in Brix (1 degree Brix = 1 g sucrose in 100 g solution), refractive index (degree to which the light is bent), and/or specific gravity. Digital equipment provides a read-out. Note: Tables are available that provide the refractive index for most common materials.

Refractometers may be used to assess urine specific gravity, serum copper sulfate, and serum protein. Sample temperature must be maintained within a prescribed temperature range for some types of refractometers.

Manual Testing

Bilirubin	Uncoagulated blood sample allowed to clot at room temperature and then centrifuged and supernatant separated immediately for examination. Dilute sample by mixing 1 mL with 4 mL saline. Label 2 tubes for direct bilirubin (DB) and serum blank (SB). Place 1 mL diluted serum and 2 mL 0.05 hydrochloric acid in each tube. Place 0.5 mL Diazo II reagent in DB and in exactly 60 seconds add 0.1 mL ascorbic acid, mix, and add 1.5 mL alkaline tartrate and read color results in 5-10 minutes. To tube SB, place 0.5 mL Diazo I reagent, 0.5 mL ascorbic acid, and 1.5 mL alkaline tartrate, and mix to use as serum blank.
Occult blood (gastric)	Sample is applied to paper reagent strip coated with guaiac, which changes color to blue in the presence of blood within 1 minute. The sample may also be applied to a slide (thin smear), which is examined microscopically.

Body Fluid Cytocentrifugation

Cytocentrifugation ("cytospin") uses a special centrifuge with slide holders that have attached funnels to hold body fluid that has been mixed with a medium in prescribed amounts. The process is able to concentrate cells that occur in small numbers in a sample. During centrifugation (usually at about 500 rpm for about 5 minutes), the fluid is wicked into a filter and onto a slide in a thin monolayer. Albumin (11% or 22%) may be added to serous fluids to preserve morphology as centrifugation may result in some distortion (although clumping patterns and ratio of nucleus to cytoplasm are unchanged). Albumin should not be added to synovial fluid. Cells in body fluids are similar to those in peripheral blood, and morphology is similar but counts are usually less. Once the slide is prepared, staining may be done to facilitate evaluation.

Amniotic Fluid Measurements

The lecithin/sphingomyelin ratio in the amniotic fluid is a good indicator for the lung maturity of the fetus. Via amniocentesis, a sample of surfactant in the amniotic fluid is removed. The lecithin/sphingomyelin ratio is then calculated. If the ratio is less than 2, then the fetal lungs are not producing enough surfactant, and this is an indicator that the fetal lungs may be immature (wet).

Determining the lecithin/sphingomyelin ratio is very important because it can help predict and/or prevent fetal respiratory distress after birth.

The concentrations of creatinine and urea nitrogen in amniotic fluid are useful for helping determine if amniotic fluid is contaminated with any maternal urine. Using amniocentesis, a sample of amniotic fluid is extracted from the mother's uterus. Because creatinine and urea nitrogen concentrations in the mother's urine are much greater (on the order of ten to fifty times greater) than those concentrations in amniotic fluid, an unexpected high concentration of creatinine and/or urea nitrogen in the amniotic fluid can indicate contamination of the amniotic fluid with maternal urine, often by bladder puncture.

Chemistry

General Chemistry

Carbohydrates

Physiology and Metabolic Pathways of Carbohydrates in the Body

Carbohydrates are complex sugars that are metabolized and converted into molecules that are the primary source of energy for cells and life processes. Through digestion, complex sugars, or **polysaccharides**, are broken down into single-molecule simple sugars known as **monosaccharides**. Carbohydrate metabolism begins in the mouth, where salivary amylase breaks down starch and sucrose molecules. The most used product of carbohydrate metabolism is the **glucose** molecule, which undergoes various metabolic processes based on the body's immediate needs. Glucose molecules absorbed in tissues through the endothelial lining of the small intestine and enters into cells with the promotion of the hormone insulin. **Glycolysis** takes place in the mitochondria of a cell by oxidizing glucose to release ATP and provide immediate energy for cellular processes. Excess glucose absorbed by the body undergoes **glycogenesis** and is converted to glycogen by insulin. **Glycogen** is stored in the liver and skeletal muscles as a reserve for energy that is converted back to glucose during periods of starvation. Long-term storage of excess sugars is accomplished through **lipogenesis**, in which insulin converts glucose molecules to protein and fat, creating adipose or fat tissue.

Abnormal States Associated with Blood Glucose Levels

Abnormal glucose levels are classified as being either too high, hyperglycemia, or too low, hypoglycemia. **Hyperglycemia** is mostly associated with diabetes, but it can also be attributed to overactivity of the adrenal, pituitary, or thyroid glands, liver disease, febrile disease, or traumatic brain injury, or it can be induced by stress. Symptoms of hyperglycemic conditions include the following: excessive urination, excessive thirst, excessive hunger, tiredness, sudden weight loss, and poor wound healing. Patients with **type 1 diabetes** are insulin dependent due to the autoimmune cell-mediated destruction of the insulin-secreting beta cells in the pancreas. **Type 2 diabetes** is an acquired disease characterized by the gradual onset of progressive hyperglycemia and insulin resistance. The combination of hyperglycemia and insulin resistance recognized during pregnancy and resolving after delivery is known as **gestational diabetes mellitus**.

Hypoglycemia is defined by a lower than normal fasting glucose with a transient decline in glucose levels within 1–2 hours following a meal. Nausea, vomiting, and muscle spasms are common symptoms associated with low blood sugar, with unconsciousness and death due to severe hypoglycemia also being possible.

Normal and Abnormal States Associated with Metabolism of Carbohydrates

Normal levels of carbohydrate metabolites indicate the proper function of various organs systems and hormones throughout the body, just as abnormal levels are associated with different imbalances and deficiencies. Although **insulin** is the only hormone that acts to decrease blood glucose levels, many hormones act in an effort to increase the release of glucose into the bloodstream. **Adrenocorticotropic hormone (ACTH)** and **growth hormone (GH)** are insulin antagonists released from the pituitary gland to increase blood glucose to normal levels. **Glucagon** in the pancreas, **T_3, T_4**, and **epinephrine** from the medulla stimulate the breakdown of glycogen into glucose, whereas **cortisol** stimulates the release of glucose from noncarbohydrate sources to regulate blood glucose levels.

Galactosemia is an inherited metabolic disorder in which the body lacks the enzymes necessary to break down galactose sugars into glucose molecules. This disorder is diagnosed in infants from newborn screening tests and the presentation of the following symptoms: loss of appetite, vomiting, diarrhea, jaundice, and failure to thrive.

Lactate or **lactic acid** is an intermediate product of carbohydrate metabolism that indicates O_2 deprivation caused by severe disease, excessive exercise, or drug abuse. Increased lactate levels can be reversed by treating the underlying cause, whereas failing to decrease lactate levels will result in lactic acidosis and may lead to life-threatening shock.

Physical and Chemical Properties of Carbohydrates

Carbohydrates are composed of carbon, hydrogen, and O_2 molecules arranged in rings or chains. Classification of carbohydrates begins with the number of simple sugar molecules they contain, **Monosaccharides**, the simplest carbohydrates, are colorless, crystalline, solid at room temperature, sweet in taste, and are highly soluble in water. **Oligosaccharides** consists of single sugar molecules joined by glycosidic linkage that yield between 2 and 10 monosaccharides upon hydrolysis. **Polysaccharides** are comprised of more than 10 monosaccharides and differ from each other by their structure and the simple sugars they are made up of.

Physically, carbohydrates can present as **isomers** that have the same chemical formula but different structural and spatial configurations. **Diastereomers** have a configuration variance in the second, third, or fourth carbon atom of glucose**. Stereoisomerism** describes the difference in spatial configurations of atoms, with varying spatial configurations of the first carbon in aldolases and the second carbon in ketones known **as annomerism**. Glucose also has optical activity that is visualized as light on a polarized plane.

Chemical properties of carbohydrates consist of the ability to form osazones, oxidize, and reduce to alcohols. Monosaccharides are deemed reducing sugars if their carbonyl groups oxidize to carbolic acids, which can be detected by Benedict's test reagent and sugars being heated together, producing a red-orange color.

Glucose Testing Using Enzymatic Reactions

Quantitative glucose testing is most commonly performed by the coupled **enzymatic reactions** using glucose oxidase and hexokinase. **Glucose oxidase** catalyzes the oxidation of glucose, which converts it to gluconic acid and H_2O_2, followed by peroxidase converting H_2O_2 to O_2. The O_2 produced, along with a chromogenic receptor, will produce a color that is measured by a spectrophotometer and is proportional to the amount of glucose present in blood. **Hexokinase** methods use the hexokinase enzyme and ATP energy to convert glucose to glucose-6-phosphate (G-6-P), which is then converted to gluconate-6-P by glucose-6-phosphate dehydrogenase and $NADP^+$. During this reaction, NADP+ is reduced to NADPH, causing an increase in absorbance and measurements taken at 340 nm. Measurements at this point in the reaction are equal to the amount of glucose present in the sample. Hexokinase methods are considered to be the reference method for glucose measurement due to their high accuracy, precision, and ability to test a variety of sample types, including blood, urine, and other body fluids.

Carbohydrate Tests

Reducing sugars are identified with **Benedict's testing method** in which glucose and other reducing sugars are converted to ions of cupric in an alkaline solution. The ions produce a visible color change that is observed as a qualitative and semiqualitative reaction.

Other carbohydrates that are commonly tested for include lactose, xylose, and lactate. **Lactose tolerance** testing includes the ingestion of lactose and a subsequent measure of blood glucose to determine the body's ability to absorb lactose and convert it to glucose**. Xylose absorption** testing is used to differentiate pancreatic-based malabsorption from intestinal malabsorption. Normal levels of xylose in urine samples indicate pancreatic malabsorption, whereas low absorption indicates an intestinal origin. **Lactic acid** measurements are used in conjunction with other lab results and the patient's clinical symptoms to assess O_2 deprivation in cells. Spectrophotometry or enzymatic methods can be used to measure lactate levels in blood and other body fluids.

Collecting, Processing, and Troubleshooting Carbohydrate Testing Samples

Blood glucose testing specimens can be collected via capillary collection or venous puncture. Capillary collection is advantageous for immediate point-of-care blood glucose testing, whereas venous samples are stable for longer periods of time. Whole blood, plasma, and serum are acceptable samples for venous collection. The preservative sodium fluoride in gray-top tubes keeps blood glucose samples the most stable by inhibiting the metabolism of glucose. Glycolysis decreases blood glucose levels in room temperature, uncentrifuged samples by approximately 10 mg/dL per hour; therefore, samples should be centrifuged and analyzed or refrigerated within 30 minutes for accurate results. Fasting glucose samples are the most accurate in evaluating glucose metabolism in patients. An 8- to 12-hour fast produces the best sample; however, a sample collected 2 hours after a meal is considered acceptable as well. Glucose levels in urine, cerebrospinal fluid (CSF), and other body fluids are most accurate in immediate analysis because the bacterial contamination in samples quickly reduces glucose levels. Capillary blood samples are considered arterial, with glucose level concentrations being 5 mg/dL higher than venous samples. Normal glucose levels in CSF are equal to two-thirds the concentration of plasma or serum samples, and glucose will not be detected in normal urine samples. High levels of ascorbic acid (vitamin C) and nonfasting specimens can falsely increase blood glucose results, whereas glucose will be falsely decreased in unspun samples due to the RBC uptake of glucose.

Glucose Tolerance Testing

Glucose tolerance testing (GTT) is a diagnostic test for diabetes that evaluates how the body responds to a measured amount of glucose intake over a set duration of time. Evaluation for types 1 and 2 diabetes is a 2-hour process, whereas gestational diabetes is evaluated at 1 hour, and repeated for 3 hours if the 1-hour test results are elevated.

In preparation for GTT, patients follow a diet of 150 g or less of carbohydrates per day for three days and an 8- to 12-hour fast immediately preceding testing. The collection of a fasting glucose specimen for baseline interpretation is followed by ingestion of a 75 g glucose drink for the average adult. Glucose tolerance challenge testing for pregnant women uses a 50 g glucose drink for a 1-hour evaluation of glucose metabolism or a 100 g drink for the extended 3-hour testing. A venous sample is collected each hour after the glucose is ingested to evaluate how well the body is metabolizing the sugar. The normal curve for GTT will display the highest glucose value approximately 140 mg/dL 1 hour after glucose ingestion, with sequential glucose levels of less than 140/dL. A 2-hour GTT result of ≥140 mg/dL indicates glucose intolerance, metabolic impairment, and prediabetes. Confirmation of a diabetes diagnosis is indicated by a 2-hour GTT result of ≥200 mg/dL.

Role of Glycated Proteins in Diabetes Diagnosis and Management

RBCs are permeable to blood glucose, allowing for glucose to bind with hemoglobin A proteins in the cell through nonenzymatic reactions taking place over the life span of the RBC to produce **glycated hemoglobin** or **hemoglobin A1C** The concentration of hemoglobin A1C molecules measured in whole blood correlates with a patient's average glucose levels over the previous 3 months. An estimated average glucose (eAG) is determined from hemoglobin A1C results with the following formula: $\mathbf{eAG = (28.7 \times A1C) - 46.71}$. A 1% change in the hemoglobin A1C results adjusts the eAG result by roughly 28 mg/dL. Hemoglobin A1C levels are used to diagnosis new cases of diabetes and to evaluate the management of current cases.

Glycated albumin measurement is based on the half-life of serum albumin and is used to estimate glucose control more rapidly than hemoglobin A1C. A ratio of glycated serum proteins to glycated albumin **(GSP/GA)** measured in blood creates a profile of the patient's glucose control for the 2–3 weeks before testing. The GSP/GA results aid in closely monitoring average glucose levels in patients with gestational diabetes, hemolytic anemia, blood loss, and those receiving hemodialysis.

Correlation of Carbohydrate Laboratory Testing with Disease States

The detection and diagnosis of **diabetes** in patients is most commonly attributed to consistently high fasting glucose, glucose tolerance, and hemoglobin A1C levels. Ranges of results that are higher than normal are designated **prediabetic** because they are not high enough to indicate a diabetes diagnosis. Diet, exercise, and other lifestyle changes may be able to lower prediabetic levels back to normal to keep the diagnosis of type 2 diabetes at bay.

Diabetic ketoacidosis is a disease state resulting in increased blood pH due to excessively high blood sugar. Laboratory findings include increased serum and urine glucose levels, increased A1C and potassium, decreased sodium and chloride, and positive blood and urine ketones.

Hypoglycemia caused by the impaired breakdown of glycogen, islet cell hyperplasia, and insulinoma creates an overproduction of insulin that drops glucose to unsafe levels that can cause cardiac and brain damage.

Normal, prediabetic, and diabetic ranges for glucose testing are as follows:

Test	Normal	Prediabetic	Diabetic
Hemoglobin A1C	<5.7%	5.7–6.4%	≥6.5%
Fasting glucose	70–99 mg/dL	100–125 mg/dL	≥126 mg/dL
Two-hour GTT	<140 mg/dL	140–199 mg/dL	≥200 mg/dL
Random glucose	—	—	≥200 mg/dL

Lipids

Physiology and Metabolic Pathways of Lipids

Fats, oils, and hormones are among the biochemical compounds that do not interact well with water and are more broadly categorized as lipids. Lipids are derived from the chemical linkage between a variety of small molecules that function as chemical messengers, energy storage molecules, or structural components of cell membranes. Fatty acids are introduced to the body from diet or from the metabolic breakdown of glucose and stored fats. Fatty acids are oxidized during lipid metabolism to create energy or to form new lipids by using small molecules. Triglycerides obtained through the diet are metabolized into smaller fatty acid chains by bile acids in the small intestine and are further digested into monoglyceride molecules by pancreatic lipases. These molecules are absorbed and resynthesized by the intestinal epithelium, combining with cholesterol and apolipoproteins to form chylomicrons. Lipid molecules play a role in the following metabolic processes: acting as hormones or hormone precursors, energy storage, metabolic fuels, cell membrane structure and functional components, and insulation for heat loss and nerve impulse conduction.

DISORDERS ASSOCIATED WITH ABNORMAL LIPID METABOLISM

Hereditary and acquired lipid disorders are caused by abnormalities in lipid metabolism leading to increased total cholesterol, low-density lipoproteins (LDLs), or triglycerides or by decreased HDL levels.

Hyperlipidemia is a generic term referring to abnormally elevated levels of plasma lipids. **Primary hyperlipidemias** are most often derived from genetic causes, whereas **secondary hyperlipidemias** are a result of underlying causes such as the following: diabetes, drug and alcohol consumption, aging, high-fat diets, physical inactivity, and obesity. Elevated LDL levels can result in plaque deposits in blood vessels, causing **atherosclerosis** and increased risk of coronary artery disease. **Familial hypercholesterolemia** is an autosomal-dominant disorder caused by a deficiency in LDL receptors on the surface of cells in the liver resulting in cholesterol being unable to move into cells. A lack of cholesterol inside of the cells promotes the production of even more cholesterol, leading to very high total cholesterol and LDL levels that bring about coronary vascular disease, strokes, and fat deposits on tendons. **Familial lecithin cholesterol acyltransferase deficiency** is an autosomal-recessive disorder that is characterized by the lack of an enzyme that esterifies cholesterol in plasma. This enzyme deficiency leads to increased levels of plasma cholesterol, phospholipids, and triglycerides that cause renal and liver failure, anemia, and lens opacities.

Hypolipidemia is characterized by abnormally low plasma lipid levels with total cholesterol below 120 mg/dL and LDL levels of less than 50 mg/dL Genetic diseases, malnutrition, malabsorption, cancer, hyperthyroidism, and liver disease are attributed to decreased plasma lipid levels.

PHYSICAL AND CHEMICAL PROPERTIES OF LIPOPROTEINS

Lipids combine with proteins in the liver and intestines to create the chemical compound known as lipoproteins. Lipoproteins serve as the mode of transport through the bloodstream for insoluble cholesterol, triglycerides, and phospholipid molecules. The structure of lipoproteins is comprised of a spherical nonpolar lipid core and a surface layer of apoproteins, phospholipids, and nonesterified cholesterol. In synthesis and circulation, lipoproteins' physical structure constantly fluctuates based on their function at the time. Hydrophobic lipids in the core of lipoproteins become hydrophilic with the assistance of the molecule's surface proteins. Ultimately, the protein components of lipoproteins determine the structure, metabolism, and interactions with liver and tissue receptor cells.

Lipoproteins are classified by their density into the following categories: chylomicrons, very low-density lipoproteins (VLDLs), low-density lipoproteins (LDLs), intermediate-density lipoproteins, and high-density lipoproteins (HDLs). Molecule densities are derived from their relative concentration of heavy triglycerides to lighter cholesterols and phospholipids, and the diameter of the molecule's spherical body. Some 60–70% of circulating lipoproteins are LDLs that transfer cholesterol from their site of synthesis in the liver to tissues in the body, whereas 20–35% are HDLs that bring excess cholesterol from tissues back to the liver to be metabolized and excreted from the body. VLDLs make up 5–12% of circulating lipoproteins that function to transport endogenous lipids, and <10% of lipoproteins are chylomicrons that transport exogenous lipids introduced to the body via dietary nutrients.

PHYSICAL AND CHEMICAL PROPERTIES OF PHOSPHOLIPIDS AND TRIGLYCERIDES

Phospholipids are composed of two fatty acid chains and one phosphate group connected to each other by one glycerol molecule. The fatty acid chains are hydrophobic, or "water fearing," whereas the phosphate group is hydrophilic, or "water loving." This unique chemical structure allows for phospholipids to line up in a double layer in the presence of water and act as the main structural component of cell membranes. Phospholipid membranes are semipermeable, only allowing small molecules that are easily dissolved in fat to pass through. This characteristic better maintains a balance between intracellular and extracellular environments.

Triglycerides are made up of a three-carbon trihydroxy alcohol glycerol molecule that is linked to a fatty acid at each of its three hydroxy groups by an ester bond. Triglycerides possess no electrical charge and are only soluble in certain organic solvents due to their hydrophobic nature. The melting point of triglycerides varies based on their fatty acid components with the melting point temperature increasing with the increase in double bonds and carbons in the hydrocarbon chains. Oils composed of unsaturated fatty acids are commonly liquid at room temperature, whereas saturated fatty acid-containing fats are solid or semisolid at room temperature. Ingested triglycerides are stored in adipose tissue, serving as insulation and padding for cells, and they are also transported to cells to be used as an energy source.

Physical and Chemical Properties of Cholesterols and Apolipoproteins

Cholesterols are an organic substance that belong to the steroid family. Approximately 30% of cholesterol in the body comes from dietary consumption, whereas the other 70% is synthesized by the liver. Cholesterols are an intermediate compound or starting material for the synthesis of steroid hormones, vitamin D, and bile acids and are an important structural component in cell membranes. Composed of one hydroxyl group, a steroid nucleus, and a hydrocarbon side chain, cholesterol is an odorless, tasteless, white, crystalline or waxy substance that is insoluble in water. Due to their insolubility, cholesterol molecules must attach to LDLs and HDLs for transport throughout the bloodstream.

Apolipoproteins are the water-soluble protein portion of lipoprotein compounds that aid in the transport of liquids. These proteins stabilize lipoprotein structures, serve as enzyme cofactors in lipid metabolic processes, and interact with lipoprotein receptors and transport proteins involved in the uptake and clearance of lipoproteins. Apolipoproteins are divided into several classes based on their genetic makeup and function, with the major apolipoproteins belonging to classes A, B, C, and E. **Apolipoprotein A** is the major structural protein of HDL, and **apolipoproteins B48** and **B100** are the major proteins in LDL. **Class C apolipoproteins** are most associated with VLDLs and aid in controlling lipid metabolism. **Apolipoprotein E** plays a role in lipoprotein metabolism and is the major lipoprotein of the central nervous system (CNS).

Lipid Testing Methods

Quantitative analysis of total cholesterol and triglyceride serum levels is achieved through enzymatic colorimetric reactions. **Cholesterol oxidase methods** measure the total cholesterol though the following process: cholesterol esterase enzymes hydrolyze cholesterol esters, cholesterol lipids are freed into a solution, and cholesterol oxidase enzymes oxidize the molecules eliciting a quantifiable, colorimetric response to the hydrogen peroxide concentrations produced. Serum or plasma triglycerides are measured by **coupled enzymatic reactions** beginning with lipase hydrolyzing triglycerides to produce glycerol and fatty acids. Glycerol is then oxidized by glycerol oxidase, and the hydrogen peroxide produced is measured by its absorbance at 500 nm.

HDL and LDL cholesterols can be measured from specimens with no pretreatment by the same enzymatic colorimetric principles. Samples can be centrifuged to remove chylomicrons, VLDL, and LDL from a sample by precipitation, and HDL can be indirectly analyzed from the supernatant of the treated sample. **Ultracentrifugation** can be used to separate and examine lipoproteins by their rates of floatation, but it is time consuming and expensive. More efficiently, LDL and VLDL serum and plasma levels can be indirectly determined by the **Friedewald method**, which calculates the concentrations from measured total cholesterol (TC), HDL, and triglyceride (TG) values. The Friedewald method formulas are as follows:

$$\text{LDL} = \text{TC} - \text{HDL} - (\text{TG}/5)$$

$$\text{VLDL} = \text{TG}/5$$

Limitations of the Friedewald method arise in samples with abnormally low triglyceride levels and samples with triglycerides measuring >400 mg/dL because they can falsely over- and underestimate LDL values, respectively.

Collecting, Processing, and Troubleshooting Lipid Testing Samples

Serum and plasma lipid samples are collected via venipuncture into tubes with no lithium heparin, EDTA, or other additives. It is highly recommended for patients to fast for 12 hours prior to collection for accurate results. The following effects may take place in a sample if 12-hour fasting is not achieved: LDL and HDL cholesterol concentrations decrease, triglyceride concentrations increase, and chylomicrons are present and cause interference for 6–9 hours after eating. For best results, samples should be centrifuged and serum or plasma should be separated from the RBCs to avoid the exchange of lipids between the sample and cells. Nonfasting samples are acceptable, and this detail should be taken into consideration when interpreting the results. Lipemia due to increased serum or plasma lipids can interfere with direct testing methodologies for cholesterol, and any free glycerol present can falsely increase triglyceride results.

Interpretation of Lipid Laboratory Results and Correlation to Disease States

Lipid test results are interpreted and correlated to disease states in the following ways:

Healthy blood cholesterol reference values

Demographic	Total Cholesterol	HDL	LDL	Triglycerides
≤19 years	<170 mg/dL	>45 mg/dL	<100 mg/dL	<150 mg/dL
≥20 years male	125–200 mg/dL	≥40 mg/dL	<100 mg/dL	<150 mg/dL
≥20 years female	125–200 mg/dL	≥50 mg/dL	<100 mg/dL	<150 mg/dL

Hyperlipidemia is the condition characterized by total cholesterol and triglyceride values above the normal ranges and can lead to plaque buildup in the blood vessels. Risk factors that increase the probability of coronary and atherosclerotic vascular diseases are the following: family history of coronary heart disease, diabetes mellitus, hypertension, current smoker, and HDL levels of <39 mg/dL. In patients with elevated LDL levels, the calculated LDL and number of risk factors present are used to determine the methods of treatment. For patients with zero and two or more risk factors, but no coronary heart disease, use low-fat diets to manage LDL levels at >100 mg/dL. Drug treatment is considered in patients with two or more risk factors and LDL levels of >160 mg/dL despite taking dietary measures and in patients with or without risk factors and LDL levels of >190 mg/dL. Maintaining an LDL level of <100 mg/dL is optimal for patients with coronary artery disease, peripheral vascular disease, or cerebrovascular disease.

Hypercholesterolemia is the most common cause of mild to moderate LDL elevations and is associated with the following disorders and factors: biliary cirrhosis, hypothyroidism, diabetes mellitus, nephrotic syndrome, menopause, oral contraceptives, hormone replacement therapy, and dietary excess.

Heme Derivatives

Heme Molecules

Heme molecules are cyclic tetrapyrroles containing iron that attach as a prosthetic group to other molecules to produce heme derivatives. The cytosol and mitochondria in liver and bone marrow cells synthesize heme molecules. To begin heme synthesis, succinyl CoA and glycine are combined by the aminolevulinic acid (ALA) synthase enzyme to form ALA. ALA dehydrase enzymes dehydrate ALA, producing porphobilinogens, that are condensed to form a linear tetrapyrrole by porphobilinogen deaminase. This compound cyclizes, forming the heme precursor uroporphyrinogen III, chlorophylls, and vitamin B_{12}. Uroporphyrinogen III is converted by uroporphyrinogen decarboxylase to coprophyrinogen III, which is then oxidized in the mitochondria to become protoporphyrinogen III. Oxidation of protoporphyrinogen III produces protoporphyrin III. In the final step of synthesis, iron is added to protoporphyrin III by ferrochelatase to create heme. The synthesis and production of heme are regulated by ALA synthase enzymes that act upon or are inhibited by levels of hemin.

When heme attaches as a prosthetic group to globulins, it forms the derivatives hemoglobin and myoglobin. Molecules of heme are also present in the cytochromes of cells to aid in cellular respiration processes. These molecules function to reversibly bind to O_2 molecules for its transport and storage. The process of heme degradation begins with the breakdown of RBCs in the spleen, where they oxidized to release iron atoms and biliverdin. Biliverdin is further degraded to form bilirubin, which is conjugated in the liver and excreted in feces and urine.

Normal and Abnormal Hemoglobin Variants

Normal hemoglobin variants function to influence normal RBC morphology and reduce the risk of hemolytic anemias, jaundice, and methemoglobinemia.

HbA is the principal hemoglobin variant circulating in adults, which contains **two α-chains** and **two β-chains.**

HbA$_2$ molecules contain **two α-chains** and **two δ-polypeptide chains**, where δ-chains vary from β-chains by only 10 amino acids, allowing the hemoglobin molecule to remain fully functional.

HbF is the major intrauterine hemoglobin present in growing fetuses and newborns. This hemoglobin contains **two α-chains** and **two γ-chains** and is quickly cleared from the body after birth as HbA production rapidly increases.

Structurally abnormal hemoglobin variants with a significant pathological role are called **hemoglobinopathies.** Single amino acid substitutions on the polypeptide chains cause structural abnormalities. Hemoglobinopathies can be inherited or can be a result of a genetic mutation on the α-chains or, more commonly, the β-chains.

HbS is the most common abnormal hemoglobin, with a valine substituting glutamic acid in the sixth position on the **β-chain.** One inherited HbS genotype causes **sickle cell trait**, whereas two inherited genotypes cause **sickle cell disease**, characterized by the "sickling" of RBCs, anemia, and reduced O_2 concentrations.

HbC occurs from lysine being substituted for glutamic acid in the sixth position on the **β-chain,** which can be inherited in a homozygous or heterozygous state, or in combination with HbS. The presence of HbC creates **target RBCs** and can precipitate **HbC crystals** in RBCs.

Hemoglobin and Bilirubin

Found in RBCs, **hemoglobin** is a conjugated protein composed of four globulin protein subunits, each linked to a prosthetic heme group. Heme groups are compounds of iron and tetrapyrrole-structured porphyrins. The pyrrole molecules of the porphyrin ring are linked together in a cyclic arrangement, with iron occupying the middle of the molecule. Hemoglobin iron molecules bind to O_2 to form oxyhemoglobin, and the amine groups of protein chains bind to CO_2. The O_2 is carried from the lungs and distributed to all tissues in the body for cellular respiration, and CO_2 is picked up from tissues as a waste product and carried back to the lungs for excretion. Oxygenated hemoglobin appears red, whereas deoxygenated hemoglobin presents with a purple-blue hue.

Bilirubin is a waste product from the breakdown of heme molecules that exists as a dark-orange to yellow open-chain tetrapyrrole structure. Biliverdin released in the breakdown of old RBCs is converted to bilirubin noncovalently bonded to albumin, known as **unconjugated bilirubin**. Unconjugated bilirubin is brought to the liver where it is **conjugated** to glucuronic acid, becomes water soluble, and can be excreted from the body in urine and bile.

Urobilinogen and Myoglobin

Urobilinogen is a colorless by-product of the bacterial reduction of bilirubin that takes place in the intestines. Approximately half of the urobilinogen formed is further reduced to urobilin in the intestines and excreted in the feces. The other half is reabsorbed by the liver, entered into the circulation, and then excreted in small amounts by the kidneys.

Myoglobin is a monomeric heme protein that is found in striated skeletal and cardiac muscles. Myoglobin molecules contain eight connected α-helix structures with attached O_2 binding sites for the transport and storage of O_2 in the cells of muscles. The O_2-bound myoglobin participates in the release of energy used for muscular contractions by transporting O_2 from the skeletal cell membrane to the mitochondria. The oxidation of iron ions in the heme portion of the molecule accounts for the red color of the muscles.

Heme-Derivative Testing Methods

Hemoglobin is measured by the **cyanomethemoglobin method** in which RBCs are lysed by a stromatolytic reagent to release hemoglobin. Ferricyanide oxidizes hemoglobin to methemoglobin, and potassium cyanide is added to form stable cyanomethemoglobin. Cyanomethemoglobin present is measured photometrically by its absorbance at 540 nm, with the color intensity being directly proportional to the concentration of hemoglobin in a sample.

Bilirubin is measured by the **diazo reaction** on a tablet, strip, or in an automated analyzer. Direct, or conjugated, bilirubin reacts with diazonium salt to form azobilirubin, which produces a blue-purple color on tablets and a red color in automated systems. Direct bilirubin concentration is directly proportional to the intensity of the color manually observed on a tablet or strip or photometrically measured in automated systems. The **total bilirubin** concentration is proportional to the photometric measurement of the red color produced from the reaction between the analyte and 3,5-dichlorophenyl diazonium.

Urobilinogen is measured on test strips based on **Ehrlich's reaction**. Ehrlich's reagent consists of *para*-dimethylaminobenzaldehyde in an acid buffer. Urobilinogen in a sample reacts with the reagent to produce a pink to red color. The intensity of color observed is directly proportional to the concentration of urobilinogen present in a sample.

Myoglobin concentrations are measured by **particle-enhanced immunoturbidimetric assays.** Myoglobin-specific antibodies are bound to latex particles and will form antigen–antibody complexes with myoglobin present in a sample. Agglutination formed by the complexes are measured turbidimetrically and are proportional to the concentration of myoglobin in a sample.

Heme-Derivative Testing Samples

Specimen sources, collection requirements, and circumstances interfering with heme-derivative testing are described below:

- Hemoglobin
  - **Specimen requirement:** EDTA whole blood, venipuncture, or capillary collection
  - Interfering substances and circumstances:
    - **Clotted samples**: clog tubing in automated analyzers, not acceptable for testing
    - **Hemolysis**: a false increase in relation to hematocrit and RBC indices, normally: $hemoglobin = 3 \times hematocrit = 3 \times RBC\ count$, known as the "rule of three"
    - **Lipemia:** a false increase in results due to abnormal light scatter, corrected with plasma replacement procedures
    - **Extremely high WBC counts**: false increase in results due to abnormal light scatter, corrected with plasma replacement procedures
    - **Abnormal hemoglobin variants**: resist RBC lysis, falsely decrease hemoglobin concentrations.
- Urine bilirubin and urobilinogen:
  - **Specimen requirement:** random urine sample in a sterile screw-cap container
  - Interfering substances and circumstances:
    - **False positive:** some medications and highly pigmented urine
    - **False negative: bilirubin,** exposure to light or ascorbic acid; **urobilinogen,** formalin.
- Bilirubin
  - **Specimen requirement:** serum or plasma, venipuncture or capillary collection, separated from cells within 2 hours of collection, and protected from light
  - Interfering substances and circumstances:
    - **Light exposure, hemolysis:** falsely decreased results due to degradation
    - **Lipemia:** falsely increased results due to abnormal light scatter.
- Myoglobin
  - **Specimen requirement:** serum or plasma, venipuncture or capillary collection, separated from cells within 2 hours of collection
  - Interfering substances and circumstances:
    - **Hemolysis:** a false increase.

Interpretation of Heme-Derivative Laboratory Results and Correlation to Disease States

Normal reference ranges for heme-derivative analytes are as follows:

Analyte	Normal Range
Hemoglobin	Males: 14–18 g/dL Females: 12–16 g/dL
Total bilirubin	7–14 days old: <15.0 mg/dL 15 days–17 years old: ≤1.0 mg/dL ≥18 years old: ≤1.2 mg/dL

Analyte	Normal Range
Direct bilirubin	0.0–0.4 mg/dL
Bilirubin, urine	Negative, 0 EU
Urobilinogen	≤1 mg/dL or 1 EU
Myoglobin	≤90 μg/L

Abnormal test results are indicative of injury or disease in the body. Listed below are the causes of abnormal **hemoglobin** results:

- Low
  - Anemias — iron or vitamin deficiency, aplastic, sickle cell, thalassemia
  - Chronic kidney disease
  - Liver cirrhosis
  - Lead poisoning
  - Cancers or myelodysplastic syndromes
- Elevated
  - Congenital heart disease
  - Chronic obstructive pulmonary disease exacerbation, emphysema
  - Dehydration
  - Polycythemia vera.

Bilirubin and urobilinogen can be used to differentiate disease states as noted below:

Disease	Bilirubin	Urobilinogen
Hemolytic disease	Normal	Increased
Liver diseases — hepatitis, cirrhosis	Normal or increased	Increased
Biliary duct obstruction	Increased	Normal

Myoglobin concentrations above normal ranges occur due to muscle and tissue damage in the following circumstances:

- Acute myocardial infarction (AMI) — rises 30 minutes after onset, peaks at 4–10 hours, returns to normal within 24 hours. Normal results exclude AMI, but an increase does not diagnose AMI
- Renal damage
- Rhabdomyolysis
- Any trauma or disease-causing muscle injury or destruction.

Proteins and Enzymes

Enzymes

Enzymes are organic protein structures that are a necessary participant in almost all reactions in the body. Enzymes increase reaction rates to yield products at speeds necessary to sustain life processes by decreasing the amount of energy needed for reaction activation. Sequences of amino acids form the globular protein structure and determine the catalytic nature of an enzyme. The amino acid sequence also determines the location of substrate and allosteric binding sites and whether or not a cofactor is necessary for catalytic activity. The substrate binding site of an enzyme is known as the active site, where attachment of a substrate signals for an enzyme to catalyze a reaction. Allosteric binding sites allow for small molecules to attach to an enzyme and create a conformational change to either increase or decrease enzymatic activity. Some enzymes do not have catalytic characteristics and are instead responsible for the binding and orientation of catalytic cofactors that act on a substrate material. Although enzymes facilitate the activation and speed of reactions, they are not altered or consumed in the reactions that they participate in. Enzymes often work together to form metabolic pathways through a chain-like process with one enzyme's product becoming the next enzyme's substrate and so on.

Normal and Abnormal Enzyme Concentrations

Normal levels of enzymes indicate that the body's organs and metabolic pathways are functioning properly. Enzyme analysis is crucial for evaluating the functionality of and damage to many organs and organ systems including the heart, liver, pancreas, muscles, bones, joints, and associated tissues such as tendons and ligaments. Low levels of enzymes may indicate certain liver or gastrointestinal dysfunctions, whereas an increase in enzymes is indicative of many other diseases and disorders. Enzyme concentrations and reactivity are also used to differentiate disease states from one another. Major enzymes used for evaluating or diagnosing disease and dysfunction are categorized as follows:

- Cardiac enzymes:
  - CK isoenzymes
  - LD isoenzymes
- Liver enzymes:
  - AST
  - ALT
  - ALP
  - 5′NT
  - GGT
  - LD isoenzymes
- Pancreatic enzymes:
  - Amylase
  - Lipase.

LD and CK Enzymes

Lactate dehydrogenase (LD) is an enzyme that catalyzes the conversion of lactate to pyruvate and pyruvate back to lactate during glycolysis. Through the transfer of a hydride from one molecule to another, lactate converts nicotinamide adenine dinucleotide (NAD) to NAD + hydrogen (NADH) to become pyruvate, whereas pyruvate converts NADH back to NAD to become lactate. An LD molecule is a tetramer composed of four subunits that is found in most cells in the body. Two different LD protein chains, M and H, combine in the subunits to create five tissue-specific isoenzyme forms of LD. The LD isoenzymes are found in the following: **LDH-1 (4H)**, heart, RBCs, and brain; **LDH-2 (3H1M),** reticuloendothelial system; **LDH-3 (2H2M),** lungs; **LDH-4 (1H3M)**, kidneys, pancreas, and placenta; and **LDH-5 (4M),** liver and skeletal muscles.

Creatine kinase (CK) is most commonly expressed in muscle, cardiac tissue, and brain tissue. CK and ATP catalyze the conversion of creatine to produce phosphocreatine and ADP in a reaction that can be reversed back to the original energy and enzyme. Two subunits, muscle (M) and brain (B), exist on the CK enzyme, which allow for three isoenzymes found in different tissues in the body. **CK-BB** is specific to smooth muscle and nonmuscle tissues in the brain, gastrointestinal (GI) tract, prostate, and uterus; **CK-MB** is specific to cardiac tissue; and **CK-MM** is expressed in cardiac and skeletal tissue destruction.

AST, ALT, AND GGT ENZYMES

Aspartate transaminase (AST) aids in amino acid metabolism by acting as a catalyst in the back-and-forth transfer of an α-amino group between glutamate and aspartate where cellular aspartate is converted to oxaloacetate. Molecules of AST consist of two identical polypeptide subunits configured in a dimeric structure. AST is present in the liver, cardiac and skeletal muscles, the kidneys, and RBCs and is released upon the disturbance of destruction of their cells.

Alanine transaminase (ALT) is most commonly found in the liver and catalyzes an amino group transfer from L-alanine to α-ketoglutarate to produce pyruvate and L-glutamate.

Gamma-glutamyl transferase (GGT) acts as a catalyst in the transfer of amino acids across the cellular membrane and in the process of glutathione and leukotriene metabolisms. The structure of GGT molecules consists of one light and one heavy polypeptide chain with the active site presenting on the light chain. GGT is present in the cell membranes of the following types of tissues: gallbladder, pancreas, bile duct, spleen, kidneys, heart, brain, and seminal vesicles.

LIPASE AND AMYLASE

Lipase is an enzyme that catalyzes the hydrolysis of ester linkages in lipids to produce fatty acids and alcohols. Most commonly found in and secreted by the pancreas, lipase aids in the digestion, transport, and processing of dietary fat molecules. As a subclass of esterase enzymes, specific lipases are also found to have activity in the liver, salivary glands, and gastrointestinal tract.

Amylase enzymes catalyze the breakdown of starches and glycogen into glucose and other simple sugars to be used by cells in the body. Secreted by the salivary glands, amylase begins the digestion process by breaking the saccharide chains of starches at random locations. Amylase continues to aid in digestion by also being secreted by the islet cells of the pancreas.

ALKALINE PHOSPHATASE, 5'-NUCLEOTIDASE, ACID PHOSPHATASE, AND CHOLINESTERASE

Alkaline phosphatase (ALP) is found in the membranes of cells in all tissues of the body and facilitates the transfer of metabolites across the cell membrane, extracellular transport of lipids, and the calcification process of bone synthesis. ALP is formed by two identical molecules each containing two zinc and three magnesium metal ions at the catalytic sites. An alkaline pH of 10 and activation of magnesium ions are essential to this enzyme's function. ALP is the most concentrated and active in the following tissues: bone, gastrointestinal mucosa, the biliary tree of the liver, renal tubule cells, leukocytes, and the placenta.

5′-Nucleotidase (5′NT) assists in metabolizing extracellular impermeable nucleotides to nucleosides that cross the membrane and enter cells. 5′NT is present in four forms, one bound to the plasma membrane and three soluble forms with affinities to different substrates. Increased serum 5′NT, along with increased ALP, aids in the differential diagnosis of hepatobiliary diseases from bone disorders.

Acid phosphatase (ACP) enzymes function in an acidic environment during digestion to release phosphoryl groups from larger molecules. ACP is a tetramer primarily found in the prostate, but it can also be found in erythrocytes, platelets, bone, liver, spleen, and kidneys.

Cholinesterase enzymes aid in keeping the nervous system functioning properly. **Acetylcholinesterase,** found in RBCs, acts in the breakdown of acetylcholine to maintain proper nerve stimulation, and plasma **pseudocholinesterase** participates in processing and metabolizing drugs.

LIPID TESTING METHODS

Spectrophotometric methods quantitatively measure an analyte by comparing the color of a solution of unknown concentration to the color of a solution of known concentration. The following enzymes are measured by spectrophotometry:

- **LD** converts pyruvate to lactate and oxidizes NADH to NAD, with the rate of decrease in NADH absorbance at 340 nm being proportional to LD enzyme activity.
- **GGT** acts on the substrate gamma-glutamyl-p-nitroanilide and the nitroaniline released measured for GGT activity.
- **ALP** converts *p*-nitrophenyl phosphate to phosphate and *p*-nitrophenylate that is measured at 404–410 nm.
- **ALT** and **AST** activity is directly proportional the rate of decrease of NADH in a coupled enzyme kinetic method, determined at 340 nm.
- **ACP** assays cleave a phosphate substrate to produce a colored product for measurement.
- **CK** activity is proportional to the photometrically measured rate of NADPH formation during a coupled enzyme reaction.

Colorimetric assays quantify the concentration of **amylase, lipase, pseudocholinesterase,** and **RBC acetylcholinesterase** by photometrically measuring the variation in the intensity of color produced by their reactions with reagent substrates.

Electrophoresis methods use charged particles in an electrical field to separate solutes based on their rate of migration through gel. **ALP** and **CK isoenzymes** are separated from one another in acrylamide gel based on their individual heat stability, molecular size, and electric charge.

Lipase is also measured by **turbidimetry**, in which the loss of light intensity transmitted through a solution is measured and light scatter is quantified.

ENZYME TESTING SAMPLES

Serum or plasma enzyme testing samples are collected via venipuncture, and their measurement reactions can be affected by a variety of environmental and biochemical changes. Serum or plasma should be analyzed or separated from cells within 2 hours because interaction with the cells can falsely decrease enzyme activity. Samples with gross hemolysis, lipemia, and icterus may be rejected or released with a disclaimer if re-collection is not an option because they can affect the enzyme results in the following ways:

- Hemolysis
  - **Falsely increased:** ACP, ALP, ALT, AST, CK, LD
  - Falsely decreased: Amylase
- Lipemia
  - Falsely decreased: LD
- Icterus
  - Falsely decreased: GGT

During the testing process, enzymes require the following specifications for accurate measurement reactions: appropriate concentration of reactant, optimal temperature of 37 °C, correct cofactors and coenzymes, proper ionic strength, and optimal pH for the individual enzyme.

Test Result Interpretations and Disease States for LD, Total CK, and CK Isoenzymes

Normal reference ranges for LD, total CK and CK isoenzymes, along with disease states associated with an influx in these enzymes, are described below:

	LD	Total CK	CK-MM	CK-MB	CK-BB
Reference range	125–243 U/L	**Males**: 40–310 U/L **Females**: 25–195 U/L	100% of total CK	0% of total CK **or** 0–3.6 U/L	0% of total CK

High **lactate dehydrogenase (LD)** levels in blood exist as a result of the following: renal infarction, myocardial infarction, some malignancies, liver disease, muscle trauma, pernicious anemia, and other hemolytic diseases. An increase in total **creatine kinase (CK)** levels is associated with damage to skeletal, cardiac, and brain muscles. Testing of CK isoenzymes further distinguishes which type of tissue is being damaged. CK-MM is the prominent isoenzyme present in a healthy individual. Increased serum of plasma total CK with CK-MB of less than 3% greater than normal indicates destruction of skeletal muscle, whereas a CK-MB increase of greater than 6% indicates cardiac muscle damage. During a myocardial infarction, CK-MB enzymes will become elevated 4–8 hours after onset, peak at 12–24 hours, and return to normal within 72–96 hours. Along with other cardiac biomarkers, this allows for optimal treatment and management of a myocardial infarction. An increase in CK-BB levels indicates injury to the brain, GI tract, colon, prostate, or uterus. Elevated CK levels are also associated with muscular dystrophy, rhabdomyolysis, and acute kidney injuries.

Test Result Interpretations and Disease States for AST, ALT, GGT, ALP, and 5′NT

Normal reference ranges for AST, ALT, GGT, ALP, and 5′NT along with disease states associated with an influx in these enzymes are described below:

	AST	ALT	GGT	ALP	5′NT
Reference range	5–45 U/L	7–55 U/L	8–60 U/L	40–130 U/L	0–15 U/L

AST enzymes are elevated in a variety of diseases and disorders due to their presence in the liver, cardiac muscles, RBCs, and other tissues. Levels of AST above normal may indicate the following: myocardial infarction, muscle trauma, renal infarction, hemolysis, hepatocellular damage, cirrhosis, and carcinomas of the liver. **ALT** is also elevated in the liver diseases mentioned and is more specific to liver tissue damage than AST. Although normally present in high concentrations in renal tissues, elevations of **GGT** in the blood is an indication of liver diseases, specifically, biliary obstructions and damage due to chronic alcoholism. **ALP** is present in bone, intestinal mucosa, renal tubule cells, the liver, certain tumors, and the placenta. A normal elevation of ALP levels is present in the third trimester of pregnancy and in growing children due to rapid skeletal growth. Diseases and disorders causing an increase in ALP include biliary obstructions due to gallstones or malignancy and bone disorders with osteoblastic activity such as Paget's disease, osteoblastic tumors, rickets, and hyperparathyroidism. Levels of **5′NT** in blood are evaluated along with ALP to differentiate bone disease (normal 5′NT) from liver disease (increased 5′NT).

Test Result Interpretations and Disease States for Amylase, Lipase, Total Acid Phosphatase, and Cholinesterase

The normal reference ranges for amylase, lipase, acid phosphatase, and cholinesterase enzymes as well as the disease states associated with these enzymes are described below:

	Amylase	Lipase
Reference range	25–125 U/L	10–140 U/L
Pancreatitis	>450 U/L	>400 U/L

Elevated concentrations of amylase and lipase are indicative of damage to the pancreas. In acute pancreatitis, **amylase** is the first enzyme to increase in concentration 2–12 hours after onset and peaks at 24 hours, whereas **lipase** increases 4–8 hours after onset and remains elevated for 7–14 days. Pancreatitis caused by an obstruction of pancreatic ducts by gallstones or malignancy and alcohol-related pancreatitis is indicated by lipase concentrations 2.5–3 times higher than amylase concentrations. Amylase concentrations <450 U/L occur due to salivary gland obstructions caused by stones, malignancy, or mumps.

	Total ACP	Prostatic ACP
Reference range	0–4.3 U/L	0–3.5 ng/mL

Increased **total acid phosphatase** indicates bone diseases and metastatic prostate, bone, and breast cancers. The tartrate-resistant portion of ACP is also elevated in cases of hairy cell leukemia. The total ACP expresses the highest elevation in metastatic prostate carcinoma, which also presents with an elevation in the **prostatic ACP isoenzyme**.

	Pseudocholinesterase	RBC Acetylcholinesterase
Reference range	5,320–12,920 U/L	30–60 U/g of hemoglobin

Cholinesterases are some of the few enzymes whose decrease in concentration are clinically significant. Significant decreases in **pseudocholinesterase** levels can result in neuromuscular effects and may alter the effectiveness of certain anesthetics. Decreased pseudocholinesterase and **RBC acetylcholinesterase** levels are used to determine and monitor organophosphate poisoning.

Proteins and Other Nitrogen-Containing Compounds

Proteins are necessary for just about every structure and process that takes place in the body. Formed by amino acids linked together, proteins serve the following purposes:

- Serving as structural components in the organization of tissue-forming cells.
- Allowing the movement and contraction of muscles.
- Acting as biochemical catalysts.
- Providing immunological responses.
- Transporting and storing important molecules throughout the body.

Proteins are synthesized in the ribosomes of various cells throughout the body by ribonucleic acid (RNA) polymerase transcribing and the DNA coding region in a cell, producing a messenger RNA (mRNA) sequence. Ribosomes then translate mRNA codons to their associated amino acids, which are linked together by peptide bonds to form chains. Finally, polypeptide chains undergo modifications and join with other chains to become fully functional proteins.

Protein metabolism begins in the gastrointestinal tract with protease enzymes hydrolyzing peptide bonds and cleaving proteins into smaller peptides or single amino acids. Protein and amino acid catabolism leads to nitrogenous waste compounds that must be excreted from the body. Uric acid and ammonia are by-products of protein and amino acid breakdown that can be toxic if they are not cleared from the body. Ammonia is carried to the liver where it is converted to urea, which is excretable by the kidneys, whereas uric acid itself is filtered and excreted by the kidneys into the urine.

Normal and Abnormal Protein- and Nitrogen-Containing Compound Concentrations

For the proper function and structure of several body systems, every protein- and nitrogen-containing compound exists in varying concentrations. Total protein concentrations less than the normal reference range can indicate malabsorption or improper digestion, or liver and kidney problems. High concentrations of nitrogenous waste products, cardiac markers, tumor markers, and other proteins can indicate a multitude of clinical disease states, as listed below:

- **Uric acid:** renal impairment or failure, gout, leukemia, chemotherapy treatments
- **Creatinine:** renal function impairment
- **Urea:** renal function impairment, high-protein diet
- **Ammonia:** advanced liver disease, viral hepatitis, cirrhosis, Reye's syndrome, renal function impairment
- **Cardiac markers**: rise, peak, and return to normal at various stages of an acute myocardial infarction allowing for more accurate diagnosis and prognosis for patients and indicate the risk of CHF
- **Tumor markers**: presence, recurrence, or failed therapy in marker specific cancers.

Amino Acids and Proteins

Amino acids link together to form peptides, polypeptides, and proteins. They consist of a carbon atom attached to a carboxyl group, an amine group, a hydrogen atom, and an "R" group side chain that is unique to each amino acid. Amino acid R groups allow them to uniquely react with other amino acids. Amino acids have melting points greater than 200 °C and are soluble in water, ethanol (ETOH), and other polar solvents. There are 11 amino acids synthesized by the body and 9 essential amino acids that must be obtained through the diet, which are classified based on their structure and chemical characteristics into the following groups:

- **Basic:** histidine, lysine, arginine
- **Aliphatic:** alanine, glycine, isoleucine, leucine, valine
- **Cyclic:** proline
- **Aromatic**: phenylalanine, tyrosine, tryptophan
- **Hydroxyl or sulfur-containing**: cysteine, methionine, serine, threonine
- **Acidic with their amide**: aspartate, asparagine, glutamate, glutamine.

Proteins are made up of 100 or more amino acids linked together by amide bonds. Each protein begins with methionine, which attaches to the amine group of the first amino acid. The amine group attaches to the carboxyl group of the second amino acid, and the trend continues for the remainder of the protein. Proteins occur in four different structure formations: primary, single amino acid chain; secondary, amino acids linked by hydrogen bonds; tertiary, attraction between alpha helix and pleated sheet amino acid chains; and quaternary, a protein with more than one amino acid chain. Chemical and physical properties are unique to each protein due to the vast variance in amino acid combinations.

Uric Acid and Urea

Uric acid is the final product of purine metabolism when xanthine and hypoxanthine are catalyzed by xanthine oxidase. As a heterocyclic compound containing carbon, nitrogen, O_2, and hydrogen molecules, uric acid forms ions and salts that have low solubility probability in water and form crystalline structures. Uric acid is filtered from the blood by the kidneys and excreted in the urine.

Urea, also known as **blood urea nitrogen (BUN),** is a product of protein metabolism produced in the liver and is the body's main source of excreting nitrogen. Protein breakdown and amino acid alterations create ammonia, which is toxic to the body in increased concentrations. In the liver, two ammonia molecules combine with CO_2 to form urea, which can be cleared from the body by the kidneys and excreted in urine. Urea molecules are composed of two amino groups attached by a carbonyl group that is colorless, odorless, and highly soluble in water.

Creatinine, Ammonia, and Serum Albumin

Creatinine is a cyclic derivative of creatine that is produced spontaneously in muscle tissue during the action of creatine kinase converting creatine to creatine phosphate. The formation and release of creatinine into body fluids occurs at a constant rate, which is determined by an individual's muscle mass. Creatinine is carried from the tissues to the kidneys, where it is filtered by the glomeruli and excreted in the urine.

Ammonia is formed by the actions of intestinal bacteria breaking down amino acids. This toxic, nitrogenous waste product is a single nitrogen atom bonded to three hydrogen atoms that is a colorless gas emitting a pungent odor. Ammonia liquefies easily due to strong hydrogen bonds, and it solidifies into a white, crystalline formation at −77.7 °C. Ammonia is carried to the liver where it is converted to the relatively nontoxic urea.

Albumin, the major protein found in blood plasma, is a globular protein synthesized in the liver. Water-soluble albumin molecules regulate the oncotic pressure of the blood by binding to and transporting various substances and ions throughout the body, including calcium, sodium, potassium, fatty acids, hormones, bilirubin, thyroxine, and pharmaceutical drugs.

Tumor Markers

Tumor markers are substances synthesized and released by tumors or by the body in response to a tumor. Markers are used to differentiate normal tissue from a tumor, screen for the presence of cancer, or monitor the recurrence or severity of certain cancers. Properties are specific to individual tumor markers, as listed below:

- **Alpha fetoprotein (AFP)** is a protein that is normally synthesized in the liver and yolk sac of a growing fetus, but it can also be secreted in small amounts in the following cancers and diseases:
    - Hepatocarcinoma
    - Endodermal sinus tumors
    - Nonseminomatous testicular cancer
    - Teratocarcinoma of the testes or ovary
    - Malignancy of the mediastinum and sacrococcyx
    - Hepatitis
    - Cystic fibrosis.

- **Beta-human chorionic gonadotropin (β-hCG)** is a subunit of the hCG glycoprotein, composed of 145 amino acids. β-hCG is produced by trophoblast cells in the placenta during normal pregnancy, molar pregnancies, or the following malignancies:
    - Endodermal sinus tumors
    - Teratocarcinoma of the testes or ovaries
    - Testicular embryonal carcinoma
    - Choriocarcinoma.
- CA 15-3 and CA27.29 antigen concentrations monitor breast cancer disease progression, response to therapy, or detect the recurrence of disease in patients previously cleared of stage II or III breast cancer.
- CA 19-9 is a carbohydrate antigen primarily evaluated for the progression of colorectal and pancreatic carcinomas. It is also elevated in malignant and nonmalignant diseases of the pancreas, liver, and gallbladder.
- CA 125 is a carbohydrate antigen that is most commonly used in monitoring ovarian and endometrial cancers.
- Carcinoembryonic antigen (CEA) is a glycoprotein produced during fetal development that ceases before birth. After birth, CEA concentrations are measured to evaluate the treatment and tumor progression of various cancers such as gastrointestinal, breast, and neck. Elevations indicate residual disease or poor response to therapy.
- Prostate-specific antigen is a protein produced by normal and malignant prostate tissues that is used to screen for prostate cancer. High blood concentrations indicate the presence of prostate cancer but must be confirmed by biopsy because increased PSA can also be caused by noncancerous prostatitis. In confirmed cases of malignancy, PSA levels are directly proportional to the volume or size of a tumor and are evaluated in disease progression and in the effectiveness of therapy.

Viral Proteins

Viral proteins are formed by linked amino acids and serve structural and nonstructural functions within a virus. **Structural proteins** are found in the capsid and viral envelope, which protect viral nucleic acids from degradation inside and on the outermost layer of the virus, respectively. Glycoproteins embedded in the viral envelope bind to receptors on host cells membranes to attach to host cells. Once attached, viral proteins undergo a structural conformation change to enable them to fuse to and enter the host's cell wall for successful survival and replication of the virus. **Nonstructural viral proteins** are responsible for the replication of viral genes inside that host cell, as well as reducing the host immune response to the virus allowing it to flourish, continuing to infect host cells and cause disease. **Regulatory** and **accessory proteins** enhance viral gene transcription in host cells and carry out specific functions to aid in viral proliferation.

Cardiac Markers

Troponin is a protein complex comprised of three regulatory subunits, C, I, and T. The troponin complex aligns itself with tropomyosin and actin along the thin filaments on cardiac and skeletal muscle fibers to regulate muscle contractions by binding to calcium, triggering the production of muscular force. Troponin C is specific to skeletal muscle and contains three calcium binding sites, of which troponins I and T contain four sites for calcium binding and are specific to cardiac muscle.

B-type natriuretic peptide (BNP) is a polypeptide hormone that is secreted from the ventricular walls in response to the stretching caused by hypertension and volume overload. The 32 amino acid molecule is cleaved from the N-terminal end of the inactive proBNP molecule. Active BNP polypeptides act against the renin-aldosterone system to increase water and sodium excretion, causing vasodilation and decreasing blood pressure.

High-sensitivity C-reactive protein (hsCRP) is a ring-shaped pentameric protein that is released into circulation in response to inflammation. Synthesized in the liver, hsCRP is attracted to and binds to the surface of dying cells flagged by macrophages and T lymphocyte cells. Increased concentrations of hsCRP are indicative of chronic inflammation and an increased risk of cardiovascular and coronary heart diseases.

Homocysteine is a product of methionine amino acid metabolism and can be recycled to synthesize new methionine molecules or converted to cysteine by B vitamins. Increased serum concentrations of homocysteine indicate an increased risk for cardiovascular diseases and renal dysfunction.

Colorimetric, Spectrophotometric, and Enzymatic Testing Methods

Colorimetric assays quantify a substance's concentration by photometrically measuring the variation in the intensity of color produced by their reactions with reagent substrates.

Spectrophotometric methods quantitatively measure an analyte by comparing the color of a solution of unknown concentration to the color of a solution of known concentration. **Enzymatic** methodologies measure the concentration of a substance based on its consumption of enzymes in a reaction. Analytes are measured via colorimetric, spectrophotometric, or enzymatic methods with the following reactions:

- **Creatinine:** Jaffe reaction — creatinine reacts with picric acid in an alkaline solution, producing a red-orange-colored complex that absorbs light at 490–540 nm.
- **Blood urea nitrogen (BUN)**: In a colorimetric reaction, urea reacts with diacetyl monoxime producing a colored complex.
- **Uric acid**: In a colorimetric reaction, uric acid is reduced to phosphotungstic acid and then to tungsten blue, which is measured spectrophotometrically. Enzymatic methods are based on a uricase reaction producing allantoin and hydrogen peroxide, where hydrogen peroxide is coupled to create a colored, quantifiable product.

Ion-Selective Electrode, Chemiluminometric Immunoassay, and Enzyme-Linked Immunoassay Testing Methods

Ion-selective electrode (ISE) methodologies use an electrode to convert the activity of a solution dissolved ion into an electrical potential. This potential is then measured by a voltmeter or pH meter, directly correlated with the ionic concentration in a solution. The following analytes are measured via ISE:

- **Ammonia**: ISE measures the pH change of an ammonium chloride solution as ammonia diffuses across a semipermeable membrane.
- **BUN**: Urease hydrolyzes urea into ammonia, which is measured by ISE.

Chemiluminometric immunoassays are used for the measurement of troponin. This method employs a sandwich antibody assay, in which troponin attached to solid phase particles competes for binding sites on monoclonal chemiluminescent antibodies with troponin in a patient sample. The amount of light detected from patient-bound antibodies is directly proportional to the amount of troponin in a sample.

The **enzyme-linked immunoassay (ELISA)** is the chief methodology for tumor marker testing. ELISA procedures include enzyme-labeled antibodies that detect and react with tumor-specific antigens in a sample. The antigen–antibody complex formed is quantified and is directly proportional to the concentration of tumor marker in a patient sample.

Protein and Nitrogen Compound Testing Samples

Specimen collection requirements, special handling procedures, and interfering substances for protein and other nitrogenous analytes are listed below:

- **Ammonia:** heparin or EDTA plasma transported on ice, centrifuged, and separated within 20 minutes of collection; assay immediately because nitrogenous constituents quickly metabolize into ammonia
    - **False increase**: nitrogen metabolism due to not placing the specimen on ice, not centrifuging and analyzing immediately, or poor venipuncture technique
- **BUN:** serum or plasma, centrifuged and separated from cells within 2 hours of collection
    - Do not use sodium fluoride as an anticoagulant for enzymatic testing samples due to the potential inhibition of enzymatic activity.
- **Creatinine, total protein, albumin, uric acid:** serum or plasma, centrifuged and separated from cells within 2 hours of collection, random or 24-hour urine collection
    - **Creatinine**: interference from noncreatinine chromogens — glucose, ascorbic acid, acetoacetate
    - **Total protein, albumin**: body fluids, CSF in a sterile container
    - **Uric acid:** lipids and several pharmaceutical drugs interfere in colorimetry
- **Tumor markers:** serum or plasma, centrifuged and separated from cells within 2 hours of collection
- Cardiac markers:
    - **Troponin, hsCRP:** serum or plasma, centrifuged and separated from cells within 2 hours of collection
        - **Troponin:** results falsely decreased due to gross hemolysis
        - **hsCRP:** falsely increased results caused by the presence of other inflammatory processes, interferences due to gross hemolysis, lipemia, and icterus
    - **BNP:** EDTA plasma or whole blood
    - **Homocysteine:** serum, centrifuged and separated from cells within 4 hours of collection, EDTA or heparin plasma centrifuged and separated from cells within 1 hour of collection.

Creatinine Clearance

Creatinine clearance testing evaluates kidney function by determining the concentration of creatinine filtered from the blood by the kidneys each minute. The creatinine clearance is a more sensitive method of estimating the glomerular filtration rate than random BUN and creatinine urine testing. A patient's creatinine clearance is calculated from creatinine values obtained from a 24-hour urine sample, serum sample, and the patient's height and weight. The 24-hour urine collection consists of voiding a first morning urine, followed by the collection of every urine sample for the next 24 hours in their entirety into one jug or container. To reduce bacterial growth and metabolite breakdown, 24-hour urine samples require refrigeration or preservatives to be added to the container. The 24 hours' worth of urine that is collected is returned to the laboratory for testing, and a serum sample is obtained to measure the patient's serum creatinine levels.

Creatinine clearance is calculated using the following equations and parameters:

Equation	Parameters
$\left(\frac{U}{P}\right) \times \left(\frac{TV}{1440}\right) \times \left(\frac{1.73}{A}\right)$	$U = \text{urine creatinine}$ $P = \frac{\text{plasma}}{\text{serum}}\text{creatinine}$ $TV = \text{24 hour urine total volume } \left(\frac{\text{mL}}{\text{24 hr}}\right)$ $1{,}440 = \text{minutes in 24 hours } \left(\frac{\text{min}}{\text{24 hr}}\right)$ $1.73 = \text{body surface area correction factor } (\text{m}^2)$ $A = \text{the patient's body surface area } (\text{m}^2)$

Correlation Between Test Result Interpretations and Disease States for Ammonia, BUN, Creatinine, Total Protein, and Albumin

Increased serum concentrations of protein- and nitrogen-containing compounds most often indicate dysfunction and disease of the kidneys and liver. The normal reference ranges and interpretations of results are described below:

Analyte	Normal Reference Range
Ammonia	0–1 day old: 64–107 µmol/L 2–14 days old: 56–92 µmol/L 15 days–17 years old: 21–50 µmol/L ≥18 years old: 0–27 µmol/L
BUN	1–17 years old: 7–20 mg/dL Males ≥18 years old: 8–24 mg/dL Females ≥18 years old: 6–21 mg/dL
Creatinine, serum	Males: 0.7–1.2 mg/dL Females: 0.5–1.0 mg/dL
Creatinine, urine	Random: no reference range established 24-hour: Males: 90–140 mL/minute Females: 87–107 mL/minute
Total protein, serum	6.0–8.0 g/dL
Total protein, urine	Random: 0–20 mg/dL 24-hour: <80 mg/24 hours
Total protein, CSF	15–45 mg/dL
Albumin, serum	3.5–5.0 g/dL
Albumin, urine	Random: Males: <17 mg/g of creatinine Females: <25 mg/g of creatinine 24-hour: <30 mg/24 hours

Hyperammonemia:

- >1,000 µmol/L in childhood can be a result of a genetic urea cycle or fatty acid oxidation defects, or organic academia
- ≤500 µmol/L indicates liver disease
- ≥500 µmol/L indicates liver and renal failure

BUN/serum creatinine ratio normally between 10:1 and 20:1. Abnormal ratios are interpreted below:

- **<10:1** — renal damage causing reduced BUN reabsorption, decreased urea formation due to liver disease, malnutrition
- **>20:1** — increased BUN reabsorption due to heart failure, dehydration, gastrointestinal bleeding, or increased dietary protein intake.

Increased CSF total protein indicates bacterial meningitis, brain tumor or abscess, neurosyphilis, or hemorrhage.

Correlation Between Test Result Interpretations and Disease States for Cardiac Markers

Normal reference ranges and interpretations of cardiac marker test results are described below:

Analyte	Normal Reference Range
Troponin I	<2.0 ng/mL
BNP	<100 pg/mL
hsCRP	<2.0 mg/L
Homocysteine	4–15 μmol/L
Uric acid	Males: 3.7–8.0 mg/dL Females: 2.7–6.1 mg/dL

Troponin I levels following the onset of an acute myocardial infarction:

- **Rise**: 3–12 hours after onset
- **Peak:** at 24 hours after onset
- **Return to normal**: 5–14 days after onset.

BNP elevations occur due to heart failure, pulmonary hypertension, acute pulmonary embolisms, and acute coronary syndromes. The following ranges aid in the evaluation of congestive heart failure (CHF) severity:

- **> Normal–200 pg/mL**: indicates compensated CHF
- **200–400 pg/mL**: indicates moderate CHF
- **>400 pg/mL**: indicates moderate to severe CHF.

Patients with an **hsCRP value ≥2.0 mg/L** have an increased risk of developing cardiovascular disease or ischemic events, and levels of >10.0 mg/L represent acute inflammation within the body.

Hyperhomocysteinemia, with levels >15 μmol/L, can be caused by deficiencies in the following B vitamins: B_6, B_{12}, and folate. Increased plasma concentrations of homocysteine can increase the risk of coronary heart disease, stroke, and peripheral vascular disease by damaging the inner lining of the arteries and promoting blood clot formation.

Uric acid concentrations increase in chronic renal failure and in response to nuclear catabolism in chemotherapy. Uric acid is also used along with other laboratory assays to assess a patient's risk of cardiovascular disease.

Acid–Base, Blood Gases and Electrolytes

Acid–Base Determinations (Including Blood Gases)

Biochemical Theory of the Henderson–Hasselbalch Equation

The Henderson–Hasselbalch equation is a logarithmic expression using the ionization constant to provide a relationship between a conjugate base and a weak acid. The laboratory uses this theory to determine the pH of the blood's bicarbonate buffer system. Carbonic and noncarbonic acid concentrations represent intake and metabolic production, whereas conjugate bases represent the body's excretion and metabolic conversion of substances in the pH buffering system. The results interpreted from the Henderson–Hasselbalch equation depict the roles of the lungs (pCO_2) and kidneys (HCO_3^-) in maintaining the pH of the blood. The general equation for determining the pH of a solution is as follows:

$$\mathrm{pH} = \mathrm{pKa} + \log\left(\frac{[\mathrm{HCO_3}^-]}{[\mathrm{H_2CO_3}]}\right)$$

pKa: the dissociation constant
HCO_3^-: a base
H_2CO_3: an acid

The goal is to have a 20:1 base-to-acid ratio.

The theory of the Henderson–Hasselbalch equation is applied to clinical chemistry in the determination of the acid–base status and the pH of the blood's bicarbonate buffer system. The pH of blood gas samples is proportional to the following modified Henderson–Hasselbalch equation:

$$\mathrm{pH} = \log\left(\frac{[\mathrm{HCO_3}^-]}{[\mathrm{pCO_2}]}\right)$$

HCO_3^-: kidney, metabolic responsibility
pCO_2: lung, respiratory responsibility

Physiology and Relationship Between pH and Hydrogen Ion Concentrations

The pH of a solution is determined by the concentration of hydrogen ions (H^+) present in a system. The hydrogen ion concentration and activity can be determined with a measured pH value using the following logarithmic equation: $[H^+] = 10^{-pH}$. The higher the concentration of H^+ ions present in a solution, the lower the pH and the more acidic a solution becomes, whereas a lower H^+ concentration creates a basic solution with a higher pH. Homeostasis of the blood's pH is maintained by mechanisms of the lungs and kidneys that control and excrete hydrogen ions based on the body's needs. Buffering systems follow as the first line of defense in maintaining pH because they act more immediately than the lungs and kidneys are able to. Buffer systems in the plasma and RBCs contain a weak acid and a corresponding weak acid of conjugate base; for example, H_2CO_3 and HCO_3^- are the weak acid and conjugate base that function within the plasma bicarbonate buffer system.

Carbon Dioxide and Oxygen Transport in the Body

The CO_2 and O_2 transport system is a continuous cycle carried out by the RBCs as they move through the lungs, heart, and tissues in the body. The O_2 is breathed into the lungs where it binds with hemoglobin molecules in RBCs to produce oxyhemoglobin. Oxyhemoglobin moves into the chambers of the heart and is distributed to all tissues of the body by the arteries and capillaries. CO_2 is the end product of cellular respiration that is picked up from the tissues by RBCs and carried back to the heart and lungs through the veins. To achieve a higher affinity for the hemoglobin molecule, CO_2 is transported in its dissolved form of bicarbonate (HCO_3^-). Deoxygenated blood flows from the right side of the heart and into the lungs where it is excreted from the body via exhalation. At this time, CO_2 is exchanged for O_2 molecules inhaled into the lungs and attached to hemoglobin molecules for cellular distribution.

Normal and Abnormal States of Acid–Base Concentrations of Blood Gases

The normal reference ranges of arterial and venous blood gases as well as the states associated with abnormal values are described below:

Arterial Blood Gas	Parameter	Venous Blood Gas
7.35–7.45	pH	7.30–7.40
35–45 mm Hg	pCO_2	42–48 mm Hg
22–26 mM/L	HCO_3^-	24–30 mM/L
85–105 mm Hg	pO_2	35–45 mm Hg

Normal arterial and venous blood gas values differ slightly from one another due to the arteries carrying oxygenated blood and the veins carrying deoxygenated blood and waste products.

Acid–base imbalances are described by blood pH values below normal in **acidemia** or above normal in **alkalemia.** The pathological disease states associated with acid–base imbalances are acidosis and alkalosis. The pH imbalances based on decreased CO_2 elimination by the lungs or increased rate and depth of respiration causing excess acid elimination are described as **respiratory acidosis** and **respiratory alkalosis,** respectively. Dysfunctions of the renal and metabolic systems causing decreased plasma bicarbonate or increased plasma base are described as **metabolic acidosis** and **metabolic alkalosis**, respectively.

Analytical Principles of Blood Gas Testing

Blood gas analysis results are achieved by a combination of measured and calculated values. Ion-selective glass electrodes are used to directly measure the hydrogen ion (H^+) concentration and partial pressures of O_2 and CO_2. The concentration of hydrogen ions present is inversely proportional to and used to determine a pH value in blood gas samples. The pressure excreted by O_2 and carbon monoxide (CO) molecules dissolved in blood is measured to determine their partial pressures. The value for bicarbonate (HCO_3^-) concentration is indirectly obtained and calculated from the pH and CO_2 partial pressure using the Henderson–Hasselbalch equation.

Collecting, Processing, and Troubleshooting Blood Gas Testing Samples

Samples collected for blood gas analysis can be collected from a vein with a syringe, straight needle, or butterfly needle or from an artery with a syringe. For analysis, blood cannot clot or be exposed to air and the samples must be collected anaerobically into tubes or a syringe containing the anticoagulant sodium heparin.

Blood gas study samples are negatively affected by air exposure and a prolonged time between collection and analysis. Air bubbles in a syringe or an uncapped specimen tube will falsely decrease the CO_2 and pCO_2 results, while falsely increasing the pH and pO_2 levels. If testing is delayed for more than 15 minutes and samples are not on ice to slow glycolysis, the CO_2 and pCO_2 values will be falsely elevated, whereas the pH and pO_2 results will be falsely decreased.

Correlation Between Blood Gas Test Result Interpretations and Disease States

Acid–base disorders are evaluated based on the following blood gas interpretations:

Disorder	pH	pCO_2	HCO_3^-	pO_2
Metabolic acidosis	Decreased	Decreased	Decreased	Decreased
Metabolic alkalosis	Increased	Increased	Increased	Increased
Respiratory acidosis	Decreased	Increased	Increased	Increased

Disorder	pH	pCO_2	HCO_3^-	pO_2
Respiratory alkalosis	Increased	Decreased	Increased	Decreased

Metabolic acidosis is caused by a primary bicarbonate deficit due to the following disease states: increased acid production in diabetic ketoacidosis, decreased H^+ excretion and HCO_3^- readsorption in renal disease, excessive HCO_3^- loss due to prolonged diarrhea, or in the late stages of salicylate poisoning.

Metabolic alkalosis arises due to a primary excess of HCO_3^- as seen in the following: sodium bicarbonate ($NaHCO_3$) infusions, citrate present in transfused blood, consumption of antacids containing HCO_3^-, gastrointestinal loss of H^+ from prolonged vomiting, potassium depletion, therapy with diuretics, or Cushing's syndrome.

Respiratory acidosis is a primary excess of CO_2 seen in emphysema, pneumonia, or rebreathing exhaled air.

Respiratory alkalosis is caused by a primary deficit of CO_2 that is observed in hyperventilation and the early stages of salicylate poisoning.

ELECTROLYTES

SODIUM, POTASSIUM, CHLORIDE, CARBON DIOXIDE, AND BICARBONATE

Sodium (Na^+) is the major cation of extracellular fluid that maintains water distribution, plasma volume, and osmotic pressure and associates with chloride and bicarbonate to maintain the body's acid–base balance. The kidneys conserve or excrete sodium ions depending on the blood volume and concentration of Na^+ in extracellular fluids.

Potassium (K^+) is the major cation of intracellular fluid that influences cardiac muscle activity, neuromuscular cell excitability, and the cellular metabolism portion of protein and glycogen synthesis. The concentration of potassium within the cell is 23 times higher than outside of the cell. Potassium participates in the acid–base balance, and the presence of adrenocortical hormones influences the Na^+ and K^+ being excreted by the kidneys.

Chloride (Cl^-) is the major anion of extracellular fluid, and it has a reciprocal relationship with **bicarbonate (HCO_3^-)**, in which the increase of one results in a decrease of the other. Chloride counterbalances Na^+ to maintain the normal anion–cation balance and electrical neutrality, while also maintaining osmotic pressure and hydration by controlling the distribution of H_2O among the cells, plasma, and interstitial fluids. Bicarbonate is the product of carbonic acid dissociation during a reversible metabolic reaction between **CO_2** and H_2O in the lungs that occurs based on the needs of the tissues. Excreted and reabsorbed by the kidneys, around 90% of the total CO_2 in blood is in the form of HCO_3^-. Therefore, measurement of the total CO_2 reflects the concentration of bicarbonate, which indicates pH and CO_2 pressure values.

CALCIUM, PHOSPHORUS, AND MAGNESIUM

Calcium (Ca^{2+}) is a cation mostly found combined with phosphate and crystalized in bone. Only 1% of calcium is present in blood and other extracellular fluids as a free or ionized cation or bound to proteins and anions. Calcium participates in the following biological processes: bone mineralization, blood hemostasis, plasma membrane stability, enzyme activity, and cardiac muscle excitability and contraction. The majority of phosphorous in the body is expressed in its oxidized form, **phosphate (PO_4^{3-})**. Phosphorus is a key component of phospholipid cell membranes and has an inverse relationship with calcium because an increase in one results in a decrease of the other. Regulatory hormones of plasma calcium and phosphorous concentrations include parathyroid hormone, vitamin D, and calcitonin in which Ca^{2+} and PO_4^{3-} are released from bone and absorbed through the small intestine.

Magnesium (Mg^{2+}) is the second most abundant intracellular cation that functions as an essential cofactor for >300 enzymes and acts against calcium as a channel-blocking agent. Only 1% of magnesium is present in plasma, with two-thirds being ionized, whereas the majority of Mg^{2+} resides in the bones.

Iron, Total Iron Binding Capacity, and Trace Elements

Iron ions in plasma are oxidized to become Fe^{3+}, which binds with transferrin. Once bound to transferrin, iron can become an enzyme cofactor, combine with heme molecules, or be stored in the liver as ferritin and hemosiderin. Approximately 65% of iron in the body partakes in the transport of O_2 within the hemoglobin molecule in RBCs, whereas some iron is transported with O_2 to muscle tissues by myoglobin. Lysed RBCs release iron ions that are salvaged and returned back to the liver by macrophages. The **total iron binding capacity (TIBC)** measures the ability for iron to bind to transferrin because it is the major carrier of iron throughout the body. TIBC measurements allow for the indirect measuring of transferrin concentration in serum or plasma.

Trace elements are organic or inorganic elements that exist in minute amounts in the body. Although they are not prominent in volume, many trace elements serve a purpose and are a necessary factor in physiological responses and biochemical reactions. Examples of important trace elements found in the human body include zinc, copper, iodine, and manganese.

Normal and Abnormal States Associated with Electrolyte Concentrations

Balanced electrolyte concentrations and normal function are indicative of a healthy system. The most common cause of electrolyte disorders is the prolonged loss of fluid from the body. Abnormalities in electrolyte concentrations can cause cardiac, neurological, and musculoskeletal symptoms. Normal serum or plasma reference ranges and abnormal electrolyte states that occur are listed below:

Electrolyte	Normal Reference Range
Sodium	135–145 mM/L
Potassium	3.5–5.0 mM/L
Chloride	98–106 mM/L
CO_2 and Bicarbonate	23–29 mM/L (venous) 22–26 mEq/L (arterial)
Calcium	8.5–10.2 mg/dL (total) 1.15–1.29 mM/L (ionized)
Phosphorus	2.5–4.5 mg/dL
Magnesium	1.7–2.3 mg/dL
Iron	65–175 µg/dL (males) 50–170 µg/dL (females)
TIBC	250–425 µg/dL

- **Hyponatremia,** decreased sodium; **hypernatremia,** increased sodium
- **Hypokalemia,** decreased potassium; **hyperkalemia,** increased potassium
- **Hypochloremia,** decreased chloride; **hyperchloremia,** increased chloride
- **Hypocalcemia,** decreased calcium; **hypercalcemia,** increased calcium
- **Hypophosphatemia,** decreased phosphorus; **hyperphosphatemia**, increased phosphorus

- **Hypomagnesemia,** decreased magnesium; **hypermagnesemia,** increased magnesium
- **Iron deficiency,** decreased iron.

Ion-Selective Electrode, Coulometric Titration, and Colorimetry as Electrolyte Testing Methods

Ion-selective electrode (ISE) methodologies dissolve ions in a solution and use an electrode to translate ion activity into an electric potential. The ion's electric potential is then measured by a voltmeter or pH meter, which directly correlates with the ionic concentration in a solution. The following electrolytes are measured with their corresponding electrodes via ISE:

- **Sodium**: Na^+ selective glass electrode
- **Potassium:** electrode for the valinomycin membrane of the K^+ transport molecule
- **Chloride:** solid-state electrode containing silver chloride, AgCl
- **Bicarbonate and CO_2**: pCO_2 electrode measures internal pH changes due to CO_2
- **Ionized calcium:** Ca^{2+} selective, pH-dependent electrode.

Coulometric titration methods for the measurement of **chloride** require an electrode to generate and release silver ions (Ag^+) into a dilute acid solution at a constant rate. In the solution, Ag^+ combines with Cl^- ions to form the insoluble precipitate, AgCl. The rate of time it takes for Ag^+ to bind with all of the Cl^- is proportional to the concentration of chloride in a sample.

Colorimetric assays quantify the concentration of chloride, calcium, iron, bicarbonate, and CO_2, by photometrically measuring the variation in the intensity of color produced by their reactions with reagent substrates.

Electrolyte Testing Methods

Volumetric and **manometric** methodologies are used to measure CO_2 and bicarbonate concentrations by measuring the amount of gas formed in a sample.

Spectrophotometric methods quantitatively measure an analyte by comparing the color of a solution of unknown concentration to the color of a solution of known concentration. **Phosphorus** is measured by spectrophotometry after molybdate combines with PO_4^{3-} ions and reduces to produce molybdenum blue.

Atomic absorption spectroscopy quantitatively determines the concentration of an analyte, such as **calcium**, based on the absorption of light by free metallic ions in a gaseous state.

Immunoturbidimetric methodologies for the measurement of **TIBC** reflect transferrin levels. An excess of ferric salts is added to a sample to saturate transferrin binding sites, and unbound iron is precipitated with magnesium carbonate. The sample is then centrifuged and the iron present in the supernatant is analyzed.

Collecting, Processing, and Troubleshooting Electrolyte Testing Samples

Samples for electrolyte testing can come from a variety of sources, with each electrolyte having specific criteria for optimal results. Specimen requirements for electrolytes are described below:

- Acceptable sample sources and additives:

Analyte	Venipuncture Specimen	Additional Specimen Sources
Sodium Chloride Potassium Calcium Phosphorus Magnesium	Lithium heparin or sodium heparin plasma Serum tubes	Urine — sodium, chloride, and potassium Other body fluids — sodium and chloride Sweat — chloride
Bicarbonate	Lithium heparin or sodium heparin plasma Serum tubes	Arterial blood gas — lithium- or sodium-heparinized syringe
Iron TIBC	Serum tubes only	—

- Unacceptable additives:
  - Sodium: Sodium heparin, Na^+ in anticoagulant falsely elevates results.
  - Potassium: EDTA, K^+ in anticoagulant falsely elevates results.
  - Calcium: EDTA and oxalate, ability to bind with Ca^{2+} falsely decreases results.
- Special requirements:
  - Sodium: Separate from cells as soon as possible to avoid results obscured by Na^+ exchange with cells.
  - Potassium: Separate from cells within 1 hour to avoid results obscured by K^+ exchange with cells. Muscle action from prolonged use of a tourniquet or excessive fist clenching and squeezing during capillary punctures falsely elevates results.
  - Bicarbonate: Keep on ice to prevent glycolysis, and analyze immediately after opening the sample to avoid loss of CO_2, which falsely decreases results.

Moderate to gross hemolysis, lipemia, and icterus **falsely** affect electrolyte results in the following ways:

Interference	Increased	Decreased
Hemolysis	Potassium, phosphorus, calcium, magnesium, iron	Bicarbonate
Lipemia	Magnesium	Sodium, potassium, chloride, bicarbonate
Icterus	Magnesium	—

Calculations for Osmolality and the Anion Gap

Osmolality calculations measure the total concentration of dissolved ions and molecules in serum or urine. A calculated osmolality greater than the reference range is indicative of dehydration. Osmolality is calculated as follows:

$$2(Na^+) + (glucose/18) + (BUN \times 2.8)$$

Reference range: 275–295 mOsm/kg.

The **osmolal gap** is the difference between the calculated and measured osmolality. An elevated osmolal gap indicates the presence of ketones or alcohol in plasma.

$$\text{Calculated osmolality} - \text{measured osmolality}$$

Reference range: 0–10 mOsm/kg.

The **anion gap** is a mathematical calculation of the differences between measured cations and anions to determine the concentration of unmeasured cations and anions. Values for measured **cations** (sodium [$\mathbf{Na^+}$] and potassium [$\mathbf{K^+}$]) and measured **anions** (chloride [$\mathbf{Cl^-}$] and bicarbonate [$\mathbf{HCO_3^-}$]) are entered into one of the following formulas to determine the anion gap:

Formula	$([Na^+] + [K^+]) - ([Cl^-] + [HCO_3^-])$	$[Na^+] - ([Cl^-] + [HCO_3^-])$
Reference range	10–20 mmol/L	7–16 mmol/L

An increased anion gap indicates an increased concentration of unmeasured anions and states of ketosis, acidosis, and increased plasma proteins. Decreased anion gaps are due to either an increase in unmeasured cations or a decrease of unmeasured anions. Anion gap calculations can be used for analytical quality control because abnormal anions gaps in multiple otherwise healthy patients is indicative of an issue with electrolyte measurement.

Correlation Between Test Result Interpretations and Disease States for Electrolytes

Disease states and their associated abnormal serum electrolyte results are listed below:

Disorder or Disease State	**Increased**	**Decreased**
Metabolic acidosis	K^+	Na^+, Cl^-, HCO_3^-
Metabolic alkalosis	HCO_3^-	K^+
Diarrhea	Cl^-	Na^+, K^+, HCO_3^-
Vomiting	HCO_3^-	K^+, Cl^-
Dehydration	Na^+, Cl^-	—
Diuretic, alcohol, or drug use	—	Mg^{2+}
Cushing's syndrome	Na^+, HCO_3^-	K^+
Cystic fibrosis	Sweat Cl^-	—
Addison's disease	K^+	Na^+
Cardiac disorders Diabetes mellitus	—	Mg^{2+}
Insulin treatment of uncontrolled diabetes	Na^+	—
Insulin injections Intravascular hemolysis Severe burns	—	K^+
Heart arrhythmias Weakness and/or paralysis*	K^+	K^+
Renal tubular diseases	—	Na^+
Renal tubular acidosis	Cl^-	—
Decreased renal reabsorption	—	PO_4^{3-}
Chronic pyelonephritis	—	Cl^-
Renal failure	K^+, Mg^{2+}, Ca^{2+}	Cl^-, HCO_3^-
Hyperaldosteronism	Na^+	K^+
Aldosterone deficiency	—	Cl^-

Disorder or Disease State	Increased	Decreased
Adrenocortical hyperfunction	Cl^-	—
Hyperparathyroidism	Ca^{2+}	PO_4^{3-}
Hypoparathyroidism	PO_4^{3-}	Ca^{2+}
Metastatic bone cancer Multiple myeloma	Ca^{2+}	—

*These symptoms can be caused by increased or decreased serum potassium.

Correlation Between Iron Study Test Result Interpretations and Disease States

Iron disorders are indicated by the following laboratory evaluation of serum iron studies:

Disease	Iron	% Saturation	TIBC	Ferritin
Iron storage depletion	Normal	Normal	Normal	Decreased
Iron-deficiency anemia	Decreased	Decreased	Increased	Decreased
Anemia of chronic inflammatory disease	Decreased	Decreased	Decreased	Increased
Thalassemia	Increased	Increased	Decreased	Increased
Hemochromatosis	Increased	Increased	Decreased	Increased
Sideroblastic anemia	Increased	Increased	Normal	Increased

Varying degrees of **fatigue** and **weakness** are symptoms of all of the iron disorders listed above. Each disease or disorder is also characterized by the following signs and symptoms:

- Iron storage depletion:
  - Loss of memory and/or attention
  - Hair loss, brittle hair, skin, and nails
  - Sore tongue
- Iron-deficiency anemia and anemia of chronic inflammatory disease:
  - Pale skin, cold hands and feet
  - Chest pain, fast heart rate, shortness of breath
  - Headache, dizziness, lightheadedness
  - Brittle nails
  - Inflamed and sore tongue
  - Cravings for nonnutritional substances such as ice or dirt
- Thalassemia:
  - Pale, yellow skin
  - Facial bone deformations
  - Slow growth
  - Dark urine
- Hemochromatosis:
  - Bronze, gray skin
  - Memory fog
  - Joint and abdominal pain
  - Diabetes, heart and liver failure
- Sideroblastic anemia:
  - Pale skin

- Headache
- Chest pain, fast heart rate, heart palpitations

Special Chemistry

Endocrinology

Hormones are chemical substances produced by a specialized endocrine gland and transported to target organs to produce effects throughout the body. In response to the body's need for hormones, the hypothalamus in the brain produces a releasing hormone that stimulates the pituitary gland to produce a stimulating hormone. Stimulating hormones are carried through the bloodstream to their "target organ," where they elicit a response and initiate a cell-specific process. The target cells' reaction is recognized by the original gland and reduces hormone stimulating production in a negative feedback loop, which aids in the regulation of hormone concentration in the body. Effects elicited by hormones include the following: growth stimulation or inhibition, induction or suppression of cell death, activation or inhibition of the immune system, fluctuations in mood, metabolism regulation, new life phase or reproduction preparation, and regulation of other hormones.

Normal and Abnormal Hormone Concentrations

Normal function and blood concentration of hormones allows for the proper function of various body processes. Conditions caused by abnormal concentrations of hormones can be due to too little (hypo) or too much (hyper) hormone production. Hormone-related diseases are classified into categories determined by location in which the synthesis, transport, or functional issue occurs:

- **Primary**: issue with the "target organ" and its cells
- **Secondary:** issue with the pituitary gland
- **Tertiary**: issue with the hypothalamus.

Common abnormal hormone conditions, their causes, and the associated signs and symptoms are listed below:

- **Primary hyperthyroidism**: weight loss, nervousness, tachycardia, and tremors
  - **Graves' disease:** autoimmune disease with thyroid-stimulating hormone antibodies, causing an overproduction of T_4
- **Primary hypothyroidism**: weight gain, fatigue, decreased mental and physical capabilities, intolerance to cold temperatures
  - **Hashimoto's thyroiditis**: thyroid autoantibodies
  - **Acquired:** radiation therapy, thyroidectomy, lithium and other medications
- **Hyperaldosteronism:** increased sodium, decreased potassium, hypertension
  - **Conn's syndrome:** overproduction of aldosterone in the adrenal gland
- **Hypoaldosteronism** and **hypocortisolism:** decreased sodium, chloride, cortisol, hemoglobin, and urinary steroids. **Primary**, increased ACTH due to adrenal cortex dysfunction; **secondary,** due to pituitary issues; and **tertiary,** due to hypothalamus problems, decreased ACTH
  - **Addison's disease:** underproduction of aldosterone in the adrenal gland

- **Hypercortisolism:** decreased plasma protein, hypertension, weight gain, fragile skin, fatigue, glucose intolerance
    - **Cushing's syndrome:** overuse of corticosteroids, pituitary gland tumors, inherited disease

Mechanism of Action for Steroid, Peptide, and Amine Hormones

Steroid hormones easily cross the cell plasma membrane of their target organ to bind and activate receptor proteins. Nuclear or cytosolic receptor proteins within target cells are ligand-dependent transcription factor that remain inactive until they bind to their specific steroid hormone. Binding of these two initiates transcription and allows the hormone to take a biological effect.

Peptide hormones cannot cross the plasma membrane into cells and act to initiate the cascade of signal transduction in target cells by binding to and activating membrane receptors.

Amine hormones can be either hydrophilic or hydrophobic. Hydrophilic amine hormones bind to and activate nuclear receptors in the same mechanism as peptide hormones because they are unable to cross their target cell plasma membrane. Hydrophobic amine hormones cross the plasma membrane of target cells and bind and activate nuclear receptors in the same mechanism as steroid hormones.

Physical and Chemical Properties of Steroid and Peptide Hormones

Steroid hormones are hydrophobic molecules comprised of fused carbon rings that are chemical derivatives of cholesterol. Due to their small size and hydrophobic nature, steroid hormones can easily cross plasma membranes. Steroid hormones are grouped into two classes based on the location of their synthesis: corticosteroids of the adrenal cortex and sex steroids made in the gonads and placenta. Each class is then further divided into the following categories based on the receptors they bind to:

- Glucocorticoids
    - **Cortisol** — primary stress hormone, production stimulated by the hypothalamic-pituitary-adrenal system
- Mineralocorticoids
    - **Aldosterone** — regulates blood pressure; is produced in the adrenal gland cortex
- Sex hormones — androgens, estrogens, and progestogens
    - **Testosterone** — male sex hormone produced in the testes
    - **Estradiol** — female sex hormone, developed in the follicles of the ovaries.

Peptide hormones are small proteins comprised of linear amino acid polymers that are synthesized by mRNA in ribosomes and stored in secretory vesicles as prohormones. Peptide hormone secretion out of the cell is highly regulated and requires specific stimuli. Before their release from cells, prohormones are cleaved by endopeptidases to form mature enzymes. The following are examples of mature peptide enzymes that are carried through the bloodstream to their target cells:

- **Adrenocorticotropic hormone (ACTH)** — stimulates cortisol secretion; produced and secreted by the anterior pituitary gland
- **Insulin** — regulates carbohydrate, fat, and protein metabolism; produced in the beta cells of the pancreatic islets
- **Prolactin** — milk production in females, secreted from the pituitary gland.

THYROID HORMONES, CALCITONIN, PARATHYROID HORMONE, LH, AND FSH

The two thyroid hormones, **thyroxine (T_4)** and **triiodothyronine (T_3)**, are produced, stored, and secreted from the thyroid gland. The synthesis of thyroid hormones requires circulating iodine being taken up by cells of the thyroid gland. In the thyroid gland, iodine becomes oxidized, combines with tyrosine components of the thyroglobulin molecule, and forms active hormones. The concentration of T_3 and T_4 release is regulated by the hypothalamus signaling the production of **thyroid-stimulating hormone (TSH)** in thyrotrope cells of the pituitary gland. TSH is taken up by thyroid gland cells and initiates T_3 and T_4 production. Thyroid hormones control and regulate the following body processes: metabolism of carbohydrates and fats, body temperature, heart rate, and protein production.

Calcitonin is a peptide hormone that is also produced by the thyroid gland. It functions to reduce the concentration of calcium in circulation, as an antagonist to **parathyroid hormone**, which is a peptide hormone secreted from the parathyroid gland to increase serum calcium levels through effects on the kidneys, intestines, and bones.

Luteinizing hormone (LH) and **follicle-stimulating hormone (FSH)** are glycoproteins with a dimeric structure composed of alpha and beta subunits that are produced in the gonadotropic cells of the anterior pituitary gland. LH acts on the ovaries to trigger ovulation and stimulates testosterone production and spermatogenesis in the testes. FSH regulates growth, development, and maturation through puberty. FSH also works synergistically with LH in reproductive processes.

HORMONE TESTING METHODS

The **electrochemiluminescent immunoassay analyzer (ECLIA)** is a quantitative method used for the measurement of various hormones. ECLIA methods use electrically charged, chemiluminescent-labeled antigens that bind to hormone antibodies present in a sample. Measurements of hormone concentrations are based on the change in the electrochemiluminescent signal emitted from the labeled antigens before and after the immunoreaction with the patient sample takes place. Thyroid hormones and ACTH are examples of hormones measured using ECLIA methods.

Liquid chromatography-tandem mass spectrometry (LC-MS/MS) combines the principles of liquid chromatography with the highly specific and sensitive capabilities of mass spectrometry. MS/MS allows for more sensitive detection and quantification of hormones such as cortisol, aldosterone, testosterones, and estrogen hormones.

The **Zimmerman reaction** is observed in the detection and measurement of androgen hormones. The 17-ketosteriods are metabolites of androgen hormones that will react in an alcoholic alkali solution with metadinitrobenze to produce a red-purple color that is detected at 520 nm. Color production measured photometrically provides a quantitative estimate of androgen hormone concentrations in a sample.

ENDOCRINOLOGY TESTING SAMPLES

Specimen collection requirements, special handling procedures, and interfering substances for endocrinology analytes are listed below:

- Thyroid hormone assays
  - TSH: serum, centrifuged and separated from cells within 2 hours of collection
  - T_3 and T_4: serum
- **Stress hormone assays** — concentrations fluctuate throughout the day; samples should be collected between 6:00 and 10:30 am when concentrations are at their highest.

- ACTH: EDTA plasma, centrifuged and separated from cells within 2 hours of collection; freeze plasma immediately to preserve specimen
- **Cortisol:** 24-hour urine collection, random urine, or serum

- Sex hormone assays
  - **Testosterone**: serum; reject specimens with gross hemolysis, lipemia, or icterus
  - **Estrone** and **estradiol**: serum; centrifuged and separated from cells within 2 hours of collection
  - **LH** and **FSH:** serum; centrifuged and separated from cells within 2 hours of collection
- **Aldosterone:** 24-hour urine, discontinue potassium-sparing diuretics 4–6 weeks prior to testing or serum, drawn between 8 and 10 am after the patient has been active for 2 hours

The following assays require the patient to not ingest multivitamins containing biotin (vitamin B_7) 12 hours prior to collection because it interferes with assay methods and falsely elevates or decreases results:

- T_3 and T_4
- ACTH
- LH and FSH

Hormone Suppression Tests

The following are common hormone suppression tests and their roles in endocrinology:

- **Dexamethasone suppression tests** assess **adrenal gland function** by measuring the change in cortisol levels in response to low- and high-dose injections of dexamethasone. Dexamethasone is a corticosteroid that acts on the pituitary gland to suppress ACTH secretion. In patients with no adrenal gland disorders, cortisol levels will decrease following high- and low-dose injections. The following disorders are indicated by abnormal dexamethasone suppression test results:

Disorder	Cortisol Level	ACTH Level
Primary hypercortisolism, Cushing's syndrome	Not suppressed by low- or high-dose injections	Low or undetectable
Cushing's disease	Not suppressed by low doses Suppressed by high doses	Normal or slightly elevated
Adrenal tumor or a different ACTH-secreting tumor	Not suppressed by low- or high-dose injections	Greatly elevated

- **Oral glucose tolerance tests** are performed as suppression tests to assess a patient suspected of having **excess GH** due to **acromegaly**, a pituitary gland disorder in which the body continues to produce too much GH in adulthood. Oral glucose tolerance tests are performed due to the inverse relationship between blood glucose and GH concentrations. Patients with acromegaly will not see a suppression of GH as glucose levels rise, whereas patients without the disease will observe GH level decrease with increasing glucose concentrations.

Hormone-Stimulation Tests

The following are common hormone stimulation tests and their roles in endocrinology:

- The **ACTH stimulation test** is performed for patients suspected of having cortisol deficiency or adrenal insufficiency. Baseline cortisol levels are determined prior to the injection of synthetic ACTH. Following the injection, the adrenal gland's stress response is evaluated based on the change in cortisol concentrations. This method is able to exclude or diagnose Addison's disease and primary or secondary adrenal insufficiencies with the following ACTH-stimulation test result interpretations:

Disorder	Cortisol Level	ACTH Level
Primary adrenal insufficiency	Low	High
Secondary adrenal insufficiency	Low	Low

- The **glucagon stimulation test** is performed for patients suspected of having a deficiency of GH or a glucagon-secreting tumor of the pancreas. In response to low blood sugar, the pancreas will release glucagon to raise blood glucose levels back to normal or safe ranges by metabolizing stored glycogen into glucose. Baseline glucose and GH levels are determined, followed by an intramuscular injection of glucagon. Failure of GH levels to rise following the injection is indicative of diabetes, pancreatic cancers, and other metabolic disorders.

Correlation Between Hormone Test Result Interpretations and Disease States

Disease states and their associated abnormal hormone results are listed below:

- Thyroid hormones
  - Primary hyperthyroidism, Graves' disease
    - **TSH:** decreased
    - **T_3** and **T_4**: normal or increased
  - Primary hypothyroidism, Hashimoto's thyroiditis
    - **TSH:** increased
    - **T_3** and **T_4**: decreased
- Adrenal cortex hormones
  - Hyperaldosteronism
- Aldosterone: increased
  - Hypoaldosteronism
    - Aldosterone: decreased
    - **ACTH:** increased in primary disease, decreased in secondary and tertiary disease
  - Cushing's syndrome
    - Aldosterone: increased
    - **Cortisol:** increased
    - **Other lab results:** increased glucose, sodium, and urine steroids
  - Addison's disease
    - Aldosterone: decreased
    - **Cortisol:** decreased
    - **Other lab results:** decreased sodium, chloride, hemoglobin, and urine steroids

- Sex and other hormones
  - Testosterone
    - **Decreased:** hypogonadism and infertility in males
    - **Increased:** infertility in females
  - **Estrogen** is increased in the following:
    - Female puberty
    - Pregnancy
    - Polycystic ovarian syndrome
    - Feminization in males
  - Estriol
    - **Increased**: fetal development during pregnancy, steadily increases in the third trimester
    - **Sudden decrease**: complications during pregnancy
  - Insulin
    - **Decreased:** types 1 and 2 diabetes mellitus, gestational diabetes, and polycystic ovarian syndrome
    - **Increased:** insulinoma — tumor of pancreatic beta cells

VITAMINS AND NUTRITION

NUTRITIONAL VITAMINS

Vitamins are nutrients that are essential to the human body, but they are not produced by human biochemical pathways. They are obtained from the diet, gastrointestinal flora, and sunlight, and they act as functional portions of enzymes that assist in converting substrates to their end products or coenzymes to catalyze all catabolic and many anabolic pathways. Catabolic pathways are the mechanism of breaking down or metabolizing molecules for the release of energy, whereas anabolic pathways use energy in the synthesis of large molecules. Fat-soluble vitamins such as A, D, and B_{12} are absorbed by the intestines and transported to the liver for use or storage. Other water-soluble vitamins are also absorbed by the intestines but require the presence of water and are more readily used upon their absorption.

NORMAL AND ABNORMAL STATES OF VITAMINS AND MINERALS

Maintaining the appropriate concentrations of vitamins and minerals is essential for the body to continue functioning properly. Vitamin excess and deficiency can lead to a variety of clinical signs and symptoms across various body systems and organs depending on the specific vitamin. **Vitamin deficiencies** can occur from lack of dietary intake, impaired absorption, and interactions with other medications. Deficiencies in vitamins can lead to important cellular processes going undone and can cause a wide range of symptoms depending on the specific vitamin and degree of deficiency. Most commonly, **vitamin excess** or **toxicity** occurs as a result of the overdosing of vitamin supplements. This leads to an accumulation of more vitamin than the body can use or excrete and has the potential to become harmful to the body.

VITAMIN D

Vitamin D functions as a prohormone to regulate levels of serum calcium and phosphorous for proper mineral metabolism for bones and other organs. There are two forms of vitamin D: D_2 and D_3. Vitamin D_2 is obtained through dietary consumption of fish, plants, and fungus, whereas vitamin D_3 can be obtained through dietary animal products or photosynthesis from the skin's exposure to sunlight. Both forms of vitamin D are broken down into the more active metabolite 1.25-dihydroxyvitamin D by a two-step process in the liver and kidneys. An increased serum concentration of this metabolite causes an increase in serum calcium and phosphorus by increasing the following mechanisms: intestinal absorption, renal reabsorption, and mineralization during bone formation.

B-Complex Vitamins

Vitamins B_{12} (cobalamin) and **B_9 (folate)** are nutrients required for cell synthesis and metabolism. Vitamin B_{12} participates in the metabolic process of every cell in the body. It is a specific cofactor in the following processes: DNA synthesis, fatty acid and amino acid metabolism, myelin synthesis for proper CNS function, and RBC maturation in the bone marrow. Folate is an important cofactor in DNA and RNA synthesis because it is necessary for the activation of B_{12}. It is also required in the metabolism of the amino acids responsible for cell division. Vitamin B_9 in the form of folic acid is pertinent during pregnancy because it reduces the risk of neural tube defects in the developing baby.

The remaining **B-complex vitamins** act as enzyme cofactors or their precursors in a variety of the body's process as described below:

- **B_1 (thiamine)** is an important nutrient for carbohydrate metabolism and digestion, and it benefits the CNS.
- **B_2 (riboflavin)** is required for cellular respiration, and it benefits the CNS, GI tract, eyes, and skin.
- **B_3 (niacin)** is an important factor to the CNS, GI tract, and skin.
- **B_5 (pantothenic acid)** is required for the synthesis of coenzyme A, which is responsible for the metabolism of fatty acids.
- **B_6 (pyridoxine)** is a necessary factor in amino acid, carbohydrate, and lipid formation in the body.
- **B_7 (biotin)** is involved in the metabolism and use of amino acids, carbohydrates, and fats, as well as numerous other metabolic reactions in the body.

Vitamins A, C, E, and K

Vitamin A functions to regulate cell differentiation and tissue growth, and it aids in maintaining healthy eyes, skin, and teeth. Vitamin A is present in foods in two main forms as **retinol** and **carotenoids**. Carotenoids are converted to retinol in the small intestine during digestion. Retinol is stored and used in the body in various forms. Retinol is important to low-light and color vision in the retina, and retinoic acid is an important growth factor of epithelial and other cells.

Vitamins C and **E** function as antioxidants to protect the body from infection and free radicals, respectively, by donating electrons to enzymatic reactions. Vitamin C as **ascorbic acid** is involved in tissue repair and neurotransmitter production, and it functions as a cofactor in enzymatic reactions related to wound healing and collagen synthesis. The mobilization and absorption of iron is also facilitated by vitamin C. **Vitamin E** molecules are composed of fat-soluble compounds that protect cells against reactive O_2 species.

Vitamin K is an important mineral in the synthesis of specific clotting factors, and it aids in maintaining strong bones by controlling calcium binding. Prothrombin proteins are dependent on vitamin K to synthesize the following clotting factors: II, VII, IX, and X. Vitamin K molecules are fat soluble and are readily found in foods.

Testing for Vitamins

The majority of vitamins and nutrients are measured by **LC-MS/MS.** This method combines the principles of liquid chromatography with the highly specific and sensitive capabilities of mass spectrometry. **High-performance liquid chromatography** separates substances by dissolving them in a fluid and forcing them through a column gradient at high pressures. Tandem mass spectrometry then ionizes molecules and further separates them by their mass-to-charge ratio in the first spectrometer, and target molecules are moved to the second spectrometer. In the second spectrometer, fragments are separated again by the mass-to-charge ratio and detected. Vitamin B_{12} and folate are measured using **immunoenzymatic** and **competitive binding receptor assays**, respectively. Immunoassay methods use enzyme-coated beads that bind with vitamin B_{12}, creating a chemiluminescent reaction for vitamin B_{12} concentration measurement. Competitive binding assays use a specific binding agent that competes for unlabeled or radioactively labeled compounds and measures the concentration of folate. Vitamin D can be measured by its total concentration in blood or for the stores of forms D_2 and D_3 present by measuring serum 25-hydroxyvitamin D. The total vitamin K concentration is not directly assessed. Vitamin K_1 can be detected via LC-MS/MS, but more frequently vitamin K deficiencies are determined by patients with prolonged prothrombin time/international normalized ratio results.

Vitamin and Nutrient Testing Samples

Specimens collected for the evaluation of vitamins concentrations present in blood are obtained via venipuncture into tubes with the appropriate additives. Vitamin testing requires a variety of sample types and handling requirements specific to each assay. Some require the use of an amber vial to protect the sample from light. Specimen requirements for vitamin testing are as follows:

Vitamin	Sample Type	Special Requirements	Rejection Criteria
A	Red-top tube or serum-separating tube (SST) serum	12-hour fast Amber vial	Gross hemolysis or lipemia
B_1	EDTA whole blood	12-hour fast Amber vial	Gross hemolysis Clots present in sample
B_2	Heparin plasma	12-hour fast Amber vial	Gross lipemia
B_3	EDTA plasma	Amber vial Centrifuge, separate, and freeze plasma within 30 minutes of collection	Gross hemolysis or lipemia
B_5	SST serum	Amber vial Centrifuge and separate serum within 2 hours of collection	—
B_6	Heparin plasma	12-hour fast Amber vial No ingestion of vitamin supplements for 24 hours before collection Centrifuge, separate, and freeze plasma immediately after collection	Gross hemolysis or lipemia
B_7	Red-top tube or SST serum	Amber vial	Gross hemolysis or lipemia

Vitamin	Sample Type	Special Requirements	Rejection Criteria
Folate and B_{12}	Red-top tube or SST serum	8-hour fast required Centrifuge and separate serum within 2 hours of collection	Gross hemolysis
C	Heparin plasma	12-hour fast Centrifuge, separate, and freeze plasma immediately after collection	Gross hemolysis
D	Red-top tube or SST serum	—	Gross hemolysis
E	Red-top tube or SST serum	12-hour fast Amber vial	Gross hemolysis or lipemia
K	Red-top tube or SST serum	12-hour fast	Gross lipemia

Correlation to Disease States

Vitamins A, C, D, E, and K

Nonspecific symptoms, such as nausea, vomiting, diarrhea, and rash, are common with any acute or chronic vitamin overdose. Vitamin normal ranges, deficiency, and toxicity symptoms are specified below:

- Vitamin A:

Age	Normal Range
0–6 years	11.3–64.7 μg/dL
7–12 years	12.8–81.2 μg/dL
13–17 years	14.4–97.7 μg/dL
≥18 years	32.5–78.0 μg/dL

  - **Deficiency:** poor immune function, night blindness, zinc deficiency
  - **Toxicity:** affects the skin with reddening, irritation, and peeling in patches.
- Vitamin C:

Normal Range
0.4–2.0 mg/dL

  - **Deficiency:** impaired immune function, easy bruising and bleeding, joint and muscle pain
  - **Toxicity:** not typically toxic, but doses greater than 2,000 mg/day can cause diarrhea, cramps, and nausea.
- Vitamin D:

Age	Male	Female
<16 years	24–86 pg/mL	24–86 pg/mL
≥16 years	18–64 pg/mL	18–78 pg/mL

- **Deficiency**:
  - Rickets — childhood disease causing softening and weakening of bones due to decreased calcium
  - Osteopenia and osteoporosis
  - Linked to hypertension, diabetes, cardiovascular disease, multiple sclerosis, colon and breasts cancers, autism, systemic lupus erythematosus, and other autoimmune diseases.
- **Toxicity:** high blood calcium levels, causing kidney stones, nausea, recurrent vomiting, constipation, excessive thirst, excessive urination, confusion, and weight loss.

- Vitamin E:

Age	Normal Range
0–17 years	3.8–18.4 mg/L
≥18 years	5.5–17.0 mg/L

  - **Deficiency:** slow wound healing, loss of coordination, muscle weakness, numbness and tingling
  - **Toxicity:** anticoagulant properties.
- Vitamin K:

Age	Normal Range
0–17 years	Not established
≥18 years	0.10–2.20 ng/mL

  - **Deficiency:** proteins C and S are present but not functional; functional deficiency of prothrombin factors II, VII, IX, X, causing unexpected or excessive bleeding, easy bruising.
  - **Toxicity:** K_1 and K_2 no known toxicity, K_3 interaction with anticoagulants varies, hemorrhagic in newborns.

B VITAMINS

Although vitamin B_{12} and folate are the most common B vitamins assessed by clinicians, the remaining B vitamins are vital to overall health. Normal ranges and symptoms of deficiency and toxicity of B vitamins are described below:

- **Vitamin B_1 (thiamine)*** 70–180 nmol/L
  - **Deficiency:** fatigue, decrease in heart function, and age-related cognitive decline
- **Vitamin B_2 (riboflavin)*** 1–19 μg/L
  - **Deficiency:** fatigue, poor iron absorption causing anemia, decreased thyroid function, B_6 deficiency
- **Vitamin B_3 (niacin)** 0.50–8.45 μg/mL
  - **Deficiency:** fatigue, digestion issues, confusion, anxiety, and scaly skin
  - **Toxicity:** early signs include skin reddening, itchiness, and burning due to vasodilation, called "niacin flush." Chronic toxicity can cause liver damage.
- **Vitamin B_5 (pantothenic acid)***
  - ≤ 1 year, 3.45–825 μg/L; >1–10 years, 3.45-229.2 μg/L; >10 years, 37–147 μg/L
  - **Deficiency:** fatigue, poor wound healing, skin problems

- **Vitamin B_6 (pyridoxine)** 3–30 μg/L
  - **Deficiency:** increased risk of heart disease, skin and sleep issues, depression
  - **Toxicity:** chronic overdosing causes extremity numbness and tingling, loss of coordination, digestion issues, and skin lesions.
- **Vitamin B_7 (biotin)** <12 years, 100–2460 pg/mL; ≥12 years, 221–3004 pg/mL
  - **Deficiency:** depression, nervous system abnormalities, hair loss, skin and nail problems
  - **Toxicity:** high blood sugar due to slower insulin release, low vitamins B_6 and C, skin rash
- **Vitamin B_9 (folate)*** ≥4.0 μg/L
  - **Deficiency:** fatigue, anemia, impaired immune function, hair loss
- **Vitamin B_{12} (cobalamin)*** 180–914 ng/L
  - **Deficiency**: fatigue, anemia, loss of appetite, weight loss, extremity numbness and tingling, depression, confusion, and mouth or tongue soreness

*These B vitamins typically do not promote symptoms of toxicity.

Therapeutic Drug Monitoring

Therapeutic States Associated with Monitoring the Pharmacokinetics of Therapeutic Drugs

The goal of **pharmacokinetics** is to determine the action of drugs in the body by evaluating the methods and rates of their absorption, distribution, metabolism, and excretion. Determination of these properties is pertinent to establishing a range of concentrations at which a drug is maximally effective with minimal toxicity, known as the **therapeutic range**. Most therapeutic ranges are based off of **trough** concentrations, which represent the lowest concentration in which the drug exists in the body. **Peak** represents the highest concentration of drug in the body after the administration of a dose. The peak and trough of drug concentrations are evaluated to establish consistent dosing of medications and monitor the clearance of therapeutic drugs. The determination of a drug's steady state in the body is necessary for maintaining therapeutic ranges for chronically administered drugs. A **steady state** in pharmacokinetics is described as the state in which drug input is equal to drug output in the body. Achieving a drug's steady state takes five and a half half-lives and results in a constant serum drug concentration.

Toxicity States Associated with Accumulation of Therapeutic Drugs

Therapeutic drug toxicity is reached when the body accumulates too much of a drug, causing adverse effects. Toxicity can occur due to too high of a dose administered, the inability to metabolize or excrete the drug, or interactions with other drugs. The half-life of a drug and the patient's age, kidney function, and hydration are all contributing factors affecting the rate of a drug's clearance and can increase the risk of toxicity. The types of toxicity and the associated adverse effects are listed below:

- **Acute toxicity** occurs 24–72 hours and up to 14 days following exposure.
- **Chronic toxicity** occurs in long-term drug therapy, emerging several weeks, months, or years after exposure.
- **Local** reactions occur at the specific area of contact.
- **Systemic** drug distribution causes reactions throughout numerous organ systems.
- **Nephrotoxicity:** damage to the kidneys
  - Fluid retention, decreased urine output, fatigue, nausea, chest pain, arrhythmias

- **Hepatotoxicity**: damage to the liver
    - Dark urine, jaundice, loss of appetite, itching, fever, fatigue, GI symptoms
- **Neurotoxicity:** damage to the CNS
    - Lethargy, weakness, vision changes, delirium, hallucinations, confusion, cognitive impairment, sedation, seizures, slurred speech, tremors, and increased muscle reflexes
- **Cardiotoxicity:** affects the electrical conduction and muscles of the heart
    - Arrhythmias, tachycardia, hypotension, hypertension, stroke, or cardiac arrest
- **Pulmonotoxicity:** damage to the lungs
    - Fast heart rate, chest pain, shortness of breath, shallow breathing, respiratory depression
- **Gastrointestinal toxicity**: damage to the GI tract
    - Nausea, abdominal pain, vomiting, diarrhea
- **Ototoxicity:** damage to the ears and sense of hearing
    - Loss of hearing, tinnitus, vertigo, balance issues

Metabolizing and Excreting Therapeutic Drugs, Drugs of Abuse, and Other Toxins

The process of drug **elimination** and the termination of drugs effects is completed through the metabolism and excretion of drugs from the body, mainly by the liver and kidneys. Drug **metabolism** is the process of transforming the structure of a drug by breaking it down into hydrophilic, excretable metabolites. The first phase of metabolism is completed by hepatic microsomal enzymes. This enzyme system is responsible for modifying drug chemicals' active group through oxidation, reduction, and hydrolysis. Conjugation of a drug or its metabolite to a polar group is the second phase of metabolism that renders the molecule possible for excretion. **Excretion** is the removal of unchanged drugs or metabolites from the body. The majority of drug chemicals are excreted from the kidneys in urine, but excretion can also take place in feces, breath, sweat, saliva, and other natural routes.

Aminoglycosides

Aminoglycosides are a category of antibiotics that are selectively active against Gram-negative bacteria including gentamicin, tobramycin, and amikacin. Molecules of aminoglycosides are composed of amino groups attached by sugar derivative glycosides. These compounds are soluble in water and are stable in solution and at a wide range of temperatures, and their activity is enhanced by an alkaline pH in comparison to an acidic environment. Aminoglycosides are used to treat severe infections caused by Gram-negative bacteria through inhibiting protein synthesis. Gram-negative bacterial cells attract aminoglycosides and facilitate the uptake of antibiotic molecules into the bacterial cells. In bacterial cells, these compounds bind to ribosomes and inhibit the synthesis of proteins, ultimately leading to the death of the bacterial cells. The bactericidal effects of aminoglycosides are dependent upon the concentration of drug in the body, meaning that the higher concentration of antibiotic that is present, the more bacteria will be killed. However, aminoglycoside toxicity is possible and peak and trough levels must be evaluated for optimal drug efficacy.

Cardioactive Drugs

Digoxin is classified as a **cardiac glycoside** with a chemical structure of a steroid molecule with a glycoside and R-group attached. Variance in cardiac glycoside activity is determined by the type of sugar and R-group attached to the steroid. Physically, digoxin demonstrates a solid, colorless or white crystalline formation that is more soluble in pyridine alcohol solutions than in water. Digoxin inhibits the sodium-potassium ATP pump, which promotes sodium and calcium exchange. Increased calcium in heart cells produces stronger heartbeats and slows the heart rate by increasing the force and velocity of heart contractions.

Quinidine, procainamide, disopyramide, and **lidocaine** are classified as **group I antiarrhythmic** drugs. These drugs inhibit sodium influx by blocking sodium channels, leading to slowed electrical conduction and the correction of irregular heart rhythms. Quinidine, procainamide, and disopyramide also have a potassium channel blocking effect that prolongs the action potential, whereas lidocaine acts to shorten the myocardial cell action potential.

Anticonvulsant Drugs

Anticonvulsant medications are used to treat epileptic seizures and act as mood stabilizers in bipolar and borderline personality disorder patients. These drugs act to suppress excessive rapid firing of neurons and prevent seizures from reaching the brain by blocking sodium channels or enhancing gamma-aminobutyric (GABA) function. Medications may be used by themselves or in conjunction with one another for increased effectiveness. Anticonvulsant drugs vary greatly in their composition and properties, with the categories of these medications described below:

- **Barbiturates** are chemical derivatives of barbituric acid that act as CNS depressants to produce anticonvulsant effects. Phenobarbital, phenytoin (Dilantin), and primidone are examples of barbiturates used as anticonvulsant therapy. Due to the high toxicity and the potential of drug overdose related to barbiturates, these drugs have mostly been replaced by benzodiazepines.
- **Benzodiazepines** have a core chemical structure of a benzene ring and diazepine fusion and act as CNS depressants by enhancing GABA neurotransmitter effects at the $GABA_A$ receptor. Short-term use of benzodiazepines is considered a safer alternative to barbiturate use with similar anticonvulsant effects.
- **Carbamazepine (Tegretol)** is a sodium channel blocker, which is effectively used to treat focal seizures and neuropathic pain.
- **Valproic acid** medications aid in the prevention of generalized, partial, and absence seizures and migraines and for treating bipolar disorder. Valproic acid is a clear carboxylic acid composed of branched short-chain fatty acids.

Antidepressants

Antidepressant or psychotropic medications are administered to treat patients experiencing major depressive and anxiety disorders, chronic pain, and in the management of some addictions. Prescribed antidepressants are chosen based on their mechanisms of action that will impact the most prominent symptoms displayed by a patient. Classes of antidepressants and their mechanisms of action are described below:

- **Selective-serotonin reuptake inhibitors:** increase extracellular levels of serotonin by limiting reabsorption into presynaptic cells and binding to postsynaptic receptors.
- **Serotonin-norepinephrine reuptake inhibitors (SNRIs):** balance inhibition of serotonin and norepinephrine uptake by their respective transporter membrane proteins.
- **Serotonin modulators and stimulators:** modulate one or more serotonin receptors at the same time and inhibit serotonin reuptake.
- **Serotonin antagonists and reuptake inhibitors:** antagonize serotonin receptors to inhibit the reuptake of serotonin, norepinephrine, or dopamine.

- **Norepinephrine reuptake inhibitors:** block the action of norepinephrine transporter membrane protein, increasing extracellular levels on norepinephrine.
- **Tricyclic:** structured with three rings of atoms, they act as SNRIs by blocking serotonin and norepinephrine transporters, elevating neurotransmitter concentrations and enhancing transmission.
- **Tetracyclic:** closely related to tricyclic medications; they are only structurally different by containing four atom rings.
- **Monoamine oxidase inhibitors:** inhibit the activity of monoamine oxidase enzymes and moderately raise serotonin neurotransmitter levels. Commonly used after the failure of other antidepressants drugs.
- **Lithium salts:** widely distributed in the CNS after they enter the body and interact with a variety of neurotransmitters and receptors to decrease norepinephrine release and increase serotonin synthesis. Commonly prescribed for bipolar disorders as mood stabilizers.

Immunosuppressants

Immunosuppressant drugs are used to suppress the strength of the body's immune system in patients with autoimmune disorders and to decrease the risk of rejection of transplanted organs. Immunosuppressant drugs of different classes are often prescribed simultaneously because they suppress different reactions using different mechanisms. The classes, their mechanisms of action, and examples of each class are described below:

- **Glucocorticoids and corticosteroids:** suppress cell-mediated and humoral immunity by inhibiting coding genes for cytokines and B cell expression of IL-1 and IL-2, reducing T cell proliferation and antibody synthesis, respectively. Induce synthesis and extracellular concentration of lipocortin-1 to inhibit inflammation.
  - **Prednisone, dexamethasone, and hydrocortisone** — reduce allergic reaction, inflammation, and autoimmune disorders. Given posttransplant to avoid acute rejection and GVHD.
- **Cytostatic:** inhibit the proliferation of T and B cells
  - **Antimetabolites**: interfere with nucleic acid synthesis
    - **Methotrexate** — rheumatoid arthritis and transplantations
    - **Azathioprine** and **mercaptopurine** — controls transplant rejections reactions
- **Monoclonal or polyclonal antibodies**: prevent transplanted organ rejection with antigen-directed antibodies and inhibited cell-mediated immunity with T lymphocyte lysis, respectively.
- **Immunophilin acting**: antirejection drugs
  - **Cyclosporine** — reduced function of effector T cells by binding to cyclophilin protein of T cells, which inhibits IL-2 transcription and release, and inhibits lymphokine production
  - **Tacrolimus** — inhibits calcineurin, preventing cell proliferation
  - **Sirolimus** — inhibits the mTOR protein, affecting the second phase to lymphocyte proliferation
- **Inosine-5′-monophosphate dehydrogenase (IMDH) inhibitors:** inhibit IMDH in a reversible, noncompetitive, and selective reaction.
  - **Mycophenolic acid** — prevents heart, kidney, and liver rejection and used for treatment of Crohn's disease.

Therapeutic Bronchodilation Drugs and Glycoprotein Antibiotics

Bronchodilator drugs are administered to treat breathing difficulties due to obstructive lung diseases such as asthma and chronic obstructive pulmonary disease. These medications dilate the bronchi and bronchioles, which decreases airway resistance and increases air flow to the lungs. **Short-** and **long-acting β_2-adrenergic antagonists** are specific to the lungs and are inhaled for reduced airway constriction for 20 minutes to 6 hours and up to 12 hours, respectively. **Theophylline** is an oral or injectable bronchodilator that is long acting and prevents asthma episodes in severe and difficult-to-control cases.

Glycoprotein antibiotics are comprised of seven peptide chains configured into three large rings with a disaccharide sugar attached. **Vancomycin** is the most commonly used of these drugs that are used to treat severe Gram-positive bacterial infections. These drugs are hydrophobic, have a moderate affinity for binding to proteins in adults, and are active in the pH range between 6.5 and 8. The bactericidal mechanism of glycoprotein antibiotics targets the synthesis of structural components in Gram-positive bacterial cell walls, weakening them, leading to lysis and death of bacteria. Peak and trough levels must be evaluated for optimal drug efficacy and to reduce the toxicity of glycoproteins.

Therapeutic Drug Monitoring Samples

Therapeutic drug monitoring (TDM) samples are collected via venipuncture with serum, plasma, and whole blood samples accepted for testing. Whole blood samples are useful in analyzing immunosuppressant drugs because they measure the medication that has accumulated in RBCs, as well as compounds in plasma. Plasma and serum should be separated from cells within 2 hours of collection, and gross hemolysis should be avoided for accurate results. TDM testing is most effective when timed as peak or trough samples, but randomly collected samples are used as well. Trough samples are collected immediately before the next dose is administered. Examples of peak collections vary as listed below:

- **Aminoglycosides**:
  - Trough
  - IV infusion peak: 30 minutes after completion
  - IM injection peak: 1 hour after injection
- **Carbamazepine, phenytoin, phenobarbital, quinidine**: Trough
- **Digoxin:** Random 6–24 hours after a dose
- **Theophylline**:
  - IV infusion: 30 minutes after a loading dose and then at 4- to 8-hour intervals during infusion
  - IV bolus: 30 minutes after completion of the infusion
  - Oral peak: 4 hours after a slow-release dose or 2 hours after a regular dose
- **Vancomycin**:
  - Trough
  - IV infusion peak: 1.5 hours after completion

Urine samples are monitored to ensure adherence to prescribed regimens or detect the misuse and abuse of therapeutic drugs. It is important to observe TDM samples for validity to ensure that clinicians receive accurate results regarding the patient's use of these medications. Urine samples for TDM evaluation must meet the following criteria to be considered valid:

- **Temperature:** 90–100 °F within 4 minutes of collection
- **pH:** 4.5–8
- **Specific gravity**: 1.002–1.030
- **Creatinine:** 20–400 mg/dL

Correlation Between Therapeutic Drug Test Results and Therapeutic, Subtherapeutic, or Toxic Ranges

The goal of therapeutic drug monitoring is to determine the concentrations that allow for drugs to provide patients with the optimal treatment while avoiding adverse effects. Therapeutic ranges vary by drug and by individual patients, but normal ranges have been established to give a general guide to follow. Some patients may exhibit adverse effects at concentrations within the therapeutic range, and some may not show signs of toxicity above this range. Drug concentrations below the therapeutic range are considered **subtherapeutic** and reflect a concentration too low to provide optimal or effective treatment. **Toxic ranges** are concentrations of medications that are known to cause adverse effects in patients. Acute toxicity is associated with short-term use of a drug and is more likely to be reversible than damage caused by chronic toxicity from long-term therapeutic drug therapy. The higher a concentration of medication that accumulates in the body, the higher the chances are for more serious and permanent toxic damages to occur. Clinical signs and symptoms must be correlated with TDM test results to determine the efficacy of treatment.

Therapeutic and Toxic Ranges of Drugs

Examples of drugs and their associated therapeutic ranges and levels of toxicity are given below:

Drug	Therapeutic Range	Toxic Level
Gentamicin	1–10 µg/mL	<12 µg/mL
Carbamazepine	4–12 µg/mL	>15 µg/mL
Cyclosporine	100–400 ng/mL	>400 ng/mL
Digoxin	0.6–2.0 nmol/L	>3.0 nmol/L
Lidocaine	1–5 µg/mL	>5 µg/mL
Lithium	0.6–1.2 nmol/L	>1.5 nmol/L
Phenobarbital	10–40 µg/mL	65–117 µg/mL — coma, with reflexes >100 µg/mL — coma, without reflexes
Phenytoin	10–20 µg/mL	>20 µg/mL
Theophylline Adults Neonates	 8–20 µg/mL 6–13 µg/mL	 >20 µg/mL >20 µg/mL
Valproic acid	50–100 µg/mL	>100 µg/mL

Toxicology

Exposure to Drugs of Abuse and Other Toxic Substances

Toxins have the ability to affect the body in a variety of ways. Understanding the absorption, distribution, metabolism, and excretion of toxins allows for more understanding of how the toxicity will present as clinical signs and symptoms. The severity of toxic effects is dependent on the chemical or compound itself, the concentration accumulated in the body, and the duration of exposure. Determining the type and severity of toxicity entails evaluating a patient for the following: vital signs, mental status, pupil size, mucous membrane irritation, lung exam for wheezing or rales, and skin exam for burns, moisture, and color. For most toxic agents, adverse effects take place at the site of their absorption. Examples of toxic chemicals and the signs and symptoms associated with toxicity are listed below:

- **Organophosphates, pesticides**: fatigue, muscle cramps and weakness, hypertension, hypoglycemia, paralysis
- **Cyanide gas:** seizures, hypotension, loss of consciousness, irregular heartbeat, potentially lethal in minutes
- **Alcohol:** slurred speech, confusion, nausea, vomiting, loss of consciousness, slowed breathing
- **Acetaminophen:** dependent on how long the drug accumulates
    - **0–24 hours**: fatigue, sweating, loss of appetite, abdominal pain, nausea and vomiting
    - **24–72 hours:** infrequent urination, dark urine, yellow skin and whites of eyes
    - **72–96 hours:** blood in urine, fever, syncope, quickened breathing, extreme fatigue, blurred vision, increased heart rate, confusion, coma
- **Lead:** symptoms vary with age
    - **Children:** irritability, loss of appetite, weight loss, abdominal pain, vomiting, constipation, lethargy, fatigue, developmental delays, hearing loss, seizures
    - **Adults:** hypertension, joint and muscle pain, memory and concentration issues, headache, abdominal pain

Alcohols

Alcohols are organic compounds containing an alkyl group and a functional hydroxyl group. Hydrogen bonds present in alcohols render most of them soluble in water and induce a higher boiling point compared to other hydrocarbon molecules. Primary alcohols contain polar hydroxide bonds that indicate their acidic nature. Secondary and tertiary alcohols become less acidic as electron donating groups attach to the hydroxyl group and increase the density on an O_2 atom.

Ethanol (ETOH), the most commonly consumed alcohol, is a simple alcohol that is naturally produced by the action of sugar fermentation by yeasts. ETOH molecules are comprised of a methyl group, attached to a methylene group, that is attached to a hydroxyl group. ETOH is a colorless liquid that mixes with water. It is also volatile and flammable, and it burns with a smokeless blue flame.

Lead, Mercury, and Arsenic

Lead (Pb) is a soft, malleable metal that is blue-gray in color and has a low melting point. It is also a poor conductor of heat and electricity, tarnishes in contact with moist air, and is highly resistant to corrosion. Oxidation of lead allows it to react and form covalent bonds with acids and bases. Lead occurs most commonly as an organic substance, but it can occur inorganically as an oxidant in highly acidic solutions.

At standard temperature and pressure conditions, **mercury (Hg)** exists as a heavy, liquid, silvery-white metal. It has the lowest freezing and boiling point of any stable metal due to its electron configuration strongly resisting electron removal. Mercury occurs naturally in water-soluble deposits of mercuric sulfide. Although it doesn't react with most acids, mercury dissolves metals such as gold and silver and can be dissolved itself by oxidizing acids.

Arsenic (As) is a metalloid that occurs naturally as a pure elemental crystal or combined with other metals and sulfur. Arsenic exists in three main structural formations called allotropes: gray, yellow, and black. The most common and stable allotrope, gray arsenic, conforms into a double-layered structure containing six membered, interlocked, ruffled rings, which gives it the property of being brittle.

Analgesics

Analgesic drugs are a group of medications that act on the peripheral nervous system and the CNS to provide pain relief, and they are chosen based on the severity and type of pain being experienced. **Acetaminophen**, or paracetamol, is used to treat mild to moderate pain and fevers with effects lasting between 2 and 4 hours. The chemical structure of acetaminophen consists of a benzene ring core with a hydroxyl group substituent and an amide group's nitrogen atom in the *para* (1,4) pattern. Acetaminophen is a water-soluble, white, crystalline solid with a boiling point >500 °C and a melting point of approximately 170 °C. By inhibiting prostaglandin synthesis and release into the CNS, acetaminophen reduces fever and pain.

Salicylates are a group of **NSAIDs** used to reduce fever, pain, inflammation, and the potential for blood clots. The active metabolite, salicylic acid, is a monohydroxybenzoic acid. The most commonly used salicylate, aspirin, binds to prostaglandin enzymes and reduces its synthesis to provide its analgesic, anti-inflammatory, and anticoagulant effects. Aspirin is a water- and alcohol-soluble, white, polymorphic, crystalline, solid analgesic drug.

Opioids are used primarily for heavy pain relief by binding to opioid receptors in the CNS, peripheral nervous system, and GI tract. Opioids range from natural to synthetically derived chemical compounds with differing structures, properties, and mechanisms of action. Agonist opioids produce a response from their receptor, whereas antagonists block their receptors response. Due to their highly addictive nature, opioids are considered a controlled substance.

Common Drugs of Abuse

Drugs of abuse are controlled substances used in a manner that is not consistent with appropriate medical use. Drug classes controlled by the government include narcotics, depressants, stimulants, hallucinogens, and anabolic steroids. These substances can be prescribed or illicit, and they have the potential to be abused by the patient developing physical and psychological dependence. Examples of each class of controlled substance and their associated properties are described below:

- **Narcotics, or opioids,** are analgesics that occur naturally in opium from a poppy plant or are synthetically produced to relieve pain.
    - **Hydrocodone** is a hydrogenated codeine derivative that presents as fine, white crystals or crystalline powder.
- **Depressants** are substances that lower neurotransmission levels to reduce stimulation in several areas of the brain.
    - **Benzodiazepines'** core chemical structure is a benzene and diazepine ring fusion. They act on GABA neurotransmitter receptors for sedative, hypnotic, antianxiety, anticonvulsant, and muscle-relaxant effects.
    - **Cannabis'** active compound, tetrahydrocannabinol, occurs naturally in the cannabis plant; it decreases alertness and induces muscle relaxation and sedation.
- **Stimulants** act to increase CNS activity to treat mood disorders.
    - **Amphetamine** drugs are a class of compounds derived from the amphetamine structure with hydrogen substituents that enhance catecholamine neurotransmission.
- **Hallucinogens** and dissociative drugs cause profound distortions in reality through altered sensations with increased energy and pleasure.

- Ecstasy or 3,4-Methylenedioxymethamphetamine (commonly known as MDMA or molly)** is a recreational psychoactive amphetamine appearing as a water-soluble white powder or crystal.

- **Anabolic steroids** are synthetic androgynous hormones that stimulate bone and muscle growth and RBC production.

Other Toxins

Carbon monoxide (CO) is a colorless, odorless gas composed of a one-carbon compound joined to a single O_2 atom. With an affinity for hemoglobin more than 200 times that of O_2, CO is toxic to humans by accumulating carboxyhemoglobin and by reducing O_2 in the blood.

Cyanide occurs in three forms as hydrogen cyanide, sodium cyanide, and potassium cyanide. At room temperature, hydrogen cyanide exists as a pale-blue transparent liquid or a colorless gas with a bitter, almond scent, whereas sodium and potassium cyanide are white crystalline solids. Inhaling hydrogen cyanide is the most common exposure to these toxic substances that interfere with cellular respiration processes in the body. Hydrogen cyanide is a linear carbon molecule with a singularly bonded hydrogen and a triple-bonded nitrogen. Cyanides are weakly acidic and partially ionize in water.

Organophosphates are a class of compounds that occur in a variety of forms with differing properties. Chemical pesticides contain organophosphates that inhibit acetylcholinesterase, causing CNS symptoms in humans. These phosphate esters with hydroxyl groups are acidic and will lose a hydrogen proton in an aqueous solution.

Immunoassay Methods for Toxicology Testing

Toxicology testing requires the use of two different testing methodologies: one as a presumptive identification of a drug and a second to confirm the presence of drugs in urine or other body fluids. Commonly, immunoassay methods are used to screen and presumptively detect drug classes. A combination of chromatography and spectrometry methods is the gold standard to confirm the presence of drugs.

Immunoassay methods screen for classes of drugs and their metabolites based on chromatographic antibody–antigen reactions. Sample pads on test cartridges are embedded with an absorbed solution containing monoclonal antibodies for each drug class. Drug conjugates for each class are immobilized at a labeled location on the membrane strip. Urine or other fluid samples are added to the test pad, and the following reactions can occur:

- When a drug is present in the sample, the antibody solution in the sample pad binds to the drug antigens in the sample. When these bind, the antigen cannot bind to the conjugate in the membrane strip and a chromatographic line does not appear. The **absence of a line** at the marked location for each drug determines a presumptive **positive** result.
- When there is no drug or metabolite present in a sample, the antibody in the sample pad will bind with its drug conjugate in the membrane strip. This binding produces a visible colored line at the location labeled for the drug. A **line produced** is indicative of a **negative** result for that specific drug class.

Thin-Layer Chromatography, Mass Spectrometry, and Gas Chromatography-Mass Spectrometry

Chromatography and mass spectrometry methods are most often used in conjunction with one another to confirm the presence of a drug or drugs in a sample.

Thin-layer chromatography is a method used to separate molecules of drug from one another in urine samples. A sheet of glass, plastic, or foil is coated with a thin layer of adsorbent material for atoms to adhere to, such as silica gel, aluminum oxide, or cellulose. A spot of the sample is added to the bottom of the thin layer plate and allowed to dry, and then it is placed into a solvent. The solvent is drawn up the plate by capillary action and pulls the chemical compounds in the sample along with it. Each drug is identifiable based on the distance traveled and migration patterns. Thin-layer chromatography methods require confirmatory testing with a second method.

Mass spectrometry is used to detect drug molecules by their mass-to-charge ratio after they have been separated and quantified by high-performance liquid chromatography or gas chromatography.

Gas chromatography-mass spectrometry is the gold standard for confirmatory drug testing due to its high rate of sensitivity and reliability. Gas chromatography uses a capillary column to separate molecules based on their chemical properties and different affinity for the column being used. Molecules are retained by the column, come off, or elute, at different times, and move to the mass spectrometer where they are detected.

Toxicology Testing Samples

Drugs remain detectable in biological samples based on their route of administration, half-life, frequency of use, and the user's state of hydration. On average, drugs of abuse remain in patients' systems for 2–4 days after use. The most widely used specimen for drug screening and confirmation is **urine**. Drug metabolites being excreted from the body can be detectable for days to weeks after use. Urine samples for drug testing can be easily collected, evaluated for potential adulteration, and stored. In order to rule out adulteration of sample collection, the same criteria as therapeutic drug monitoring samples must be met. Urine samples are considered valid based on the following criteria:

- **Temperature:** 90–100 °F within 4 minutes of collection
- **pH:** 4.5–8
- Specific gravity: 1.002–1.030
- **Creatinine:** 20–400 mg/dL

A collection of 100–120 **hairs** cut closely from the scalp can be analyzed to evaluate long-term drug use. Hair samples can detect drugs for up to 90 days after use and provide a lessened risk of adulteration due to the entire collection and transport process being supervised by lab staff. **Saliva** samples or swabs can be selected for detection of recent drug use in the hours and days prior to testing. **Plasma** and **serum blood** samples can be collected via venipuncture to determine if someone is actively under the influence of certain drugs and alcohol and to evaluate toxicity due to heavy metals, CO, and other toxins. Blood alcohol levels can also be determined by the person exhaling into a breathalyzer.

Laboratory Test Results for Toxic Substances and Associated Disease States

Described below are the laboratory test results and disease states associated with toxic substances:

Substance	Normal Range	Toxic Range	Symptoms/Disease
Lead, blood	All ages: <5.0μg/dL	0–15 years old: ≥20.0μg/dL ≥16 years old: ≥70.0μg/dL	Newborn: premature birth, low birth weight, slowed growth Child: GI issues, seizures, hearing loss, developmental and learning delays Adult: hypertension, mood disorders, infertility in men and pregnancy complications in women
Mercury, blood	<10 ng/mL	Mild exposure: 15 ng/mL Significant exposure: 50–200 ng/mL	Peripheral neuropathy, itching or burning sensations, tremors, irritability, vision changes, lack of coordination
Arsenic, urine	<20 μg/mL organic and inorganic	>20 μg/mL of inorganic arsenic, organic not typically toxic	GI tract, skin, and CNS involvement.
Acetaminophen, serum	10–25 μg/mL	>200 μg/mL	Disease depends on the duration that the toxin accumulates in the body
Salicylate, serum	<30.0 mg/dL	≥50.0 mg/dL	Nausea, vomiting, tinnitus, vertigo, seizures, hyperthermia, acid–base disturbance
CO, blood	Nonsmoker: 0–2% Smoker: ≤9%	≥20%	Headache, weakness, dizziness, nausea, vomiting, shortness of breath, blurred vision, confusion, loss of consciousness
Cyanide, blood	≤0.05 μg/mL	Toxic: ≥0.50 μg/mL Potentially lethal: ≥2.0 μg/mL	Acute: dizziness, headache, vertigo, confusion, difficulty breathing Chronic: paralysis, hypothyroidism, mild liver and kidney damage
Organophosphates, RBC acetylcholin-esterase	31.2–61.3 U/g of hemoglobin	<31.2 U/g of hemoglobin	Fatigue, muscle weakness and cramps, hypoglycemia, hypertension

Laboratory Test Results for Classes of Drugs of Abuse and Alcohol and Associated Clinical Signs and Symptoms

Acute ETOH intoxication signs and symptoms generally manifest in patients with an **average blood alcohol concentration of ≥0.20%.** Intoxication symptoms include the following: confusion, vomiting, seizures, slow and irregular breathing, pale or blue-tinged skin, hypothermia, and unconsciousness. The clinical presentation varies among individuals because those who frequently consume alcohol require a higher blood alcohol concentration to present with symptoms. **Long-term excessive consumption** of alcohol leads to the following **chronic conditions**: fatty liver disease, liver cirrhosis, increased risk of heart disease, nerve damage, depression, dementia, ulcers, and certain cancers.

Drug classes commonly screened for in urine samples and clinical presentations associated with their use or overdose are listed below:

- **Amphetamines and methamphetamines:** restlessness, tremors, muscle twitches, pain or weakness, rapid breathing, hostility, panic, dark urine, seizures, or coma
- **Cannabis:** increased heart rate, hypotension, muscle relaxation, dizziness, distorted perception, loss of coordination and motor skills, agitation, anxiety, confusion, dry eyes or mouth
- **Cocaine:** heart arrhythmias, headache, stomach pain, nausea, chest pain, seizure, respiratory failure, stroke, or heart attack
- **Opiates:** cold and clammy skin, pinpoint pupils, severe muscle weakness, drowsiness, very slow breathing, or coma
- **Barbiturates:** clammy skin, dilated pupils, weak and rapid pulse, shallow breathing, respiratory failure, or coma
- **Benzodiazepines:** irritability, memory issues, slower thinking, drowsiness, anxiety, muscle weakness, slurred speech, confusion, or coma
- **Phencyclidine**:
  - **Low to moderate dose:** profuse sweating, increased heart and breath rates, shallow breathing, hypertension
  - **High dose:** decreased respiration, heart rate, and blood pressure; nausea; vomiting; drooling; blurred vision; dizziness; loss of balance; possibly violence or suicide.

Hematology

Physiology

Hematology Terminology

Nucleated RBC (NRBC)	Immature red blood cell that contain a nucleus, abnormal when found in peripheral blood.
Hematocrit	Percentage of erythrocytes in whole blood.
Reticulocyte	Immature erythrocyte that shows a basophilic reticulum under vital staining.
Hematopoiesis	Formation and maturation of blood cells.
Differential	Different types of leukocytes by percentage (monocytes, lymphocytes, neutrophils, basophils, and eosinophils.)
Plasma	Liquid portion of blood or lymph.
Leukemia	Malignancy of blood-forming organs with abnormal proliferation and development of leukocytes and precursors.
Buffy coat	In centrifuged blood, the layer of leukocytes above the packed red blood cells.
Hypertonic	A solution with greater osmotic pressure than the solution to which it is compared.
Hypotonic	A solution with lower osmotic pressure than the solution to which it is compared.
Sodium citrate	Crystalline compound used as an anticoagulant and retains coagulation factors.

Hematopoiesis

The process of production and differentiation of blood cells is known as hematopoiesis. The process works as follows: bone marrow produces stem cells, which in turn differentiate into colony forming units and then, subsequently, into monocytes, granulocytes, erythrocytes, thrombocytes, T lymphocytes, and B lymphocytes. Bone marrow also produces progenitor cells and precursor cells. Precursor cells develop into blasts, while progenitor cells differentiate into a single cell line, either granulocyte, thrombocyte, or erythrocyte.

Hemoglobin

Hemoglobin is an iron-containing protein that is used to transport oxygen from the lungs to other body tissues. The iron in the hemoglobin is what gives blood its characteristic red color. Hemoglobin contains 4 iron atoms, 4 heme groups, and 4 globin chains (or protein groups). Hemoglobin contains approximately 94% globin and 6% heme. In addition, hemoglobin is produced in the bone marrow by erythrocytes. The most common form of hemoglobin in an adult is hemoglobin A.

Structure of Hemoglobin Types

- Fetal hemoglobin (Hb F): Two gamma globin chains and two alpha globin chains
- Hemoglobin Barts: Four gamma globin chains and no alpha globin chains
- Hemoglobin A: Two alpha globin chains and two beta globin chains
- Hemoglobin A_2: Two alpha globin chains and two delta globin chains

Erythrocytes

A erythrocyte is a red blood cell (RBC). Red blood cells are cells that carry oxygen from the lungs to the rest of the body's tissues. These cells are red because of the hemoglobin that they contain. RBCs are produced by the bone marrow, especially of the long bones, and stored in the spleen.

Erythrocyte Maturation Series, Production and Destruction

Erythrocyte maturation series:

	College of American Pathologists Terminology	American Society for Clinical Pathologists Terminology
1.	Hemocytoblast	
2.	Pronormoblast	Rubriblast
3.	Basophilic normoblast (erythroblast)	Prorubricyte
4.	Polychromatophilic normoblast	Rubricyte
5.	Orthochromic normoblast	Metarubricyte
6.	Reticulocyte	
7.	Erythrocyte	

The first 5 stages of both classification systems contain a nucleus, which gets smaller and disappears from reticulocytes or mature erythrocytes. The first 4 stages are found in the bone marrow but the immature cells of stage 5 and stage 6 (reticulocytes) may enter the peripheral blood when production is high. **Erythrocyte production (erythropoiesis) and destruction**: Kidneys produce erythropoietin in response to decreased oxygen level in the blood, stimulating the bone marrow to produce erythrocytes. The lifespan of an erythrocyte is about 120 days with 2–3 million circulating in an average adult. Production falls when oxygen levels rise. Aging erythrocytes are removed in the spleen and liver by macrophages. Some component parts are reused: Iron returns to the bone marrow, heme is broken down into bilirubin for excretion, and globin is reused or reduced to amino acids.

Reticulocytes

The last stage before maturity in the development of an erythrocyte is the appearance of the reticulocyte. These bodies do not contain a nucleus, although they do feature mitochondria and ribosomes. For adults, a normal range of reticulocytes is 0.5–1.5%, while for newborns the normal range is 2.5–6.5%. The reticulocyte count can be used as a gauge of bone marrow function and erythropoietic activity. These bodies can be viewed using a reticulocyte stain or a Wright stain.

Types of Erythrocytes

- Macrocytes: Erythrocytes with a mean corpuscular volume greater than 100 fL; indicates certain kinds of anemia
- Echinocytes: Erythrocytes with evenly-distributed spikes or bumps; may be caused by an elevated number of platelets
- Keratocytes: Erythrocytes with spiny extensions on the surface; possibly indicative of renal problems, ulcers, or liver disease
- Acanthocytes: Erythrocytes with irregularly-spaced spikes on the surface; possibly indicative of liver disease
- Microcytes: Erythrocytes with a mean corpuscular volume of less than 80 fL; may indicate certain kinds of anemia or thalassemia

- Codocytes: Erythrocytes consisting of a cell surrounded by successive concentric rings of hemoglobin, transparent material, and hemoglobin; may indicate liver disease, anemia, or another hemoglobinopathy
- Spherocytes: Small erythrocytes with no pale spot in the center; these also have an elevated mean corpuscular hemoglobin concentration; symptomatic of burns and hereditary spherocytosis
- Schistocytes: Erythrocytes fragments generated by movements through damaged blood vessels; symptomatic of burns
- Dacrocytes: Erythrocytes shaped like tears, and smaller than normal

Abnormal Erythrocyte Inclusions

- Howell-Jolly bodies: Fragments of DNA between 1 and 2 μm in size, and found in clusters among red blood cells; these bodies will test positive for the Feulgen stain, and will stain bluish-red to purple; typical of individuals with missing or damaged spleen, megaloblastic anemia, or sickle cell anemia
- Pappenheimer bodies: Clusters of iron granules found in an erythrocyte, typically at one end; turn dark blue or violet with Wright or Prussian Blue stain; caused by an aggregation of ribosomes, mitochondria, and iron fragments; characteristic of megaloblastic anemia, sideroblastic anemia, and thalassemia
- Heinz bodies: Denatured hemoglobin not usually included in an erythrocyte; 0.3–2.0 μm; identified with cresyl blue or crystal violet stains; typical of G6PD deficiency
- Basophilic stippling: Ribosomal RNA not usually included in an erythrocyte; inclusions may be fine or coarse, small or large; stains dark blue or purple; characteristic of lead poisoning, megaloblastic anemia, and thalassemia

Leukocytes

Granulocytes

A granulocyte is a type of white blood cell that has granules in its cytoplasm. There are three types of granulocytes: basophils, eosinophils, and neutrophils. Approximately 75% of all white blood cells are granulocytes.

Lymphocytes

Lymphocytes are a special type of white blood cell that play an important role in the immune system. B cells and T cells are the two types of lymphocytes.

Monocytes

A monocyte is another type of white blood cell. These cells are characterized by a well-defined nucleus. They play an important role in the body's immune response to pathogens. These cells are also produced in the bone marrow.

Basophils, Eosinophils, and Neutrophils

These three types of granulocytes are distinguished by their ability to be stained with various types of stains in the laboratory. Basophils are stained black by basic stains, eosinophils are stained red by acid stains, and neutrophils are stained pale lilac by neutral pH stains. Basophils play an important role in allergies and allergic reactions, as well as in inflammation. Eosinophils play an important part in the defense against infection by parasites, and neutrophils take part in the defense against infection from microorganisms.

LEUKOCYTES MATURATION SERIES

Granulocytes (neutrophils, eosinophils, basophils) with lobed nuclei and granules	Agranulocytes (monocytes, lymphocytes) with single-lobe nuclei and no granules
1. Myeloid progenitor 2. Myeloblast (10-20 μm): oval nucleus with no granules evident in cytoplasm. 3. Promyelocyte (10-20 μm): Granules in cytoplasm. 4. Myelocyte (10-18 μm): Large oval nucleus. Primary granules evident but secondary more prevalent. 5. Metamyelocyte (10-18 μm): Kidney-shaped nucleus with primary and secondary (most prevalent) granules. 6. Band: U-shaped nucleus, secondary or neutrophilic or basophils granules most common. 7. Segmented cells (14 μm): 2-5 joined lobes.	**Monocyte**: 1. Myeloid progenitor 2. Monoblast (12-20 μm) with large oval nucleus and lymphoid dendritic cells 3. Promonocyte (from monoblast) 4. Monocyte 5. Macrophage and myeloid dendritic cell. **Lymphocyte**: 1. Common lymphoid progenitor 2. Lymphoblast (10-20 μm) with large round nucleus. 3. Prolymphocyte 4. Small lymphocyte and natural killer cell 5. B and T lymphoctyes (from small lymphocyte)

T LYMPHOCYTES AND B LYMPHOCYTES

T lymphocytes are white blood cells responsible for the body's cell-mediated immune system response to a viral or bacterial infection. This response is accomplished through the antigens on specific T lymphocytes that have the ability to destroy cells that have been infected by a virus, bacteria, other microbe, or cancerous cells. B lymphocytes, on the other hand, are a type of lymphocyte that combats infection or viruses through the use of antibodies, called humoral immunity. In humoral immunity, B lymphocytes secrete specific antibodies into the blood plasma, and these antibodies attach themselves to specific antigens. Antigens can be located on viruses, bacteria, or other microbes. The binding of the antibodies to the antigens then signals to the body that these are the cells that should be lyzed or subjected to phagocytosis.

FUNCTIONS OF T CELL SUBSETS

- T-helper cell: Takes information about antigens from macrophages and monocytes and delivers that information to other cells; identified by cluster differentiation four-membrane proteins
- T-suppressor cell: Manages response of immune system; divided into three types: inducer, mediator, and effector; identified by the presence of cluster differentiation eight (CD8) membrane proteins
- Cytotoxic T cell: Contributes to the rejection of organs and the promotion of viral infections
- T memory cell: over a long period of time, these cells respond to previously-introduced antigens

THROMBOCYTES AND COAGULATION

Thrombocyte is another word for platelet. A platelet is a type of blood cell that is small in size, irregular in its shape, and colorless. Platelets play an important role in the clotting and coagulation of blood, and they can also aid in helping to repair injured blood vessels. Platelets are produced by the bone marrow and are stored in the spleen.

THROMBOCYTE MATURATION SERIES

The **thrombocyte maturation series** is as follows:

1. Hemocytoblast (able to produce all cell types)
2. Myeloid stem cells
3. Megakaryoblast (21-50 μm) with irregular-shaped nucleus.
4. Promegakaryocyte (20-80 μm) with 2-4 small nucleoli.
5. Megakaryocyte (≤100 μm) with multi-lobed nucleus.
6. Thrombocyte

Count increased in polycythemia vera, RA, acute infections, anemias, cirrhosis, chronic leukemia, splenectomy, TB, ulcerative colitis, and trauma.

Count decreased in aplastic anemia, megaloblastic anemia, iron-deficiency anemia, idiopathic thrombocytopenia, severe hemorrhage, bone marrow replacement, radiation, multiple infections, lymphoma, aplastic anemia.

APPEARANCE OF CELLS IN THE DEVELOPMENT OF A PLATELET

- Megakaryoblast: The first stage in platelet development; 20–50 μm; nucleus contains nucleoli; no visible chromatin; irregularly shaped cytoplasm with no granules; cytoplasm stains blue
- Promegakaryocyte: Slightly larger, 20–80 μm; contains double nucleus; cytoplasm as tags and granules; demarcating membrane system emerges
- Megakaryocyte: Between 30 and 100 μm; several nuclei; coarse chromatin; visible granules of blue and red
- Metamegakaryocyte: Largest cell in the human body; smaller nucleus to cytoplasm ratio; at this stage, platelets begin to detach from the demarcating membrane system

PLATELET COAGULATION GROUPS

- Contact group: Contains the coagulation factors XI, XII, high molecular weight kininogen, and prekallikrein; all of these factors are created in the liver and serve to activate fibrinolysis, intrinsic coagulation activation, and the activation of the complement system
- Prothrombin group: Contains coagulation factors II, VII, IX, and X; these factors are produced in the liver and require vitamin K; anticoagulation therapies and antibiotics may decrease the activity of these coagulation factors
- Fibrinogen group: Contains coagulation factors I, V, VIII, and XIII; these factors do not require vitamin K, and, with the exception of factor VIII, are located in platelets; these factors are substrates for the fibrinolytic enzyme plasmin

FIBRINOLYSIS AND COAGULATION INHIBITORS

- Alpha 2-antiplasmin: Inhibits fibrinolysis; not affected by heparin
- Alpha 1-antitrypsin: Alters coagulation factor XI; not affected by heparin
- Alpha 2-macroglobulin: Alters the function and development of plasmin; not affected by heparin
- Antithrombin III: Obstructs the function of factors IX, X, XI, XII, plasmin, and kallikrein; made more effective by heparin
- C1 inactivator: Obstructs the function of factors XI, XII, and plasmin; not affected by heparin

Disease States

Vitamin K and Newborn Babies

Vitamin K is a very important vitamin because it is related to proper clotting of the blood. It helps form prothrombin to make a clot. If there is a lack of Vitamin K, there will be a corresponding decrease in the production of prothrombin. Adults with decreased prothrombin have increased PT/PTT times, broken capillaries and bruising. Vitamin K is synthesized in the intestines of newborns, and since their intestinal flora are often underdeveloped at birth, there may not be enough Vitamin K synthesized. This can lead to hemorrhagic disease or navel bleeding in newborn babies. An intramuscular injection of Vitamin K at birth can help ward off such problems by supplying the newborn with the Vitamin K that he/she needs until the newborn is able to synthesize enough Vitamin K independently.

Aplastic Anemia

Aplastic anemia is a disorder in which the bone marrow does not produce enough erythrocytes (red blood cells), leukocytes (white blood cells), and platelets. This disease can be caused by an autoimmune disorder, or by exposure to certain chemicals, drugs, or radiation. However, approximately half of all cases have no known cause. Because of the decreased amount of granulocytes, patients with aplastic anemia are susceptible to infections. And, because of the abnormally low amount of platelets produced, hemorrhaging, prolonged PT/PTT, and bruising are often seen. The disease is ultimately diagnosed by a bone marrow biopsy, and the best course of treatment is a bone marrow transplant.

Sickle Cell Trait and Sickle Cell Disease

Patients with sickle cell trait have inherited from their parents one abnormal hemoglobin gene, hemoglobin S. Hemoglobin S is responsible for turning red blood cells into abnormal sickle shaped (curved) cells. Patients with sickle cell trait, however, also have one gene for normal hemoglobin, hemoglobin A. Because these patients do have some hemoglobin A, they rarely exhibit any adverse symptoms. However, they can pass the sickle cell trait onto their children. Patients with sickle cell disease, on the other hand, have inherited two genes for hemoglobin S, and no genes for hemoglobin A. Therefore, the latter will exhibit the adverse symptoms of the disease, like severely debilitating joint pain during sickle cell crisis. They also will pass the gene for hemoglobin S onto any children they may have (who may or may not develop sickle cell disease).

Acute Leukemia and Chronic Leukemia

Acute leukemias are characterized by an extremely rapid growth of immature white blood cells (leukocytes) in the bone marrow. These new cells are unable to kill invaders because of their immaturity. Immature leukocytes may crowd out normal leukocytes in the bone marrow. Acute leukemias occur most often in young adults and children. Acute leukemias progress very rapidly, and so treatment of the disease needs to be started immediately after diagnosis. Chronic leukemias, on the other hand, are characterized by the growth of abnormal (but relatively mature) leukocytes. The abnormal leukocytes are produced at a higher rate than the production of normal leukocytes in the bone marrow. This disease can take a long time to progress, on the order of months to even years. Chronic leukemia is most commonly found in the elderly, and unlike with acute leukemias, treatment does not need to begin immediately after diagnosis, because chronic leukemias do not progress very rapidly.

Review Video: Leukemia
Visit mometrix.com/academy and enter code: 940024

Hairy Cell Leukemia

Hairy cell leukemia is a rare, chronic disease that is characterized by the presence of hairy cells in the bone marrow. Hairy cells are leukocytes (white blood cells) that have hair like projections. They are found in the bone marrow, the spleen, and in some cases, the liver. B lymphocytes are the most often affected by this type of leukemia. Hairy cell leukemia occurs most often in the elderly, and is often associated with enlargement of the spleen. Some symptoms of hairy cell leukemia include: Fatigue, excessive bruising, abdominal pain, infections, and anemia. The cause of hairy cell leukemia is unknown, but there may be a genetic component to the disease. In the laboratory, when hairy cells are exposed to acid phosphatase, they stain positive. When they are exposed to tartaric acid, however, they do not destain.

Basophilic Stippling, Heinz Bodies, Howell-Jolly Bodies, Rouleaux, and Schistocytes

Basophilic stippling could be seen in a patient with lead poisoning. Heinz bodies are characteristic of hemolytic anemia, and Howell-Jolly bodies are characteristic of megaloblastic anemia. Rouleaux of erythrocytes is seen in patients with myeloma, and schistocytes can be seen in patients that have high blood pressure (hypertension).

Possible Causes for Abnormal Leukocyte Counts

Neutrophilia: Neutrophils count is increased, probably because of inflammation, leukemia, exercise, bacterial infection, or inflammation

Neutropenia: Neutrophil count is decreased, probably because of damaged spleen, vitamin B12 or folate deficiency, or infection

Eosinophilia: Eosinophil count is increased, probably because of scarlet fever, hay fever, parasitic infection, hives, asthma, or chronic myelocytic leukemia

Eosinopenia: Eosinophil count is decreased, probably because of high stress or acute inflammation

Basophilia: Basophil count is increased, probably because of hypothyroidism, chronic hemolytic anemia, hypersensitivity reaction, or another myeloproliferative disorder

Basopenia: Basophile count is decreased, probably because of infection or hypothyroidism

Atypical Lymphocytes

Atypical lymphocytes are larger in size than normal lymphocytes, and typically have less nucleus relative to cytoplasm. The cytoplasm in an atypical lymphocyte is dark blue, owing to elevated production of RNA. Nucleoli will be visible, and the Golgi apparatus will be larger than usual. A distinctive transparent area in the Golgi apparatus, known as the Hof area, will appear under the microscope.

Leukemia or Lymphoma Associated with Philadelphia Chromosome, Reed-Sternberg Cells, and Howell-Jolly Bodies

- Philadelphia chromosome: Also known as Ph1 chromosome; associated with chronic myelocytic leukemia, adult T cell leukemia, and acute lymphocytic leukemia
- Reed-Sternberg cells: Associated with Hodgkin's lymphoma
- Howell-Jolly bodies: Associated with acute be erythroleukemia; these bodies are small and round, and are found in the nuclei of red blood cells

Thalassemia

Thalassemia is a condition in which there is a deficiency in the synthesis of at least one globin chain in the hemoglobin molecule. Thalassemia major is a condition in which there are neither alpha nor beta globin chains in the hemoglobin, while thalassemia minor is a condition in which there are simply decreased amounts of alpha and beta globin chains. The standard test for diagnosing this condition is hemoglobin electrophoresis. If the test shows increased fetal hemoglobin and Hb A_2, then thalassemia is indicated.

Porphyria

In the condition known as porphyria, an individual has a diminished production of heme resulting from an enzyme deficiency. Such individuals may manifest microcytic or hypo-chronic anemia, and will display decreased mean corpuscular volume, mean corpuscular hemoglobin, and mean corpuscular hemoglobin concentration. Abdominal pain, sensitivity to light, and disorders of the central nervous system are common symptoms. This condition may be either inherited or acquired. Two examples of inherited porphyrias are erythrohepatic protoporphyria and acute intermittent porphyria. One example of an acquired porphyria is porphyria cutanea.

Platelets

A platelet is a cell fragment is derived from a megakaryocyte. Platelets form in bone marrow, are stored in the spleen, and then move to blood plasma to assist with blood clotting after an injury. Platelets are small, colorless, and irregularly shaped. They have no hemoglobin, no nucleus, and no DNA. Platelets also transport and store several chemicals. A normal platelet count for a healthy adult is between 150,000 and 400,000 per microliter of blood. Platelets are also called thrombocytes.

Platelet Disorders

- Thrombocytopenia: Decrease in the production of platelets; may be the result of ineffective thrombopoiesis, loss of platelets due to hemorrhage or hemolytic uremic syndrome, spleen conditions, or megakaryocyte hypoproliferation
- Primary thrombocytosis: Wild elevation in the production of platelets; may be caused by chronic granulocytic leukemia, polycythemia vera, or essential thrombocythemia
- Secondary thrombocytosis: Increase in the production of platelets, slightly less than that of primary thrombocytosis; often caused by chronic inflammatory disease, acute inflammatory disease, acute blood loss, iron deficiency, hemolytic anemia, or malignant disease

Hematology Lab Testing

Red Blood Cell Indices

- Mean corpuscular volume (MCV): Calculated as hematocrit divided by red blood cell count; indicates average volume of individual red blood cells; normal range between 80 and 95 femtoliters (fL); a low MCV is sometimes the result of anemia or liver disease
- Mean corpuscular hemoglobin (MCH): Calculated as hemoglobin divided by red blood cell count; indicates average weight of hemoglobin in each red blood cell; normal range is 26–34 picograms; a low MCH is sometimes the result of microcytic anemia, while a high MCH is sometimes the result of macrocytic anemia

- Mean corpuscular hemoglobin concentration (MCHC): Calculated as hemoglobin concentration divided by hematocrit, and multiplied by 100; indicates average concentration of hemoglobin in grams per deciliter (g/dL) of red blood cells; normal range is 32–36%; low levels may be the result of thalassemia or anemia, while high levels may indicate spherocytosis
- Hematocrit (HCT): The volume of packed red blood cells; the ratio of red blood cells in whole blood; normal range is 40–52%

Blood Smear for Platelets

Blood smear for platelets may be carried out if the automated blood count shows an abnormally high or low. For the smear, a slide is treated with a stain and a drop of blood spread thinly across the slide. A microscopic examination or digital analyzer may be used to analyze the smear and determine the size and shape of the platelets. For example, if the platelets are exceptionally large ("giant") (the size of RBCs), this may be an indication of myeloproliferative neoplasm or immune thrombocytopenic purpura. A blood smear can also help to differentiate clumps of platelets from enlarged platelets.

Determining Concentration of Particular Cells in a Sample Using a Hemocytometer

Use a Neubauer-ruled hemocytometer to manually count blood cells or other microscopic particles in blood. The hemocytometer is a glass microscope slide with rectangular indentations that create a chamber with a depth of 0.1 mm. This chamber is scored with a series of perpendicular lines that form a grid (fields). Dilute a blood sample and pipette 10 microliters inside the chamber. Cover it with a glass coverslip. The diluted sample spreads across the chamber. Wait 10 minutes for cells to settle. Examine the chamber at 10x magnification under the microscope. Differentiate and count the cells in 9 large fields. Report the total WBC count per cubic millimeter as the (number of cells counted ×1000)/9.

Osmotic Fragility Test

The osmotic fragility test is based on the ability of a red blood cell to hold up when exposed to variances in salt concentration of a solution. Certain cells, such as spherocytes (spherical shaped red blood cells), will swell and eventually burst (hemolyze) as the salt concentration in the solution decreases. As the salt concentration decreases, more water will enter the red blood cell because of the principle of osmosis. If the cell has accepted the maximum amount of water that it can, but water is still trying to enter the red blood cell and the pressure inside the cell keeps increasing, the cell will burst, releasing hemoglobin (hemolysis). The reason that spherocytes are susceptible to hemolyzing in this test is because they have a low ratio of surface area to volume, as opposed to normal erythrocytes that are donut-shaped. Spherocytes are osmotically fragile -- not as resilient to pressure as are normally shaped erythrocytes.

Stains Related to Hematology

- Nonvital polychrome stains: Also known as Romanowsky stains; DNA and RNA turn blue, acid components turn orange or red, red blood cells turn pink
- Nonvital monochrome stains: Used to stay in histocytes, iron granules, and other particular cellular parts in a red blood cell; Prussian blue is a common example
- Vital monochrome stains: Used to stay in the nature to hemoglobin and other specific cellular parts; Heinz body stains and reticulocyte stains are two common examples

NORMAL HISTOGRAMS

A normal erythrocyte histogram will be between 36 and 360 femtoliters, with a peak representing mean corpuscular volume between 70 and 110. A normal leukocyte histogram, meanwhile, will be between 45 and 450 fL, with the three peaks. The first peak, 45–90 fL, is the normal range of lymphocytes; the second peak, 90–160 fL, is the normal range for immature leukocytes and monocytes; the third peak, 160–450 fL, is the normal range for granulocytes. A normal thrombocyte histogram will be between 2 and 20 femtoliters, and will not have any peaks.

ABNORMAL HISTOGRAMS

If the curve on a red blood cell histogram is especially wide, it may be that there has been an elevation in the red blood cell distribution width. If the red blood cell histogram has two peaks, this may be an indication of the presence of both microcytic and macrocytic erythrocytes. A shift to the left or to the right indicates a decrease or increase, respectively, in mean corpuscular volume. As for white blood cell histograms, an overlap of peaks at approximately 90 fL may indicate an elevated number of immature cells or bands, while values over 450 fL may indicate a high granulocyte count. Values lower than 50 fL suggest the existence of nucleated red blood cells, sickle cells, or large clumps of platelets.

PRECAUTIONS/PROCEDURES FOR COAGULATION TESTING

Lab technicians need to be especially careful when handling, collecting, and processing coagulation test samples. The drawing of the blood should be nontraumatic, so that coagulation is not activated. Samples should be placed into silicon-coated glass tubes or plastic tubes; the use of glass tubes without silicon coating may activate factors XI, XII, and prekallikrein. Samples must contain a sufficient amount of blood and must be processed within two hours. All testing must be performed at a temperature of 37 °C, lest factors VII and XI be activated by cold temperatures or factors V and VIII break down at room temperature.

POSSIBLE ERRORS WHEN MANUALLY COUNTING BLOOD CELLS

Lab technicians must guard against several kinds of common error when manually counting blood cells. Equipment that is not properly cleaned and dried may contribute to counting errors. A failure to dilute samples appropriately or follow the correct procedures in counting may lead to error. If the sample is not maintained at the appropriate temperature, it may develop clots, which will skew the count.

Hemostasis

Hemostasis is the cessation of bleeding. There are four main steps involved in hemostasis: 1. A damaged blood vessel narrows (vasoconstriction) and the reduced diameter helps slow down any bleeding. 2. Platelets that are present in the blood attach themselves to the collagen in the walls of the blood vessel to create a hemostatic plug within seconds. This process is sometimes referred to as primary hemostasis. After the formation of a hemostatic plug, secondary hemostasis occurs. The clotting factors help fibrin form from fibrinogen. The fibrin then aids in the formation of blood clot at the wound site. Secondary hemostasis takes a few minutes. 3. The newly-formed blood clot helps the wound site create new smooth muscle cells to repair the wound. The clot can then be lyzed (destroyed) when it is not needed any longer.

Coagulation Terminology

Coagulation	Formation of a clot. Four stage process: (1) damaged vessel constricts; (2) platelets adhere to damaged area (platelet adhesion) to form a platelet plug; (3) Extrinsic and intrinsic pathways lead to common pathway in which prothrombin activator reacts with calcium ions to form prothrombin, which forms thrombin, which causes fibrinogen to form fibrin monomers that react with fibrin stabilizing factor and calcium ions to form fibrin polymers that attract platelets and phospholipids to form a clot; (4) Fibrinolysis (clot breakdown) occurs when plasmin breaks fibrin into fragments, which are then removed by phagocytes
Sodium citrate	Anticoagulant (crystalline compound) that prevents clotting but preserves coagulation factors.
Thrombin	Clot activator that converts fibrinogen into fibrin.
Platelet function test	Tests the ability of platelets to form a clot and helps to diagnose bleeding disorders.
Warfarin (Coumadin®)	Warfarin (Coumadin®) is an anticoagulant that interferes with the formation of vitamin K–associated clotting factors (II, VII, IX, X) and C and S anticoagulant proteins.

Fibrin, Heparin, and Plasmin

Fibrin is a protein that aids in blood clotting. Along with platelets, fibrin helps form blood clots. Fibrin is made from the glycoprotein fibrinogen, in the liver.

Heparin is a polysaccharide anticoagulant that helps prevent blood clotting. Heparin is concentrated in the vessels surrounding the liver and the lungs. It can also be found in the spleen and various other muscles. Heparin is also a drug that can be given to patients that need to take advantage of its anticoagulant properties, such as in the case of a pulmonary embolism.

Plasmin is an enzyme that helps dissolve (lyze) fibrin that is present in blood clots. Lyzing a clot turns coagulated blood into liquid blood again. Plasmin is derived from plasminogen in the blood plasma.

Coagulation Procedures

Prothrombin time (PT)	10–14 seconds	Collect 1 mL blood in sodium citrate blue-capped tube (completely filled).
		Increased: Anticoagulation therapy, vitamin K deficiency, decreased prothrombin, DIC, liver disease, and malignant neoplasm. Some drugs may shorten time.
Partial thromboplastin time (PTT)	30–45 seconds	Collect 1 mL blood in sodium citrate blue-capped tube (completely filled).
		Increased: Hemophilia A & B, von Willebrand disease, vitamin deficiency, lupus, DIC, and liver disease
	21–35 seconds	Collect 1 mL blood in sodium citrate blue-capped tube (completely filled).

Activated partial thromboplastin time (aPTT)		Similar to PTT but an activator added that speeds clotting time. Used to monitor heparin dosage. Increased: Hemophilia A & B, von Willebrand disease, vitamin deficiency, lupus, DIC, and liver disease Decreased: Extensive cancer, early DIC, and after acute hemorrhage
D-dimer	0.5 mcg/mL FEU*	Collect 1 mL blood in sodium citrate blue-capped tube (completely filled) for immunoturbidimetry. Transport frozen.
		D-dimer is a specific polymer that results when fibrin breaks down, giving a marker to indicate the degree of fibrinolysis. Increased: DIC, pulmonary embolism, DVT, late pregnancy, neoplastic disorder, preeclampsia, arterial/venous thrombosis
Fibrinogen (Factor I)	100-400 mg/dL	Collect 1 mL blood in sodium citrate blue-capped tube (completely filled) for photo-optical clot detection.
		Synthesized in liver, converts to fibrin, which combines with platelets in coagulation sequence. Increased: Acute MI, cancer, eclampsia, multiple myeloma, Hodgkin disease, nephrotic syndrome, tissue trauma Decreased: DIC, liver disease, congenital fibrinogen abnormality
Fibrin degradation product (fibrin split products [FSPs])	<5 mcg/mL FEU*	Collect 1 mL blood in sodium citrate blue-capped tube (completely filled) for latex agglutination test. Transport frozen.
		FSPs occur as clots form and more breakdown of fibrinogen and fibrin occurs, interfering with blood coagulation by coating platelets and disrupting thrombin, and attaching to fibrinogen so stable clots can't form. Increased: DIC, liver disease, MI, hemorrhage, pulmonary embolism, renal disease, obstetric complications, kidney transplant rejection
Heparin assay (Antithrombin III)	1-3 mo: 48-108%	Collect 1 mL blood in sodium citrate blue-capped tube (completely filled) for chromogenic immunoturbidimetry.
	1-5 y: 82-139% 6-17 y: 90-131% >18 y: 80-120%	Utilized to diagnose heparin resistance in patients receiving heparin therapy and to diagnose hypercoagulable conditions. Increased: Acute hepatitis, kidney transplantation, vitamin K deficiency Decreased: DIC, liver transplantation, nephrotic syndrome, pulmonary embolism, venous thrombosis, liver failure, cirrhosis, carcinoma

Platelet aggregation	Results vary according to laboratory.	Collect 4-5 mL sample in sodium citrate tubes for analysis with light transmission aggregometer. Must be processed within 60 minutes of collection.
		Test measures the ability of platelets to aggregate and form clots in response to various activators. Decreased: Myeloproliferative disorders, autoimmune disorders, uremia, clotting disorders, and adverse effects of medications. Drugs that affect clotting should be avoided before test for up to 2 weeks (on advice of physician).

FEU* = fibrinogen equivalent units

Hemophilia

Hemophilia is an inherited disease in which the body has trouble forming blood clots because it lacks a clotting factor. People afflicted with hemophilia have the tendency to hemorrhage and have episodes of uncontrolled bleeding. The bleeding can either be external or internal. Hemophilia is a sex-linked disease (recessive on the X chromosome), and because of this, males are more likely to be hemophiliacs than are females. Many royal families in Europe inherited hemophilia from Queen Victoria. Hemophilia is passed from mother (the carrier) to son. There are three types of hemophilia, A, B, and C. These types are all defined by a different deficiency in a clotting factor necessary for the formation of blood clots and for the control of bleeding.

Hemophilia A is also referred to as "classic hemophilia". This is the most common form of hemophilia, and it is due to a deficiency in Factor VIII. Females are carriers. This disease affects males and leads to a prolonged clotting time and bleeding episodes. Less than 10 IU of factor VIII is characteristic of hemophilia A. Hemophilia A is 7 times more prevalent than Hemophilia B (Christmas disease), a deficiency or mutation of Factor IX. Christmas disease is also X-linked, and affects mostly males. People with Hemophilia B are at increased risk of hemorrhage. Finally, Hemophilia C is identified by the deficiency of Factor XI. This disease affects both sexes, and is an autosomal recessive disorder affecting primarily Jews of Ashkenazi descent. People with Hemophilia C often do not require treatment, and the disease is usually not severe. There is also no bleeding at the joints, as seen with Hemophilia A and B.

Bernard-Soulier Syndrome

Bernard-Soulier syndrome is a disease that is due to the lack of glycoprotein Ib, which is normally present in the membranes of platelets. Glycoprotein Ib is the protein that reacts with the von Willebrand factor, and its absence causes problems in platelet aggregation and in the forming of blood clots. Platelets in a person with Bernard-Soulier syndrome are larger and more spherical than normal platelets, and their membranes are not as strong. This disease is inherited, and affects both males and females with an equal frequency.

Von Willebrand's Disease

von Willebrand's disease is a hereditary defect on Chromosome 12 that causes the von Willebrand factor, necessary for clotting, to either be absent or defective. Unlike Hemophilia A and B, both females and males can have von Willebrand's disease, and it especially targets people with blood type O. The von Willebrand factor (vWF) is a protein that aids in platelet aggregation and blood clotting, and it helps control platelet activity. Without the von Willebrand factor, or with a deficient factor, patients have menorraghia (heavy menstruation), epistaxis (nosebleeds), and bruising. Type I and II cases of von Willebrand's disease are mild and require no treatment, except when patients are undergoing surgery or dental work. Type III is severe, with spontaneous bleeding into their joints. Patients use Demoprexin, Cyklokapron, Amicar, and thrombin powder on cuts to control bleeding.

ABO Discrepancies

ABO discrepancies often occur during crossmatching:

- **Rouleaux formation**: Should disperse with serum dilution with normal saline. If still evident, aggregation represents hemagglutination. Note: Dilution may result in inability to detect weak antibodies.
- **Autoagglutination**: Reaction occurs in auto-control tube and may indicate the presence of cold agglutinins, autoantibodies, and alloantibodies. **Cold agglutinins** (anti-I, H, M, N, P, and Lewis) cause hemoagglutination at room temperature, but the reaction ceases at 37 °C (confirming cold agglutinins). Complete antibody screen, and warm plasma and reagent RBCs for 15 minutes at 37 °C and then carry out reverse ABO testing to eliminate interference of autoantibodies and **alloantibodies** (of foreign RBCs). **Autoantibodies**, most often produced in response to hemolytic anemias, frequently result in a positive direct antihuman globulin (AHG) test because of the autoantibodies coating the RBCs. The presence of autoantibodies is confirmed by washing the cells with NS, eluting the RBCs, and testing antisera. No agglutination should be noted.

Immunology

Immunology and Serology Terminology

Thermostable	Unaffected by heat.
Thermolabile	Easily affected by heat.
Physiologic	Related to body functions.
Inactivation	Destruction of biological activity, such as by heat or other agent.
Complement	A group of blood proteins that go through a cascade of interactions as part of immune response.
Reagin	Complement-fixing antibody, IgE immunoglobulin that attaches to tissue cells in the species it derives from and interacts with antigen to cause release of histamine and other vasoactive amines.
Amboceptor	Old term for hemolysin.
Hemolysin	Antibody that binds to red blood cells and lyses them to release hemoglobin.
Cardiolipin	Phospholipid that increases with some disorders, such as autoimmune and coagulation disorders.
Monoclonal	Referring to a single clone; derived from a single cell.
Polyclonal	Referring to multiple clones; derived from multiple cells.

HLA System

HLA stands for human leukocyte antigen. The human leukocyte antigens are part of the major histocompatibility complex (MHC), a region found on chromosome 6. HLAs are found in all nucleated cells in the body. HLAs are inherited from one's parents and are practically unique to a particular individual. There are four main types of human leukocyte antigens, HLA-A, HLA-B, HLA-C, and HLA-D. Human leukocyte antigens help encode proteins on the surfaces of nucleated cells, and they play an important role in helping the body distinguish its own cells from foreign cells. Therefore, HLAs are very important when it comes to human organ transplant rejection or acceptance. In the laboratory, HLA-A, HLA-B, and HLA-C antigens can be identified using blood serum, however, HLA-D antigens can only be identified by the use of a mixed lymphocyte culture.

Immunogen, Antigen, Hapten, Adjuvant, and Antibody

- Immunogen: Any substance that produces an immune response
- Antigen: Any substance that reacts with substances in the immune system; antigens do not always produce an immune response
- Hapten: A molecule with a low molecular weight, which combines with another molecule to produce an antibody response
- Adjuvant: A substance that magnifies immune responses
- Antibody: A protein that fixes itself to an antigen; also known as immunoglobulins, and divided into five classes: IgA, IgD, IgE, IgG, and IgM

Classes of Antibodies

Every antibody has two heavy polypeptide chains and two light polypeptide chains. The identity of the heavy chains depends on the class of antibody. The light chains will be either kappa or lambda chains. Each polypeptide chain has a variable region, which identifies the particular antibody, and one or more constant regions. All of the chains are joined by disulfide bonds.

Testing and Disease States

Progesterone and Human Chorionic Gonadotropin

Progesterone is a steroid hormone that is necessary to successfully maintain a pregnancy. After a woman ovulates, the level of progesterone in her blood increases dramatically. The progesterone helps prepare the uterine wall for a fertilized egg to implant, in the case of a pregnancy. The high levels of progesterone also help prevent an early spontaneous miscarriage of the pregnancy. During pregnancy, the main source of progesterone is the placenta. Progesterone also helps in the production of milk in the woman's mammary glands.

Human Chorionic Gonadotropin (hCG) is a protein hormone that is released by the placenta. hCG is released very soon after conception during a pregnancy, and it is the hormone that is often tested for with a home pregnancy test to determine the existence of a pregnancy. The level of hCG in a woman's blood is at its highest level during the first trimester of pregnancy. It drops off after that, so that a woman in her seventh month may test negative for pregnancy.

Chronic Granulomatous Disease

Chronic granulomatous disease (CGD) is a hereditary, X-linked disease in which phagocytes cannot kill pathogens. Mostly boys under 10 years old are affected, and will likely die by the age of 30. Phagocytes cannot produce superoxide anions to destroy invaders because they lack NADPH oxidase. Therefore, a patient with chronic granulomatous disease has recurrent fungal and bacterial infections, which can be fatal. This lack of NADPH enzyme also allows for oxidative products, such as hydrogen peroxide, to build up and cause death. In the laboratory, the nitroblue tetrazolium test can be used to determine the existence of chronic granulomatous disease. Patients with CGD will have neutrophils with greatly reduced nitroblue tetrazolium activity.

Autoimmune Disease

Any condition in which a person creates antibodies for their own antigens is an autoimmune disease. There are a couple of different theories that seek to explain autoimmune disease. The immunologic deficiency theory asserts that all of the antibodies produced by B lymphocytes are suppressed by T lymphocytes, and so antibodies are produced any time there is a decrease in T lymphocyte activity. The forbidden-clone theory asserts that occasionally lymphocytes erroneously fail to destroy autoantigens during fetal development. The theory of sequestered antigens asserts that some antigens can remain invisible to the immune system until tissue is damaged.

Type I Hypersensitivity

An immediate hypersensitivity is referred to as a type I hypersensitivity. This is simply an allergic reaction that occurs within minutes of contact with the allergen or antigen. An individual experiencing such a reaction is producing an increased level of IgE immunoglobulin. There are a few different laboratory tests that can be used to determine allergies by measuring total serum IgE: ELISA, RIST, RIA, and RAST.

Febrile Agglutination Tests

Febrile agglutinins are antibodies that are active at normal body temperature and can cause their antigens (such as RBCs, proteins) to clump when exposed to each other, resulting in a fever. Febrile agglutinins are present in some disorders, such as systemic lupus erythematosus, hemolytic anemia, inflammatory bowel disease, and lymphoma. They may also occur in response to some infections (salmonella, brucellosis, typhoid fever) and when taking some medications (penicillin, methyldopa), so these medications may interfere with test results. To identify an infection, a blood sample is taken when a patient is actively infected (with fever and symptoms) or during convalescence, diluted (20-40 times), and mixed with antigens of a specific infectious microorganism. This sample is then examined to determine if an antigen-antibody reaction has occurred. Increased IgM usually indicates a new infection and increased IgG indicates a chronic infection or history of infection.

C-Reactive Protein Agglutination Slide Tests

C-reactive protein (CRP) agglutination slide tests can be used to screen patients for CRP (qualitative test) or to determine the titer (quantitative test). A number of different test kits are available, so procedures may vary.

Qualitative test	Quantitative test
Add latex solution to positive and negative controls and serum (or diluted and undiluted serum), mix, and agitate for 2 minutes to observe for agglutination (clumping) in serum, a reaction indicating the presence of C-reactive protein.	Mix serum samples to different dilutions in saline and conduct test similar to qualitative method to determine the highest dilution that shows agglutination (positive reaction).

Antistreptolysin Screen and Titer

Antistreptolysin O screen and titer (ASO) identifies the presence of streptolysin O antibodies, which form in response to the streptolysin O enzyme (antigen) secreted by group A β-hemolytic streptococci. The antibodies are present within one week and peak at 2-3 weeks after onset of streptococcal infection. Increased titer is present with strep-associated rheumatic fever, scarlet fever, endocarditis, and glomerulonephritis.

Rheumatoid Arthritis (RA) Tests

Rheumatoid factor (RF)	Normal value 0-20 IU/mL. Assesses for macroglobulin type antibody that is present in connective tissue disease. Non-specific for RA
Anti-citrullinated protein antibody (ACPA)	Normal values: Negative: <20. Weakly positive: 20-39. Moderately positive: 40-59. Strongly positive: >60. Assesses for autoantibodies against citrullinated proteins, to which those with RA react.
Erythrocyte sedimentation rate (ESR)	Normal values: Age <50: 0-15 mm/h males and 0-25 mm/h females. Age >50: 0-20 mm/h males and 0-30 mm/h females. Inflammation causes increased globulins or fibrinogens, and these cause RBCs to clump and fall to the bottom of a vertical test tube. ESR is nonspecific for RA, but increased ESR may indicate increased inflammation.
C-reactive protein (CRP)	Normal value <1 mg/dL. Assesses for abnormal glycoproteins, which are produced by the liver when inflammation is present. CRP is non-specific for RA.

Polyclonal Hypergammaglobulinemia and Monoclonal Hypergammaglobulinemia

Polyclonal hypergammaglobulinemia: A broad spike in the gamma region of the protein electrophoresis performed on a serum; indicates elevated levels of specific antibodies; the result of infectious disease, liver disease, or inflammation

Monoclonal hypergammaglobulinemia: A narrow peak in the gamma region of a protein electrophoresis performed on a serum; due to malignant transformation of a B lymphocyte clone; the results of multiple myeloma, immunoglobulin heavy chain diseases, or Waldenström's macroglobulinemia

Microhemagglutination Test for Treponema Pallidum

The **microhemagglutination test for *Treponema pallidum* (MHA-TP),** a gram-negative spirochete, is a nontreponemal antibody tests that assesses serum for antibodies to syphilis although this particular test has been generally replaced by other tests that are more specific, such as fluorescent treponemal antibody absorption (FTA-ABS), immunoassays, and molecular testing. MHA-TP can be used to confirm a positive diagnosis of syphilis on other tests. MHA-TP is able to detect antibodies to *T. pallidum* and is used for all stages of syphilis except during the first month of infection. One of the problems with MHA-TP is that false positives may occur in the presence of other infections, so it is not specific to syphilis: mononucleosis, Lyme disease, malaria, relapsing fever, leptospirosis, and leprosy. Patients with systemic lupus erythematosus may also have a false-positive on the test.

Immunofluorescence Reactions

Direct immunofluorescence: Reagent antibody labeled with fluorescent dye reacts to a specific antigen, forming an antigen-antibody complex, and thereby suggesting the existence of a particular antigen

Indirect immunofluorescence: Unlabeled antibody reacts with antigens and a sample, forming an antigen-antibody complex; at this point, the antigen-antibody complex reacts with another labeled antibody, forming an antibody-antigen-antibody complex

Biotin-avidin immunofluorescence: A form of indirect immunofluorescence in which a labeled antibody and a labeled fluorochrome react with an antigen

Terms Related to Transplant Immunology

- Allograft: Tissue is transplanted from one place to another on the same individual
- Isograft: Tissue from one individual is transplanted onto a genetically identical individual
- Autograft: tissue from one individual is transplanted onto an individual from the same species
- Graft acceptance: The condition in which healing and revascularization signal the acceptance of a tissue graft or transplant
- Hyperacute graft rejection: Rejection of a graft or transplant in the first 24 hours
- Acute graft rejection: Rejection of a graft or transplant within weeks
- Chronic graft rejection: Rejection of a graft or transplant within months or years

Microbiology

Preanalytic Procedures

Specimen Labeling and Collection

For the best chance to recover and identify the causative organism for an infection, microbiology specimens should be collected before antibiotics are administered and collected from the site where the suspected infection is located. In addition to two patient identifiers (name, date of birth, or medical record number), the source, or where the sample was collected, should be noted on the specimen label. Specimen collection procedures vary depending on the source, but all microbiology samples must be collected into sterile containers to prevent contamination. To avoid contamination from normal flora, alcohol wipes or iodine may be used to disinfect the area above or around the source of microbiology specimens.

Common Transport Systems and Conditions Required for Specimens

There are a variety of disposable culture containers that are ideal for microbiological specimen transport. Sterile swab systems with a plastic shaft are ideal for the safe transport of aerobic and anaerobic samples. Anaerobic swab systems contain gel in the bottom of the tube to support the viability of any anaerobic organisms that are present. If transport to the laboratory is delayed for more than 2 hours, most microbiology specimens can be refrigerated at 4–6 °C for temporary storage. Genital cultures and **CSF** samples should never be refrigerated, and they require immediate culturing because they are susceptible to degradation at low temperatures and contain **fastidious** organisms requiring special handling conditions. Urine, feces, and sputum may be refrigerated because the cool temperatures will help prevent the overgrowth of normal flora present in the samples.

Prioritization, Rejection Criteria, Biosafety Cabinets, and PPE

All microbiology specimens should be collected prior to antibiotic administration for the best chances of cultivating pathogenic organisms for identification. Blood culture samples must be collected from two different sites to confirm septicemia and avoid false diagnosis due to contamination. Genital and CSF samples targeted for gonococcal organisms must be cultured immediately due to their fastidious nature.

Samples submitted in inappropriate collection containers or transport media meet the criteria for rejection. Anaerobic cultures cannot be set up from aerobic swab collection systems due to the exposure to air inhibiting the growth of these organisms. Any sample with leaks or risk of outside contamination cannot be accepted for culture due to the risk of false identification of organisms that have infiltrated a sterile container.

Lab coats and gloves are always necessary PPE when handling biological specimens, and biosafety cabinets provide additional protection from aerosol-inducing specimens. Sputum samples and other respiratory specimens must be handled under biosafety hoods due to the risk of aerosols being introduced into the air. These cabinets provide additional protection to eyes and the respiratory tract of lab personnel, with a glass shield and mechanisms that direct airflow up and into the hood instead of out toward lab staff.

Sample Preparation and Media Types

Samples are added to various types of media to aid in the growth and identification of pathogenic organisms present in a sample. Inoculating the appropriate media related to the source of the specimen and knowledge of organisms' growth requirements are imperative to providing accurate information for patient diagnosis and treatment.

Categories of media and examples are given as follows:

- **Supportive**: contain nutrients that allow most nonfastidious organisms to grow based on their metabolism
    - **Sheep blood agar** — an all-purpose, general medium used for primary inoculations and subculturing
- **Selective:** contains dyes, antibiotics, and other compounds that inhibit some bacteria, effectively allowing others to grow
    - **Colistin plus nalidixic acid** — selective for Gram-positive, inhibits growth of Gram-negative organisms
    - **MacConkey agar and eosin methylene blue agar** — selective for Gram-negative, inhibits Gram-positive growth
- **Enrichment:** allow for the growth of one bacterium by providing nutrients specific to that organism
    - **Chocolate** — contains X and V growth factors, ideal for fastidious organisms
    - **Selenite** — favors *Shigella* and *Salmonella*
- **Differential:** contain factors that give particular organisms distinct, recognizable features
    - **Sheep blood agar and colistin plus nalidixic acid** — differentiation of organisms by hemolytic properties
    - **MacConkey agar and eosin methylene blue agar** — differentiation of Gram-negative organisms by their ability/inability to ferment lactose.

Inoculation Techniques and Objectives

To inoculate for **colony counts**, a sterile 10 μL loop is placed into a sample, and then it is struck down the middle of the plate in a straight line. The loop is then dragged left and right over the center line for the entire area of the plate. This allows for a standard of quantification of colonies growing on media and a clue as to how strong of an infection is present.

Inoculating media for **isolation** consists of transferring inoculum from a sterile pipette or loop and streaking it into quadrants on a plate with the goal of successively fewer colonies in each quadrant. This is achieved by heavily placing a small amount of specimen inoculum on one edge of a plate and using a loop to streak the inoculum over the first quarter or quadrant of the media. With a quarter turn of the plate, streak from quadrant one into the second quadrant, and repeat for the third and fourth quadrants. This allows for colonies to grow isolated from one another in the third and/or fourth quadrant of the plate, providing the ability to obtain pure samples of bacteria for further testing and identification.

Incubation Conditions

Common incubation and bacterial growth requirements are as follows:

Temperature	Oxygen (O_2)	Other Atmosphere
Psychrophiles Thrive in cold temperatures. Optimal temperature: 15 °C.	Aerobes require the presence of O_2 to grow.	Microaerophiles prefer lower amounts of O_2 than is present in "normal" or room air.
Mesophiles The most pathogenic organisms, which thrive at moderate temperatures, such as the human body temperature of 37 °C.	Facultative anaerobes are able to grow with or without O_2 present.	Capnophiles prefer a higher CO_2 content than regular air provides.
Thermophiles grow best in heat with optimal temperatures between 50 and 60 °C.	Obligate anaerobes are harmed by the presence of O_2 and require O_2-free environments to grow.	Aerotolerant organisms do not require the presence of O_2 to grow, but they are not harmed if O_2 is present.

Slide Preparation Using Stains

Techniques used for microbiology slide preparation are determined by the type of sample submitted. Commonly used techniques are described below:

- **Fluid/Liquid**: Using a sterile pipette, place one drop of body fluid or other liquid samples onto the slide and swirl or spread it into a thin layer.
- **Swabs**: Roll the swab directly onto the surface of a slide. If two swabs are submitted, use one to inoculate the media and the second for slide preparation. If only one swab is submitted, inoculate all media first and roll the swab onto the slide last to avoid contamination of the media.
- **Organism colony**: Slide preparation for organism colonies requires a drop of sterile water or saline to first be added to the slide. Place the colony on the slide and mix it with the water to create a suspension.

A circle may be drawn with a wax pencil around the sample to aid in identifying where to examine on the slide. Allow the sample to air dry. Once the sample dries, slides will need to be fixed to keep the specimens from washing off during the staining process. One minute of heat fixing or the same duration fixing with 95% methanol is appropriate.

Gram Stain

The Gram stain is a differential stain that separates bacteria into two groups based on their reaction to the primary stain and the counterstain. This stain works by targeting the cell wall of bacteria and how they differ. The cell wall of Gram-positive organisms is made of a peptidoglycan layer with teichoic acid crosslinks, whereas the cell wall of Gram-negative organisms is comprised of a thinner peptidoglycan layer and additional outer membranes.

The Gram stain procedure consists of four elements that produce a differentiation in bacteria present on a slide. Crystal violet is used as the primary stain that stains every organism equally. Gram's iodine is then added to form a complex with the crystal violet within Gram-positive bacteria cell walls. An alcohol/acetone decolorizer then flushes away the purple color from the Gram-negative bacteria. Finally, a counterstain of safranin is introduced to stain the colorless Gram-negative organisms and allows them to be observed.

Procedure and Interpretation of Gram Stain

Gram stain procedure:

1. Flood the slide with crystal violet for 10 seconds*.
2. Rinse the slide with water.
3. Flood the slide with Gram's iodine for 10 seconds*.
4. Rinse with water.
5. Quickly add decolorizer until the slide runs clear (no color) for ~10 seconds.
6. Rinse with water.
7. Flood the slide with safranin for 10 seconds*.
8. Rinse with water.
9. Allow the slide to air dry.
10. Examine under an oil immersion lens.

*Time increments may vary; 30- or 60-second intervals are common as well.

Outcome:

- Gram-positive bacteria will stain purple/blue.
- Gram-negative bacteria will stain pink.

Along with the color of the bacteria, the shape and morphology are able to be determined with a Gram stain. Information provided from this stain is helpful in determining subsequent tests, culture, and means for identification. It may also guide treatment because some antibiotics work better toward Gram-positive or Gram-negative organisms specifically.

Acid-Fast Stain

The acid-fast stain, also called the **Ziehl–Neelsen** stain, is performed to detect organisms that cause tuberculosis. These bacteria are deemed acid-fast bacilli (**AFB**) due to their ability to be visualized by the acid-fast staining process. This is a differential stain for mycobacterium that will retain the primary stain, whereas all other bacteria, without a cell wall containing mycolic acid, will decolorize and counterstain.

The acid-fast procedure consists of the primary stain, carbolfuchsin, with heat to facilitate penetration of the stain into the cell walls of mycobacterium with high lipid content. A 3% hydrochloric acid, 97% ETOH decolorizer is then used to leach the primary stain from the cell walls of bacteria that do not contain high contents of mycolic acid. Methylene blue is used as a counterstain to make all of the other bacteria a visible blue color.

Acid-fast/Ziehl–Neelsen procedure:

1. Heat fix stain/slide for 2 hours at 65–70 °C or 15 minutes at 80 °C.
2. Flood stain with heated carbolfuchsin at 60 °C for 5 minutes.
3. Rinse with water.
4. Decolorize with 3% HCl/97% ETOH ~2 minutes (for an average-thickness slide).
5. Rinse with water.
6. Flood with methylene blue 1–3 minutes.
7. Rinse with water.
8. Allow to air dry.
9. Examine under an oil immersion lens.

Interpretation:

- Mycobacterium (AFB) will stain red.
- All other bacteria will stain blue.

Modified Acid-Fast Stain

The modified acid-fast stain, or **Kinyoun** stain, is performed to detect organisms that cause tuberculosis by differentiating **AFB** from all other bacteria in a microbiology specimen. This achieves the same outcome as the acid-fast stain, without the use of heat. The modification of heat requirements means that the Kinyoun stain is also referred to as "cold" acid-fast staining.

This method uses a carbolfuchsin stain prepared with phenol to facilitate the penetration of stain into the lipid-rich cell walls of mycobacteria. An acid/alcohol solution, comprised of 3% HCl and 97% ETOH, is used to decolorize nonmycobacterium organisms by removing the primary stain from their cell walls. A counterstain of methylene blue or malachite green is used to allow decolorized bacteria to become visible again upon examination, allowing for differentiation to occur.

Modified acid-fast/Kinyoun procedure:

1. Heat fix stain/slide for 2 hours at 65–70 °C or 15 minutes at 80 °C.
2. Flood stain with Kinyoun carbolfuchsin at room temperature for 5 minutes.
3. Rinse with water.
4. Decolorize with 3% HCl/97% ETOH for ~2 minutes (for an average-thickness slide).
5. Rinse with water.
6. Flood with methylene blue or malachite green for 1–3 minutes.
7. Rinse with water.
8. Allow to air dry.
9. Examine under an oil immersion lens.

Interpretation:

- Mycobacterium (AFB): red
- All other bacteria: blue (methylene blue) or green (malachite green).

Potassium Hydroxide (KOH) Reagent

Potassium hydroxide (**KOH**) reagent is used to aid in the direct examination of yeast and fungal elements present in samples, including, but not limited to, vaginal discharge, skin, hair, and nails. Presence of fungal elements upon visualization aids in the diagnosis and treatment process of suspected fungal infections.

The 10–20% KOH reagent that is added to specimens clears debris and breaks down keratin in hair and nail samples. The breakdown of keratin and the clearing of other debris allows for fungal elements to be more readily observed with a light microscope on a clean glass slide.

KOH procedure:

1. Place the specimen on a clean glass slide — use clean forceps for hair/skin/nail or roll a swab with vaginal discharge/wound sample onto the slide.
2. Add one drop of KOH reagent to the sample on the slide.
3. Place a glass coverslip over the area of the slide; press gently to reduce the presence of bubbles.

4. Place the slide on the microscope stage and examine on low (10×) power to visualize the presence of any fungal structures, such as hyphae or budding yeast.
5. If fungal structures are observed, examine the slide at 40× magnification for further identification and verification of fungi.

Calcofluor-White Stain

Calcofluor-white is a nonspecific chemifluorescent stain that binds to the cellulose and chitin in cell walls of fungal and parasitic organisms, allowing for visualization via a fluorescent microscope. KOH may be added to the white stain to clear the sample of debris and allow for better visualization. With this method, chitin-containing structures will fluoresce white on a dark background with ultraviolet (UV) light. Evans blue is used as a counterstain to create a dark field, and it allows cells and tissues to be fluoresced and visualized under blue light. Fungal and parasitic elements will fluoresce a bright apple-green color, and all of the other elements will fluoresce at a red-orange color for differentiation between them.

Calcofluor-white procedure:

1. Place the specimen on a clean glass slide.
2. Add one drop of calcofluor-white stain and one drop of KOH (optional) to the slide.
3. Place a glass coverslip over the slide, and press gently to reduce the presence of bubbles.
4. Let the specimen stain, and stain for 1 minute.
5. Examine under UV light at 100× to 400× magnification for the presence of yeast, fungi, or parasitic elements.

Trichrome Stain

The trichrome stain is a permanent stain that allows for visualization of and morphological distinguishing of parasitic cysts and trophozoites in clinical specimens. The most common specimens submitted for trichrome staining are fresh or preserved stool fecal samples; however, other clinical specimens are able to be stained with polyvinyl alcohol (PVA) fixation.

The trichrome stain consists of chromotrope 2R, light green SF, phosphotungstic acid, glacial acetic acid, and distilled water. Stain preparation is necessary, by adding 1 ml of acetic acid to the dry components, allowing the mixture to stand for 30 minutes, and then adding 100 ml of distilled water. The stain should be purple in color and should be protected from light. Proper fixation of slides is included in the trichrome procedure because it is necessary for quality staining and optimal use of this method.

Trichrome procedure:

1. Prepare a fresh fecal smear or PVA smear.
2. Place the slide in 70% ETOH for 5 minutes — for PVA smears, skip this step.
3. Remove the slide and drain off the excess liquid.
4. Place the slide in 70% ETOH with added iodine (dark reddish-brown color) for 2–5 minutes.
5. Remove the slide and drain off the excess liquid.
6. Place the slide in 70% ETOH for 5 minutes.
7. Remove the slide and drain off the excess liquid.
8. Place the slide in clean/new 70% ETOH for 2–5 minutes.
9. Remove the slide and drain off the excess liquid.
10. Place the slide in a prepared trichrome stain solution for 10 minutes.
11. Remove the slide and drain off the excess stain.
12. Dip the slide in 90% ETOH acidified with 1% acetic acid up to 3 seconds (no longer).

13. Dip once in 100% ETOH.
14. Place the slide in 100% ETOH for 2–5 minutes.
15. Place the slide in clean/new 100% ETOH for 2–5 minutes.
16. Place the slide in xylene for 2–5 minutes.
17. Repeat the slide in xylene for 2–5 minutes.
18. Mount the slide with a cover glass, and allow it to dry overnight at 37 °C.
19. Observe with a fluorescent microscope.

Outcome:

- Background debris — green
- Protozoa — blue-green to purple; the nuclei and inclusions of parasites will show red to purple-red.

GIEMSA STAIN

Giemsa stain is used in the visualization, differentiation, and identification of parasites in clinical specimens. Most commonly, Giemsa stains are performed on blood smears, but they may be performed on specimens from other sources as well, such as lesion biopsies and various aspirates. Thin-film smears allow for RBC inclusion and extracellular morphologies to be more easily observed, whereas thick smears allow a larger volume of sample to be surveyed for potential parasites. Giemsa-stained blood films are used as diagnostic testing for malarial infections, due to the *Babesia* parasite present demonstrating the characteristic "Maltese cross" ring formation.

Prepared from a powder containing azure, methylene blue, eosin dye, and methanol, Giemsa stock stain is diluted with buffered water to properly stain slides for observation. In blood smears, the Giemsa stain color in parasites will mimic the color of the stained WBCs. This acts as an internal quality control for the method. The morphologic characteristics of parasites observed with this stain are used for differentiation and subsequent identification.

Giemsa stain procedure:

1. Place a slide into absolute methanol for 30 seconds to fix a thin sample to the slide. (Skip this step for thick slides; methanol fixation is not needed.)
2. Allow the slide to air dry.
3. Place the slide in 1 part Giemsa stock stain to 20 parts buffered water for 20 minutes*.
4. Remove the slide and drain off the excess stain.
5. Dip the slide in buffered water one to two times to wash the slide.
6. Remove the slide and allow it to air dry, propped in a vertical position.
7. Observe the slide under a 40× lens and then under an immersion lens with a light microscope.

*Dilutions of Giemsa stock stain may vary between 10 and 50, depending on the preparation. The staining time must be adjusted for the different stain concentration present. Typically, the dilution factor will correspond to the appropriate duration of staining (e.g., 1:10, 10 minutes; 1:30, 30 minutes).

Outcome:

- Parasitic forms: blue to purple with reddish nuclei
- RBCs: pale gray-blue
- WBC nucleus, cytoplasm: purple, pale-purple, respectively

- Eosinophilic granules: bright purple-red
- Neutrophilic granules: deep pink-purple.

Analytic Procedures—Bacteriology

Blood and Bone Marrow

Specimen Sources and Collection to Check for Infection in Bloodstream

To diagnose an infection in the bloodstream, or **sepsis**, the most common samples collected are blood cultures. **Blood cultures** consist of blood being added to aerobic and anerobic bottles containing a broth that supports microbial growth. Ideally, two sets of blood cultures will be collected from separate sites to compare results and more easily determine false positives due to contamination from true-positive results. If infection originating from a port or intravenous catheter is suspected, draw one set of cultures from the port or catheter line and the other set peripherally. Intravenous catheter tips may cause infection from opportunistic skin flora at the time of insertion or removal of the device. After removal, the catheter tip itself may be cultured if it is a suspected source of infection.

The procedure for peripheral collection of blood cultures is as follows:

1. At the site chosen to draw, aseptically cleanse the skin in a circular motion with 70% alcohol, and allow it to dry.
2. Repeat cleansing of the site with iodine, allow it to dry for 1 minute.
3. Following proper phlebotomy practices, insert the needle into the vein and withdraw the blood. Do not change the needle before injecting the blood into the blood culture bottle. The necessary volume for blood culture bottles to achieve a 1:10 dilution of blood to broth is 10 mL for adult aerobic or anaerobic and 5 mL for pediatric patients.
4. Repeat the procedure at a second draw site.

Continuous Blood Culture Monitoring Systems

Blood culture monitoring systems continuously assess blood culture bottles for the presence of bacterial growth. Cultures are incubated at 35–37 °C for 5–7 days in a chamber that is constantly rocking to promote the growth of any potential pathogens that are present. Gas sensors in the chamber use fluorescence to detect any CO_2 production within the blood culture bottles. The CO_2 gas production, turbidity, lysis of RBCs, and visual observation of bacterial colonies in a blood culture bottle are indicative of bacterial growth. If bacterial growth is detected, the system will alarm to notify lab staff that the presumptively positive blood culture bottle should be subcultured and Gram stained for organism detection and identification.

Continuous monitoring systems are advantageous because they monitor bacterial growth without the need to visually inspect bottles each day or blindly subculture and Gram stain every blood culture collected. Monitoring systems can also be interfaced with laboratory information systems (LIS) to allow for easier reporting of results and for reducing the risk of clerical errors.

Rapid Identification and Antibiotic Resistance Detection of Microorganisms

Rapid identification of microbial agents and their relationship to antibiotics allows for patient treatments to begin more quickly and aids in finding the most effective means to fight against an infection. Organisms can be evaluated for specific **biochemical reactions** that can aid in the presumptive identification of an infectious agent. The following biochemical tests are used in differentiating bacteria from one another: catalase, coagulase, oxidase, indole, L-pyrrolidonyl-β-naphthylamide (PYR), urease, motility, and results of various stains. **Automated instrumentation** allows for microdilutions of an isolate to be identified and evaluated for antibiotic susceptibility or resistance. An inoculum of a pure colony grown from culture media is added to sterile water or saline to create a 0.5 McFarland standard. The inoculum is added to panels of microwells with a specific reaction taking place in each well. Automated instruments are able to produce quantitative results for antibiotic susceptibility and resistance in 3–8 hours, along with a definitive identification of the organism. **Molecular techniques** are available for the rapid detection of antibiotic-resistant organisms, such as methicillin-resistant *Staphylococcus aureus* (MRSA), vancomycin-resistant *Enterococcus* (VRE), extended-spectrum beta-lactamases (ESBLs), and carbapenem-resistant *Enterobacteriaceae* (CRE). Molecular methods are able to detect the presence or absence of a gene that is specific to the antibiotic resistance; for example, PCR methods are used to detect and amplify the mecA gene responsible for MRSA strains.

Skin Flora

The skin's normal flora is comprised of organisms that inhabit the skin and are routinely **commensal**, meaning they don't cause harm to a healthy host. Although skin flora can be beneficial, they can also become pathogens under certain circumstances by displacement to another part of the body or **opportunistic** infection in an immunocompromised host. Species of skin flora inhabit different areas of the body based on the environment that part of the body produces. Common skin flora grow in the axilla, perineum, toe webs, hands, face, trunk, and upper arms and legs.

Skin flora commonly include the following organisms:

- ***S. aureus*** — colonizes in the nasal passages, most common to become pathogenic
- ***Staphylococcus epidermidis*** — most prevalent skin flora, attach to the outer layer of skin, the epidermis, and inhibit overgrowth of potential pathogens
- ***Corynebacterium*** (diphtheroid) and ***Propionibacterium acnes*** — typically found in the sebaceous glands.

S. Aureus and Coagulase-Negative Staphylococci

S. aureus react and present in the following ways:

- Biochemical reactions:

Catalase	+
Coagulase	+

- **Gram stain**: Gram-positive cocci in "grape-like" clusters
- **Growth requirements**: aerobic and facultative anaerobe, grows= best at 35 °C in ambient air or a CO_2-rich environment
- **Colony morphology**: soft, opaque or pale gold, and circular on sheep blood agar, most colonies are beta-hemolytic, and colonies present with a yellow halo on mannitol salt agar

Coagulase-negative *Staphylococci* react and present in the following ways:

- Biochemical reactions:

Catalase	+
Coagulase	–

- **Gram stain**: Gram-positive cocci in clusters
- **Growth requirements**: aerobic and facultative anaerobe, grow best at 35 °C in ambient air or a CO_2-rich environment
- Colony morphology:
  - ***S. epidermidis*** — white, cohesive, raised circular colonies on tryptic soy agar, opaque, gray, smooth, raised colonies with no hemolysis on sheep blood agar
  - ***S. saprophyticus*** — white-yellow, opaque, smooth, raised colonies with a butter-like texture on sheep blood agar.

BETA-HEMOLYTIC STREPTOCOCCI

Beta-hemolytic *Streptococci* react and present in the following ways:

- Biochemical reactions:

Catalase	−
Gas production	−
Motility	−
Optochin	R
Bile solubility	−
Leucine aminopeptidase	+
Vancomycin	S

- **Gram stain:** Gram-positive cocci in chains
- **Growth requirements:** 5–10% CO_2 with vertical stabs in agar to promote beta-hemolysis
- **Colony morphology**: the groups of beta-hemolytic strep present on sheep blood agar as follows:
  - **Group A** — grayish-white, transparent to translucent, matte or glossy, large zone of hemolysis
  - **Group B** — larger than group A colonies, translucent to opaque, flat, glossy, narrow zone of beta-hemolysis, and some strains are nonhemolytic
  - **Group C** — grayish-white, glistening, wide zone of beta-hemolysis
  - **Group F** — grayish-white, small, matte, narrow zone of beta-hemolysis
  - **Group G** — grayish-white, matte, wide zone of beta-hemolysis.

ENTEROCOCCUS SPECIES

Enterococcus species react and present in the following ways:

- Biochemical reactions:

Catalase	−
PYR	+
Gas production	+
Optochin	R
Bile solubility	−
Bile esculin	+
6.5% NaCl	+
Leucine aminopeptidase	+

- **Gram stain:** Gram-positive cocci in chains or diplococci
- **Growth requirements:** aerobic and facultative anaerobe, able to grow in temperatures ranging between 10 °C and 45 °C
- **Colony morphology:** large white colonies on sheep blood agar, may be alpha- or beta-hemolytic, blackens medium of bile esculin agar during growth.

Candida Species

Candida species present in the following ways:

- **Gram stain**: Gram-positive single yeast buds, pseudohyphae constricted but connected at the ends, or true septate hyphae
- **Growth requirements**: aerobic and facultative anaerobe, grow best at 25–37 °C
- **Colony morphology**: creamy, white, dull, grows upward with foot-like projections from the bottom of the colony on sheep blood agar and cream-colored, smooth, pasty colonies on Sabouraud dextrose agar.

Streptococcus Pneumoniae

Streptococcus pneumoniae react and present in the following ways:

- Biochemical reactions:

Catalase	–
Bacitracin	R
Na Hippurate	–
Optochin	S
Bile solubility	+
Bile esculin	–
6.5% NaCl	–

- **Gram stain**: Gram-positive diplococci, lancet shaped
- **Growth requirements**: facultative anaerobe, grow best at 35–37 °C in a 5% CO_2 environment
- **Colony morphology**: alpha-hemolytic, mucoid or "water drop" colonies with a convex middle on sheep blood agar.

Acinetobacter Baumannii

Acinetobacter baumannii react and present in the following ways:

- Biochemical reactions:

Oxidase	–
Growth on MacConkey agar	+
Motile	–
Glucose oxidation	+
Maltose oxidation	–
Esculin hydrolysis	–
Lysine decarboxylase	–
Nitrate reduction	–
Urea	V

- **Gram stain**: Gram-positive/variable coccobacilli
- **Growth requirements**: aerobic and facultative anaerobe, grow best at 35 °C in ambient air or a CO_2-rich environment
- **Colony morphology**: smooth, creamy, opaque, raised on sheep blood agar, purplish hue on MacConkey agar.

ENTEROBACTERIACEAE

Enterobacteriaceae react and present in the following ways:

- Biochemical reactions:

Oxidase	–
Catalase	+
Nitrate reduction	+

- **Gram stain**: Gram-negative bacilli
- **Growth requirements**: aerobic and facultative anaerobe, grow best at 35 °C in ambient air or a CO_2-rich environment. MacConkey and other selective agars are incubated in ambient air only. *Yersinia pestis* grow best at 25–30 °C.
- **Colony morphology**: large, smooth, and gray on sheep blood and chocolate agars.
  - Lactose fermenting species, pink on MacConkey agar:
    - Citrobacter
    - Escherichia
    - Enterobacter
    - Klebsiella
  - Lactose nonfermenting species, colorless to pale on MacConkey agar:
    - Shigella
    - Yersinia
    - Proteus
    - Salmonella.

PSEUDOMONAS SPECIES

Pseudomonas species react and present in the following ways:

- Biochemical reactions:

Motility	+
Oxidase	+
Indole	+
Lysine decarboxylase	–

- **Gram stain**: Gram-negative bacilli
- **Growth requirements**: obligate aerobe, grow best at 35 °C in ambient air or a CO_2-rich environment
- **Colony morphology**:
  - ***P. aeruginosa*** — grayish white, translucent to opaque, circular with irregular edges on sheep blood agar. Colorless, transparent, circular, on MacConkey agar. Colonies are smooth or mucoid, if swarming occurs. Produce a grape, or corn tortilla-like odor.

Bacteria Commonly Responsible for Infective Endocarditis

Infective endocarditis results in inflammation and damage to heart valves and the inner lining of the heart, the **endocardium**. Endocarditis occurs when bacteria are introduced to the bloodstream and settle in this portion of the heart, creating acute or subacute infections. **Acute** infections typically cause great damage to a healthy heart and require more aggressive treatment, whereas **subacute** infections are less virulent and generally attack weaker hearts with preexisting conditions.

The following bacteria are common agents of endocarditis:

- *Staphylococcus aureus:*
    - Most common cause of acute endocarditis — damage to a healthy heart
    - Normal skin flora introduced through broken skin barrier
        - Intravenous drug abuse
        - Infected abscess
        - Contamination during surgery or catheterization procedures
- *Streptococcus viridans:*
    - Most common cause of subacute endocarditis — damage to a weak heart with congenital heart defects
    - Normal oral flora introduced by a breach in the oral mucosa
        - Dental procedures
        - Poor oral hygiene
- *S. epidermidis* (coagulase-negative *Staphylococci*):
    - Most associated with infections of prosthetic heart valves
    - Normal skin flora introduced through broken skin barrier
        - Cardiac catheterization procedures
    - Often requires surgical intervention to treat
- *Enterococcus* and *Streptococcus bovis*:
    - Subacute, nosocomial infections
    - Normal GI/genitourinary flora introduced via exacerbated infection or malignancy.

Cerebrospinal Fluid (CSF)

CSF Collection

A **lumbar puncture** procedure consists of a needle being inserted through a patient's back between two lower vertebrae and moved into the space surrounding the spinal cord. The space surrounding the spinal cord is filled with cerebrospinal fluid (CSF) that will drip from the needle once properly inserted. Fluid will then be collected into sterile containers for laboratory testing.

CSF collection from a **ventricular shunt** is accomplished through the placement of a catheter behind the ear that will drain excess spinal fluid from the brain. A shunt is inserted into the ventricles of the brain to relieve pressure caused by an accumulation of CSF. Catheter tubing is placed to divert excess CSF either outside of the body for sterile collection or to other parts of the body, such as the pleural or peritoneal cavities, to be absorbed by blood vessels.

A catheter may be placed into a lateral ventricle that is attached to a **reservoir** implanted under the scalp for external access to a shunt system. The reservoir is often used to deliver drugs directly to the CSF and CNS or to aspirate CSF for testing with a syringe in a minimally invasive manner.

Haemophilus Influenzae

Haemophilus influenzae react and present in the following ways:

- **Biochemical reactions**:

Catalase	+
Oxidase	+
X factor (hemin)	+
V factor (NAD)	+
Beta-hemolytic on sheep blood agar	–
Lactose fermentation	–
Mannose fermentation	–

- **Gram stain:** Gram-negative bacilli
- **Growth requirements**: aerobic and facultative anaerobe, grow best on chocolate agar in 5–10% CO_2 at 35–37 °C
- **Colony morphology**:
    - **Unencapsulated strains** — small, smooth, and translucent on chocolate agar
    - **Encapsulated strains** — larger, mucoid, with a mouse nest odor on chocolate agar.

Neisseria Meningitidis

Neisseria meningitidis react and present in the following ways:

- **Biochemical reactions**:

Catalase	+
Oxidase	+
Nitrate reduction	–
Maltose fermentation	+
Glucose fermentation	+
Lactose fermentation	–

- **Gram stain:** Gram-negative diplococci
- **Growth requirements**: aerobic and facultative anaerobe, grow best in a humid, 5–10% CO_2 environment at 35–37 °C
- **Colony morphology:** a green hue may be present on agar underneath colonies
    - **Unencapsulated strains** — medium, round, smooth, gray to white, moist on chocolate and sheep blood agar
    - **Encapsulated strains** — more mucoid appearing.

Escherichia Coli

Escherichia coli react and present in the following ways:

- **Biochemical reactions**:

Indole	+
Citrate	–
Hydrogen sulfide (H_2S)	–
Lysine decarboxylase (LDC)	+
Lysine deaminase (LDA)	–

Urease	–
Motility	+
Voges–Proskauer	+
Triple sugar iron (TSI) agar	A/A
Gas production	+

- **Gram stain**: Gram-negative bacilli
- **Growth requirements**: aerobic and facultative anaerobe, grow best at 37 °C
- **Colony morphology**: circular, convex colonies, dull gray, smooth on sheep blood agar, pink to red, surrounded by dark-pink precipitate on MacConkey agar, and yellow on Hektoen and xylose lysine deoxycholate agar (XLD) agars.

Listeria Monocytogenes

Listeria monocytogenes react and present in the following ways:

- **Biochemical reactions**:

Catalase	+
Motility at 20–25 °C	+
Esculin	+
Nitrate reduction	–
Christie–Atkins–Munch–Petersen (CAMP) test	+
Hippurate	+
Glucose fermentation	+

- **Gram stain:** Gram-negative bacilli or coccobacilli
- **Growth requirements:** aerobic and facultative anaerobe, grow best at 35–37 °C in ambient air or 5–10% CO_2
- **Colony morphology:** white, translucent, smooth, moist, with a narrow zone of beta-hemolysis on sheep blood agar.

Corynebacterium and Propionibacterium Species

Corynebacterium species react and present in the following ways:

- **Biochemical reactions**:

Catalase	+
Motility	–
Esculin	–
Mycolic acids	+

- **Gram stain:** Gram-positive bacilli, slightly curved, with rounded ends — some species are pleomorphic, presenting a Chinese letter formation appearance
- **Growth requirements:** aerobic and facultative anaerobe, grow best at 35–37 °C in ambient air or 5–10% CO_2
- **Colony morphology**: on sheep blood agar
    - ***Corynebacterium diphtheriae***: varying morphology from small, gray, and translucent to medium, white, and opaque; black or gray colonies on cystine-tellurite blood agar
    - **Less virulent *Corynebacterium* species:** small to medium, gray, white, or yellow, nonhemolytic colonies

Propionibacterium species react and present in the following ways:

- **Gram stain:** Gram-positive bacilli, pleomorphic, diphtheroid-like, may be club shaped or in palisade arrangements
- **Growth requirements**: anaerobic, grow best at 35–37 °C for 48 hours
- **Colony morphology:** small white to gray on anaerobic blood agar. More mature colonies will be larger and yellow colored.

Correlation of CSF Culture and Gram Stain Results with Other Test Results in Diagnosis of Meningitis

Correlating the appearance, microbiology, cell count, and chemistry testing of a CSF sample will provide evidence for determining the presence of a meningitis infection, as well as differentiate the causative agent. The expected results of a **normal CSF** sample free of infection are as follows:

- Appearance: clear and colorless
- Protein: 15–45 mg/dL
- Glucose: 60–70% plasma glucose levels
- Cell count: 0–5 WBC/μL
- Differential: 70% lymphocytes, 30% monocytes.

Abnormalities in the color and clarity of a CSF sample can be indicative of the following: a traumatic tap; current, recent, or previous subarachnoid hemorrhage; and infection. Evidence of a **traumatic tap** will show blood in collection tubes, with a successive clearing in each tube, a clear supernatant when spun, and clots from the presence of fibrinogen. Samples will contain blood in every collection tube during a current **subarachnoid hemorrhage**, appear pale-pink to pale-orange in a recent hemorrhage, and appear yellow in a past hemorrhage. A cloudy sample, maybe due to increased WBCs, can be indicative of an infection.

Bacterial infections can be detected and a presumptive causative organism can be seen on a Gram stain of CSF and correlated with the cell count and chemistry results.

The correlating CSF results and their etiology are as follows:

Etiology	CSF Protein	CSF Glucose	WBC Population	Lactate
Bacterial	Greatly increased	Decreased	Neutrophils	Increased
Viral	Increased	Normal	Lymphocytes	Normal
Fungal	Increased	Normal to decreased	Lymphocytes Monocytes	Increased

Direct and Molecular Methods Used in Detection of CSF Infections

Direct detection methods for the evaluation and diagnosis of CSF infections includes stains, rapid latex antigen testing, and serological testing. Bacterial meningitis can be detected by the presence of bacteria found on a Gram stain. India ink and acid-fast stain preparations allow for the direct detection of *Cryptococcus* and tuberculosis pathogens, respectively. Rapid latex antigen tests are useful in the immediate detection of classic meningitis causing bacteria such as *S. pneumoniae, H. influenzae,* group B strep, *E. coli, Neisseria meningitides,* and *Cryptococcus neoformans.* Latex beads coated with sensitized monoclonal IgG antibodies for each bacterium are added to a test card with a CSF sample, mixed, and mechanically rotated for 5 minutes. Agglutination of the latex determines the presence of bacterial antigens, thus indicating a bacterial infection. Serological methods are also used in determining syphilis infections of the CNS. The fluorescent treponemal antibody absorption test is very sensitive but less specific in CSF samples than serum. Molecular methods aid in detecting pathogens that do not grow on routine media or in patients who have already had antibiotic treatments. PCR testing is available for the detection and amplification of nucleic acids in the RNA or DNA of various CSF pathogens including bacteria, virus, fungi, and parasites.

Common Meningitis-Causing Pathogens

Bacterial meningitis is caused by opportunistic bacteria that enter the bloodstream, are carried across the blood–brain barrier to the meninges, and spread throughout the spinal fluid. The etiology, transmission, and virulence of common meningitis-causing bacteria are listed below:

S. pneumoniae, H. influenzae, and ***N. meningitidis*** are normal flora of the upper respiratory tract and are spread from person to person by respiratory droplets. The most susceptible population are children younger than 5 years of age, and pneumonia or bacteremia are commonly the initial infection in a host prior to meningitis.

- *S. pneumoniae*
  - Pneumolysin: antiphagocytic capsular protein
  - Several adhesion factors and immunogenic cell wall membrane
- *H. influenzae* and *N. meningitidis*
  - Encapsulated strains: resistant to phagocytosis and complement-mediated lysis
  - *H. influenzae*: B strain, most likely to cause meningitis
  - *N. meningitidis*: most common meningitis causing strains: A, B, C, Y, W.

E. coli and ***L. monocytogenes*** are transmitted via the ingestion of contaminated food. Along with ***Streptococcus agalactiae,*** they are common pathogens of neonatal meningitis due to transmission from mother to baby at birth.

- *S. agalactiae* (group B strep)
  - Polysaccharide capsule: prevents phagocytosis
  - Pore-forming toxins: promote entry into host cells and facilitate organism survival
- *E. coli*
  - K1 strain: inhibits phagocytosis and resists bactericidal activity of serum antibodies
- *L. monocytogenes*
  - Escape phagocytic vacuoles due to listeriolysin O, phospholipase A, and phospholipase B.

Common Pathogens of CSF Shunt Infections

The following are normal skin flora organisms that act as opportunistic pathogens when introduced into the CNS at the shunt surgical site, in the shunt itself, or in the CSF fluid. Contamination of the shunt can occur during surgery to implant the device or during the aftercare and maintenance of the shunt. Virulence factors are as follows:

- Coagulase-negative *Staphylococcus*
  - Encapsulated serotypes: resistant to phagocytosis
  - Several adhesion factors and biofilm producing the cell wall membrane
- *Corynebacterium*
  - Toxigenic strains are lysogenic due to exotoxin production

- *Propionibacterium*
  - Acquired resistance to the following antibiotic classes:
    - Macrolides: erythromycin and azithromycin
    - Lincosamides: clindamycin
    - Tetracyclines: doxycycline and minocycline.

Body Fluids from Normally Sterile Sites

Sources and Collection of Specimens for Body Fluids of Normally Sterile Sites

Sterile fluids in several cavities of the body are necessary for protection and normal function of the organs they surround. During disease or infection, these fluids can accumulate and become harmful. Collection of these fluids for analysis requires an aseptic surgical needle puncture into a membrane or cavity where fluid is then aspirated and placed into sterile collection containers. The following are sources of normally sterile fluids able to be collected for analysis:

- **Serous fluids** surround the pericardial, pleural, and peritoneal cavities.
  - **Pericardial** fluid exists in the space surrounding the heart.
  - **Pleural** fluid is present around the lungs in the thoracic cavity.
  - **Peritoneal** fluid, or **ascites,** resides in the abdominal and pelvic cavities.
- **Synovial fluids** surround and lubricate the joints in the body.
- **Vitreous** liquid fills the space between the lens and retina of the eye, whereas the **aqueous humor** fills the anterior and posterior chambers of the eye.
- **Amniotic fluid** surrounds the fetus in the uterus during pregnancy.

Indigenous Organisms Associated with Skin and Mucosal Surfaces

The mucous membrane is composed of layers of tissue that line the cavities in the body and cover the surfaces of internal organs. Mucosal surfaces and their associated indigenous organisms function together to protect exogenous pathogens from entering the body. Colonization of commensal normal flora inhibits the growth of potential pathogens by competing for nutrients on the surface of mucous membranes. Most indigenous species have a commensal or mutualistic relationship with the mucous membrane by coexisting or equally benefiting from one another. The following mucosal surfaces are home to the associated organisms:

- **Skin** — *S. aureus, S. epidermidis, Corynebacterium,* and *Propionibacterium acnes*
- **Conjunctiva (eyes)** — *S. aureus, S. epidermidis, S. pneumoniae, H. influenzae, Neisseria species, Candida, Aspergillus,* and *Penicillium*
- **Oral cavity and nasal passages** — *S. aureus, S. epidermidis, S. pneumoniae, S. pyogenes, S. mitis, S. salivarius, S. mutans, Enterococcus faecalis, H. influenzae, Neisseria species, E. coli, Proteus, Corynebacterium, Lactobacillus, Actinomycetes, Candida, Mycoplasmas,* and *Cryptococcus*
- **Lower respiratory tract** — *Staphylococcus, Streptococcus, Fusobacterium, Acinetobacter, Pseudomonas, Sphingomonas, Prevotella, Megasphaera, Candida,* and *Aspergillus* species
- **Gastrointestinal tract** — *Lactobacillus, Clostridium, Bacteroides, Enterococcus, Streptococcus, Corynebacterium, Enterobacter,* and *Helicobacter* species
- **Genitourinary tract (vaginal)** — *Lactobacillus, S. aureus, S. epidermidis, E. faecalis, S. pneumoniae, S. pyogenes, Neisseria species, E. coli, Proteus species,* and *Corynebacterium.*

NEISSERIA AND ACINETOBACTER SPECIES

Neisseria species react and present in the following ways:

- **Biochemical reactions**:

Catalase	+
Oxidase	+
Nitrate reduction	+

- **Gram stain:** Gram-negative diplococci
- **Growth requirements**: aerobic and facultative anaerobe, grow best in a humid, 5–10% CO_2 environment at 35–37 °C
- **Colony morphology:** small, white to gray-brown, smooth, butter-like, and translucent on sheep blood agar with a green hue on agar underneath colonies possible

Acinetobacter species react and present in the following ways:

- **Biochemical reactions**:

Oxidase	–
Catalase	+
Motile	–
Nitrate reduction	–

- **Gram stain**: Gram-negative coccobacilli
- **Growth requirements**: aerobic and facultative anaerobe, grows best at 35 °C in ambient air or a CO_2-rich environment
- **Colony morphology**: smooth, round, mucoid, opaque to white colonies on sheep blood agar.

PSEUDOMONAS AERUGINOSA

Pseudomonas aeruginosa react and present in the following ways:

- **Biochemical reactions**:

Motility	+
Oxidase	+
Catalase	+
Urease	–
Indole	–
Methyl red	–
Voges–Proskauer	–
Tryptic soy agar	K/K

- **Gram stain**: Gram-negative bacilli
- **Growth requirements**: obligate aerobe, grow best at 35 °C in ambient air or a CO_2-rich environment
- **Colony morphology**: grayish white, translucent to opaque, circular with irregular edges on sheep blood agar. Colorless, transparent, circular on MacConkey agar. Colonies are smooth or mucoid, if swarming occurs. Produces a grape, or corn tortilla-like odor.

CLOSTRIDIUM PERFRINGENS

Clostridium perfringens react and present in the following ways:

- **Biochemical reactions**:

Indole	–
Urease	–
Lecithinase	+
Nagler test	+
Reverse CAMP test	+
Vancomycin	S
Kanamycin	S
Colistin	R

- **Gram stain:** Gram-positive to Gram-variable bacilli, straight rods with blunt ends, boxcar shape. Some strains are spore forming.
- **Growth requirements:** anerobic, grow best at 35–37 °C
- **Colony morphology:** gray to grayish yellow, circular, dome-shaped, translucent, and glossy, with a double zone of beta-hemolysis on anaerobic sheep blood agar.

BACTEROIDES FRAGILIS GROUP

Bacteroides fragilis react and present in the following ways:

- **Biochemical reactions**:

Nitrate reduction	–
Urease	–
Motility	–
Growth on bile	+
Reverse CAMP test	+
Vancomycin	R
Kanamycin	R
Colistin	R

- **Gram stain:** Gram-negative bacilli, pleomorphic with rounded ends — commonly resemble a safety pin
- **Growth requirements:** anaerobic, grow best at 35–37 °C
- **Colony morphology:** convex, circular, white to gray, and translucent with no hemolysis on anaerobic sheep blood agar. At 48 hours of growth, colonies are >1 mm, circular, and gray, surrounded by a gray zone on Bacteroides bile esculin agar.

MOLECULAR TECHNIQUES TO PROCESS BODY FLUID SAMPLES

Although microscopic and culture techniques are still the main source of body fluid infection detection, molecular methods are continuing to be developed for more rapid detection of disease. PCR techniques for the detection of bacteria or fungi are available for the improved management of immunosuppressed or high-risk patients. Most available PCR techniques rely on the amplification and sequencing of the 16SrRNA gene in bacteria and the internal transcribed region 2 in fungi.

Amniotic fluid is often sent for molecular analysis for the presence of specific genetic markers linked to diseases, such as Down syndrome and cystic fibrosis, or infection, such as cytomegalovirus. PCR methods focus on the amplification of gene sequences unique to the disease being tested for.

Common Pathogens of Normally Sterile Body Fluids

Infections of normally sterile body fluids occur by the introduction of bacteria to a body cavity during an invasive procedure, from a traumatic injury, or from the bloodstream. Common body fluid pathogens and their virulence factors are listed below:

- *Neisseria* species
    - Outer membrane pili: enhance adhesion and inhibit phagocytosis
    - Lipopolysaccharide endotoxin and IgA proteases
    - Encapsulated strains: resistant to phagocytosis and complement-mediated lysis
- *S. aureus*
    - Exotoxins: hemolysins, leukocidins, spreading factor by coagulase and hyaluronidase, nuclease, protease, and lipase
    - Most strains; penicillin resistance due to beta-lactamase
    - MRSA: methicillin-resistant strain
- Beta-hemolytic *streptococcus*
    - O_2-stable streptolysin S, O_2-labile streptolysin O
    - Streptococcal pyrogenic exotoxin B: inhibits action of immunoglobulins, cytokines, and complement
    - Hyaluronidase acts as a bacterial spreading factor
- *Enterococcus*
    - Adhesion factors facilitating binding to host cells, inducing cell and tissue destruction
    - Intrinsic antibiotic resistance of various species:
        - Beta-lactam antibiotics: penicillin, cephalosporin, carbapenem
        - Aminoglycosides: vancomycin-resistant *Enterococcus* (VRE)
- *Enterobacteriaceae*
    - All species release lipopolysaccharide endotoxin; some also produce exotoxins
    - H, K, and O antigens
    - Some strains express resistance to carbapenem antibiotics
- *P. aeruginosa*
    - Lipopolysaccharide endotoxin, hemolysins, protease
    - Exotoxin A: toxic to macrophages, prevents phagocytosis
    - Encapsulated: inhibits phagocytosis and actions of complement
- *C. perfringens*
    - *C. perfringens* enterotoxin, alpha and beta toxins: damage tissues, blood vessels, and blood cells
    - Hemolysins, proteases, lipases, collagenase, and hyaluronidase: aid in invasive processes
- *B. fragilis*
    - Polysaccharide encapsulation: protects from phagocytosis, stimulates abscess formation
    - Penicillin resistance due to beta-lactamase

Lower Respiratory

Sources and Collection of Lower Respiratory Tract Samples

Lower respiratory tract specimens can be collected from the sources and with the methods described below.

Ideal **sputum** specimen collection occurs first thing in the morning, with no food ingestion for 1–2 hours prior. Rinsing the mouth with water before collection and collecting directly into a sterile specimen container aid in avoiding contaminating the sample with saliva. Sputum is collected through the following methods:

- **Expectorated** sputum is expelled by a deep cough by the patient.
- **Induced** sputum collection uses an aerosol spray that reaches the lungs, inducing a deep cough.
- **Endotracheal aspirate** samples are collected via mechanical suction from patients with a tracheostomy tube.

Bronchoscopy procedures visualize the lungs by passing a tube with a light source and camera down a patient's throat and into the lungs. Bronchoscopes are used for collection of the following lower respiratory tract specimens:

- **Bronchial washings** are collected from the bronchial tubes. A measured amount of sterile saline is passed through the scope, and then it is gently suctioned back out. The suctioned saline is placed into a sterile container because it contains the cells and fluids needed for analysis.
- **Bronchoalveolar lavage** samples are collected from the smaller bronchoalveolar pathways via the same process as bronchial washings. Multiple lavage samples may be collected from several sites during one procedure.
- **Bronchial brushings** are collected by passing a brush through the bronchoscope and gently abrading the surface of the airway mucosa and bronchial lesions to collect cells for analysis.

Quantitative and Semiquantitative Result Reporting of Lower Respiratory Tract Specimens

Quantitative and semiquantitative results from Gram stains of lower respiratory tract specimens are used to evaluate the quality of samples before culture and aid in the diagnostic and treatment process for patients suspected of lower respiratory tract infections. Expectorated and induced sputum samples must meet specific Gram stain criteria to be considered acceptable for culture. Observed in 10–20 fields under low power, the following criteria indicate an acceptable specimen: <10 squamous epithelial cells and ≥10 WBCs per field. Regardless of the number of white cells present, samples with more than 25 epithelial cells per low-power field will be rejected. These results indicate that a sample did not originate in the lower respiratory tract and is contaminated by saliva and oral flora. Gram stains of acceptable lower respiratory tract samples are examined further under the oil immersion lens. Under this lens, any bacteria present are evaluated for their Gram stain reaction and morphologic characteristics and are semiquantitatively enumerated as rare, few, moderate, or many. Physicians interpret semiquantitative results for bacteria in conjunction with quantitative WBC and epithelial cell results to determine the following: the presence or absence of infection, the presumptive cause of infection, and the severity of infection.

ORAL FLORA

The oral cavity is home to a variety of organisms whose Gram stain and colony morphology on sheep blood agar are described below:

- Gram-positive cocci:
  - Staphylococcus
    - *S. aureus*: soft, opaque or pale gold, and circular
    - *S. epidermidis*: opaque, gray, smooth, raised, with no hemolysis
  - Streptococcus
    - *S. pneumoniae*: alpha-hemolytic, convex, mucoid or "water drop"
    - *S. pyogenes*: grayish-white, transparent to translucent, matte or glossy, large zone of hemolysis
    - *S. mitis*: alpha-hemolytic, broken glass appearance
    - *S. salivarius*: small, colorless, smooth or rough, nonhemolytic or weakly alpha-hemolytic
    - *S. mutans*: small white to gray, rough, nonhemolytic or alpha-hemolytic
  - *E. faecalis*: circular, smooth, nonhemolytic
- Gram-positive bacilli:
  - *Corynebacterium*: small to medium, gray, white, or yellow, nonhemolytic
  - *Actinomycetes*: white, rough, crumbly texture, occasionally pigmented red
  - *Lactobacillus*: small to medium, gray, alpha-hemolytic
- Gram-positive buds, hyphae, or pseudohyphae:
  - *Candida*: creamy, white, dull, grows upward with foot-like projections
- Gram-negative cocci:
  - *Neisseria*: small, white to gray-brown, smooth, butter-like, translucent, possible green hue underneath
- Gram-negative bacilli:
  - *H. influenzae*: on chocolate agar
    - Unencapsulated strain — small, smooth, and translucent
    - Encapsulated strain — larger, mucoid, with a mouse nest odor
  - *E. coli*: circular, dull gray, smooth, convex.

COMMON LOWER RESPIRATORY TRACT PATHOGENS

Infections of the lower respiratory tract are caused by the following organisms whose Gram stain and colony morphology on sheep blood agar are described below:

- Gram-positive cocci:
  - *S. aureus*: soft, opaque or pale gold, and circular
  - *S. pneumoniae*: alpha-hemolytic, convex, mucoid or "water drop"
- Gram-negative bacilli:
  - *H. influenzae*: on chocolate agar
    - Unencapsulated strain — small, smooth, and translucent
    - Encapsulated strain — larger, mucoid, with a mouse nest odor

- *K. pneumoniae*: small to medium, grayish-white, translucent or opaque. circular, dome shaped, mucoid, nonhemolytic
- *Legionella*: green or iridescent pink, circular with entire edge, convex, glistening, with a ground-glass appearance on buffered charcoal yeast extract agar

- Mycoplasma pneumoniae:
  - Organisms do not stain well due to the lack of a rigid cell wall.
  - Pinpoint, granular, "fried egg" appearance on media enriched with cholesterol and fatty acids.
- Mycobacterium tuberculosis
  - Mycolic acid in the cell wall resists Gram stain. Appear as slim rods, gram variable or bright red using an acid-fast stain.
  - Off-white to buff, dry, rough, raised, and wrinkled on Löwenstein–Jensen medium.
- Fungi
  - Yeasts: Gram-positive buds, hyphae, or pseudohyphae
    - *Candida*: creamy, white, dull, grows upward with foot-like projections
  - Other fungi: fluorescent white buds, hyphae, or pseudohyphae with KOH reagent and calcofluor-white stain
    - Variable growth on Sabouraud's dextrose agar for up to 6 weeks after inoculation.

Legionella and M. Tuberculosis

Legionnaires' disease and Pontiac pneumonia are lower respiratory infections caused by ***Legionella*** bacteria. *Legionella* bacteria's natural habitat is freshwater lakes and ponds, and it becomes pathogenic when it is able to grow in human-made water systems such as air conditioners, shower heads, hot water heaters, and large plumbing systems. Water aerosols containing the bacteria are inhaled and can cause disease.

Legionella

- Heat shock protein 60: aids in invasion
- Outer membrane protein: prevents phagocytosis
- Type IV pili: entry into macrophages for spread and survival.

Primary infections caused by ***M. tuberculosis*** take place in the lungs causing pneumonia-like symptoms. If left untreated, tuberculosis can become disseminated and spread to other organ systems in the body.

M. tuberculosis

- No endotoxins or exotoxins, toxic effects on cells from lipids and phosphatides
- Cord factor: destroys cell mitochondria, inhibits leukocyte migration
- Waxy layer and mycolic acid cell wall: delay hypersensitivity, induce multidrug-resistant variants.

Opportunistic fungi such as ***Aspergillus*** and ***Cryptococcus*** species aspirated into the lungs can cause pneumonia and lead to sepsis in immunocompromised patients. Bacterial lung abscesses are commonly a polymicrobial infection predominantly comprised of **anaerobic oropharyngeal or gastric normal flora** aspirated into the lungs.

Direct and Molecular Techniques for Detecting Respiratory Pathogens

S. pyogenes, or group A *Streptococcus*, is the respiratory pathogen responsible for upper respiratory infections including strep throat and pharyngitis, whereas *B. pertussis* is responsible for whooping cough. These infections are very contagious, and quick, accurate detection is vital to reduce the spread of these organisms.

Rapid test kits have been created for the detection of *S. pyogenes* using **immunochromatographic** or **immunofluorescent assays**. Positive results are enough evidence to diagnose infection, whereas negative results need to be confirmed with a throat culture. **Direct-fluorescent antibody testing** is a serologic test for the presence of IgG antibodies to *B. pertussis.* Although helpful in diagnosing an infection of *B. pertussis,* a diagnosis will be delayed because this method is best when a patient is tested between 2 and 8 weeks of symptom onset. Traditional culture or molecular methods allow for a timelier diagnosis for *B. pertussis* than antibody testing.

The most common molecular method used to detect *S. pyogenes* and *B. pertussis* is **real-time PCR**, with specific nucleic acid probes of <200 base pairs for each organism. **Multiplex PCR** methods are also used to detect *B. pertussis,* along with multiple other respiratory pathogens. The highly specific **isothermal loop-mediated amplification** method can also be used in detecting *B. pertussis* infections between 0 and 3 weeks of symptom onset.

Common Pneumonia-Causing Pathogens

Lower respiratory tract infections can manifest into various disease states including tracheitis, acute or chronic bronchitis, and community- or hospital-acquired pneumonia. The mode of transmission for these pathogens is through the inhalation of respiratory droplets from an infected person. Common pneumonia-causing pathogens and their associated virulence are described below:

- *S. aureus*
    - Exotoxins: hemolysins, leukocidins, spreading factor by coagulase and hyaluronidase, nuclease, protease, and lipase
    - Beta-lactamase: penicillin resistance, MRSA: methicillin resistance
- *S. pneumoniae*
    - Pneumolysin: antiphagocytic capsular protein
    - Several adhesion factors and immunogenic cell wall membrane
- *H. influenzae*
    - Encapsulated strains: resistant to phagocytosis and complement-mediated lysis
- *Klebsiella pneumoniae*
    - Encapsulated to inhibit phagocytosis and complement-mediated lysis
    - Lipopolysaccharide endotoxin causing inflammation
    - Fimbriae for adhesion and siderophores that acquire host iron for organism survival
- *M. pneumoniae*
    - P1 membrane protein: acts as a cytohesin to ciliated epithelial cells
    - Community-acquired respiratory distress syndrome toxin: damages respiratory epithelium and ciliary activity by releasing cytokines and inflammatory mediators.

Upper Respiratory

Upper Respiratory Tract Samples

Upper respiratory tract samples collected with a swab require a plastic shaft flocked swab and the appropriate transport media for the potential pathogens, whether aerobic, anaerobic, or viral. Specimens collected to evaluate for such infections include the following:

- **Throat** swabs are placed in the back of the throat, and the tonsillar area is vigorously swabbed in patients suspected of strep throat infections.
- **Nasal** swab collection consists of a swab inserted at least a half inch into the nostril, firmly rotated, and left in place for 10–15 seconds. Repeat the process in the other nostril using the same swab.
- **Nasopharyngeal** swab collection requires a thin, flexible swab that is more easily inserted into the nasopharyngeal passage. The patient's head should be tilted back slightly at a 70° angle to straighten the passage from the nares to the nasopharynx. Gently insert the swab through the nose, to the posterior nares, rotate it several times, and remove.
- **Sinus** exudate samples are collected via direct needle aspirate of the sinus or with a swab during surgical procedures of the sinuses.
- **Middle ear** samples are collected with a swab or needle aspirate. If the patient's eardrum has ruptured, the fluid released into the outer ear can be collected by inserting a sterile swab into the ear using an auditory speculum. Neonates, the elderly, or patients with persistent, chronic, or recurrent otitis media may have middle ear fluid collected via tympanocentesis, requiring a sterile needle puncture through the tympanic membrane to aspirate the middle ear fluid.

Major Pathogens of Upper Respiratory Tract

Infections of the upper respiratory tract are caused by the following organisms whose Gram stain and colony morphology on sheep blood agar are described below:

- Gram-positive cocci:
    - *S. pyogenes*: grayish-white, transparent to translucent, matte or glossy, large zone of hemolysis
    - *S. pneumoniae*: alpha-hemolytic, convex, mucoid or "water drop"
- Gram-positive bacilli in a "Chinese letter" formation:
    - *C. diphtheriae*: small, circular, convex, white to gray
- Gram-negative coccobacilli:
    - *B. pertussis*: small, round, shiny, silver colored, becoming whitish gray with age on charcoal blood agar
- Gram-negative bacilli:
    - *H. influenzae*: on chocolate agar
        - ❖ Unencapsulated strain — small, smooth, and translucent
        - ❖ Encapsulated strain — larger, mucoid, with a mouse nest odor
    - *P. aeruginosa*: grayish-white, translucent to opaque, circular with irregular edges

Common Throat, Oropharynx, and Ear Pathogens

Upper respiratory infections caused by ***S. pyogenes, C. diphtheriae, B. pertussis,*** and ***H. influenzae*** are transmitted by inhaling respiratory droplets of an infected individual or touching the mouth and nose with a contaminated hand or object. Throat and oropharynx pathogens' virulence factors are described below:

- *S. pyogenes*
    - O_2-stable streptolysin S, O_2-labile streptolysin O
    - Erythrogenic toxin: causes scarlet fever rash
    - Streptococcal pyrogenic exotoxin B: inhibits immunoglobulins, cytokines, and complement actions
    - M protein: prevents phagocytosis
    - Hyaluronidase: bacterial spreading factor
- *C. diphtheriae*
    - Diphtheria toxin: inhibits protein synthesis, leading to the death of host cells, and is carried in the bloodstream to other organs causing paralysis and CHF
    - Pili structures and proteins for adherence and colonization
        - SpaA, B, and C: selective to pharyngeal epithelial cells
        - SpaD and H: selective for lung and laryngeal epithelial cells
- *B. pertussis*
    - Adhesion and colonization factors
        - Filamentous hemagglutinin
        - Pertussis toxin: specific to tracheal endothelium; S2 adheres to ciliated epithelial cells and S3 adheres to phagocytes
    - Lipopolysaccharide endotoxin
    - Invasive adenylate cyclase: reduces local phagocytic activity
    - Lethal toxin: localized inflammation, issue necrosis
    - Tracheal cytotoxin: kills ciliated respiratory epithelium

Ear infections are not contagious; they manifest from upper respiratory infections. ***P. aeruginosa*** cause swimmer's ear, developing from moisture in or damage to the ear canal. Middle ear infections, otitis media, occur along with or following other upper respiratory symptoms caused by ***S. pneumoniae*** or ***H. influenzae.***

Gastrointestinal

Salmonella Species

Salmonella species react and present in the following ways:

- **Biochemical reactions**:

Indole	–
Citrate	+
H_2S	+
LDC	+ *
LDA	–
Urease	–
Ornithine decarboxylase (ODC)	+
Motility	+
TSI agar	K/A
Gas production	Variable

*Key differentiating characteristics.

- **Gram stain**: Gram-negative bacilli
- **Growth requirements**: mainly aerobic but facultative anaerobe as well, 37 °C with growth in 16–24 hours of inoculation.
- **Colony morphology**: opaque or translucent, smooth, 2–4 mm in diameter on supportive media, green or transparent with black center on Hektoen enteric agar, transparent or red with black centers on xylose-lysine-deoxycholate agar.

Shigella Species

Shigella species react and present in the following ways:

- **Biochemical reactions:**

Indole	Variable
Citrate	–
H_2S	– *
LDC	–
LDA	– *
Urease	–
ODC	Variable
Motility	– *
TSI agar	K/A
Gas production	–

*Key differentiating characteristics.

- **Gram stain**: Gram-negative bacilli
- **Growth requirements**: aerobic and facultative anaerobe, 35 °C with growth 18–24 hours after inoculation
- **Colony morphology**: clear or slightly pink on MacConkey agar, green or transparent on Hektoen agar, transparent or red on xylose-lysine-deoxycholate agar

Toxigenic Escherichia Coli

Toxigenic *Escherichia coli* react and present in the following ways:

- **Biochemical reactions:**

Test	Result
Indole	+
Citrate	–
H_2S	–
LDC	+
LDA	–
Urease	–
ODC	+
Motility	+
TSI agar	A/A
Gas production	+

- **Gram stain**: Gram-negative bacilli
- **Growth requirements**: aerobic and facultative anaerobe, grow best at 37 °C
- **Colony morphology**: circular, convex colonies, gray, translucent to opaque on sheep blood agar, pink, opaque on MacConkey, green with a metallic sheen, opaque on eosin methylene blue agar.

Campylobacter Species

Campylobacter species react and present in the following ways:

- **Biochemical reactions:**

Test	Result
Catalase	+
Oxidase	+
Hippurate	+

- **Gram stain**: Gram-negative bacilli, small curved rods, "seagull appearance"
- **Growth requirements**: Microaerophilic, *Campylobacter*-selective agar at 42 °C
- **Colony morphology**: mucoid, flat, grayish colonies with irregular edges, potentially swarming.

Vibrio species react and present in the following ways:

- **Biochemical reactions:**

Test	Result
Catalase	+
Oxidase	+

- **Gram stain**: Gram-negative bacilli, curved rod with polar flagella
- **Growth requirements**: aerobic and facultative anaerobe, require media with increased salt concentration, sodium chloride, and acidic pH, 35–37 °C for 6–8 hours for APW or 35–37 °C 18–24 hours to TCBS and all other media.
- **Colony morphology**: creamy white, smooth and convex; yellow-green on TCBS, colorless on MacConkey agar.

Yersinia Enterocolitica

Yersinia enterocolitica react and present in the following ways:

- **Biochemical reactions:**

Indole	V
Citrate	–
H_2S	–
LDC	–
LDA	–
Urease	V
ODC	+
Motility	V*
TSI agar	K/A
Gas production	–
Catalase	+
Oxidase	–

*Motile at 22–25 °C; nonmotile at 37 °C (body temperature).

- **Gram stain**: Gram-negative bacilli
- **Growth requirements**: aerobic and facultative anaerobe, grow optimally at room temperature (22–25 °C)
- **Colony morphology:** translucent or opaque or gray-white, slightly mucoid (after 24 hours of growth) on sheep blood agar, flat, colorless or pale pink on MacConkey agar, "bulls-eye" appearance with deep-red center and translucent outer zone on cefsulodin irgasan novobiocin (CIN) agar.

Aeromonas Species

Aeromonas species react and present in the following ways:

- **Biochemical reactions:**

Indole	+
Citrate	+
H_2S	V
LDC	+
Urease	–
ODC	–
Motility	V
TSI agar	K/A
Gas production	V
Catalase	+
Oxidase	+

- **Gram stain**: Gram-negative bacilli, single, in pairs, or short chains
- **Growth requirements**: aerobic and facultative anaerobe, grow best at 35–37 °C
- **Colony morphology:** circular, gray on sheep blood agar, dark green on sheep blood agar after 72 hours due to beta-hemolysis, deep-red center surrounded by translucent outer zone of colony on CIN agar.

Plesiomonas Shigelloides

Plesiomonas shigelloides react and present in the following ways:

- **Biochemical reactions:**

Test	Result
Indole	+
Citrate	
H_2S	
LDC	+
LDA	
Urease	
ODC	–
Motility	
TSI agar	K/A
Gas production	–
Catalase	+
Oxidase	+

- **Gram stain**: Gram-negative bacilli
- **Growth requirements**: aerobic and facultative anaerobe, grow best at 35–37 °C
- **Colony morphology:** clear and colorless on MacConkey, CIN, and XLD agars, clear and green on Hektoen agar.

Direct and Molecular Techniques for Detecting Clostridium Difficile- and Shiga Toxin-Producing Organisms

Due to their ability to cause life-threatening infections, the rapid detection of *C. difficile*- and Shiga toxin-producing *E. coli* organisms is pertinent for prompt patient care. Although exclusion of these organisms is possible, current methodologies alone cannot provide a definitive diagnosis for active infections and require interpretation along with clinical and epidemiological findings.

Direct immunochromatographic *C. difficile* testing methods simultaneously target the glutamate dehydrogenase (GDH) antigen and toxins A and B produced by toxigenic strains. Similarly, rapid tests for Shiga toxins 1 and 2 use antibody-labeled assays to determine the presence or absence of toxigenic strains of *E. coli.* Evaluations of these tests are as follows:

- *C. difficile*:
  - GDH antigen and toxin absent: no *C. difficile* infection
  - Both GDH antigen and toxin present:
    - Symptomatic: consistent with active infection
    - Asymptomatic: consistent with *C. difficile* colonization
  - Either GDH antigen or toxin present: inconclusive; molecular testing recommended
- Shiga toxin (ST1 and ST2):
  - ST1 and ST2 absent: no Shiga toxin-producing *E. coli* present
  - Either ST1 or ST2 or both present: Shiga toxin-producing *E. coli* present.

PCR and nucleic acid amplification testing molecular methods provide a definitive rule-out or supportive diagnosis of toxigenic infections. Nucleic acid amplification testing targets genes specific to toxigenic *C. difficile* strains including toxins A and B and 16S ribosomal RNA. Genes for ST1, ST2,

E. coli 0157:H7, and *Shigella dysenteriae* type 1 are targeted for detection of Shiga toxin-producing organisms.

Serotyping E. Coli, Salmonella, and Shigella Organisms

Serotyping allows for the differentiation of species and subspecies of organisms that otherwise have indistinguishable physical and biochemical properties. Determining the serotype of enteric pathogens allows for further insight on disease manifestations and proper treatment methods. Serotyping can be completed using the following test methodologies: bacterial, latex, or coagglutination, and fluorescent or enzyme-labeled immunoassay.

E. coli, Salmonella, and *Shigella* species and subspecies are differentiated from one another by the antigenic properties of their O, K, and H antigens. Present in the outermost layer of the bacterial cell wall, the **O antigen** is a polymer of immunogenic repeating oligosaccharides. The **K antigen** is present in the capsular polysaccharides, and a threadlike structure portion of the flagella in motile organisms contains the **H antigen**. More than 2,000 *Salmonella* serotypes have been detected and are determined by their individual expression of the O and H antigens. Based on their O antigenic properties, *Shigella* organisms are organized into four main species, or serogroups: A (*S. dysenteriae*), B (*S. flexneri*), C (*S. boydii*), and D (*S. sonnei*), which can be further divided further into several serotypes. *E. coli* subspecies are differentiated based on the composition and immunogenic properties of the O, K, and H antigens; for example, *E. coli* 0157:H7 is the extremely dangerous subspecies that produces a *Shigella*-like toxin that causes an enterohemorrhagic response.

Major Gastrointestinal Pathogens

Gastrointestinal infections occur from humans ingesting bacteria present in raw, undercooked, or unpasteurized products or human to human via the fecal–oral route. Reservoirs and virulence mechanisms of major gastrointestinal pathogens are described below:

Pathogen	Reservoir	Virulence Factors
Salmonella	Poultry	Lipopolysaccharide endotoxin: intracellular survival O and H antigens: immunogenic, motility Adhesion, colonization, and antiphagocytic properties Type III secretion system for survival in macrophages
Shigella	Human	Endotoxins: invasion, multiplication, and antiphagocytic properties Adhesion factor: colonization O antigen, Shiga toxin: immunogenic, inhibits cell protein synthesis causing life-threatening disease Type III secretion system: invading macrophages
P. shigelloides	Soil, water, seafood	Enterotoxins, invasins, and hemolysin
***Aeromonas* species**	Amphibians, reptiles, fish; more prevalent during warm-weather months	Lophotrichous flagella: motility Various toxins, proteases, hemolysins, lipases, adhesins, and agglutinins
Y. enterocolitica	Swine	Lipopolysaccharide endotoxin Protein capsular antigen: protects against phagocytosis Proteins to promote adhesion and invasion

Pathogen	Reservoir	Virulence Factors
***Campylobacter* species**	Poultry, cattle, and sheep	Lipopolysaccharide endotoxin and exotoxins Superoxide dismutase: harmful to cells' DNA or membrane factors Siderophores: iron sequestering
E. coli	Cattle	O, K, and H antigens: immunogenic, encapsulation, motility K1: inhibits phagocytosis, resists serum antibody activity O157:H7: hemorrhagic effects
***Vibrio* species**	Water, oysters, other seafood	Adhesion factor, pili: colonization, mucosa adherence Hemagglutination protease: intestinal inflammation and degradation Cholera toxin: quickly causes severe dehydration Siderophores

Skin, Soft Tissue, and Bone

Skin, Soft-Tissue, and Bone Cultures

Skin, soft-tissue, and bone cultures are collected from sites of suspected infection due to trauma, irritation, bites, burns, natural openings, or poor postoperative healing. Wound culture specimens are collected from **superficial wounds** of the epidermis and dermal layers of skin such as rashes, dermatitis lesions, or pustules. The wound surface should be free of debris and disinfected, and then a swab should be used to collect material from the deepest available area of the wound to avoid contamination from normal flora. **Deep-wound** specimens are collected from abscesses, ulcers, and boils in the subcutaneous tissue. The area can be debrided and a specimen collected using the same method noted for superficial wounds. An abscess or boil may also have purulent material expressed and can be collected with a swab or aspirated with a sterile syringe for culture. **Surgical extraction** and **biopsy** may be necessary for collecting deep-tissue samples for culture because they hold the greatest potential to cause a systemic infection. Portions of bone or infected tissue can be debrided, removed, and placed in a sterile cup with a small amount of sterile fluid. Samples suspected of infections caused by anaerobic organisms should be transported in media that reduce O_2 exposure and support the viability of such organisms.

Indigenous Organisms and Major Pathogens of Skin, Soft Tissue, and Bone

Soft tissues of the body comprise various structures including muscles, tendons, ligaments, fascia, nerves, fibrous tissues, fat, blood vessels, and synovial membranes. These soft tissues, located deep in the body, and bones are normally sterile. Indigenous skin flora, their Gram stain, and colony morphology on sheep blood agar are described below:

- Gram-positive cocci:
    - *S. aureus*: soft, opaque or pale gold, and circular
    - *S. epidermidis*: opaque, gray, smooth, raised, nonhemolytic
- Gram-positive bacilli in a "Chinese letter" formation:
    - *Propionibacterium acnes*: pigmented white or red, semiopaque, convex, and glistening

Major pathogens and their colony morphologies are described below:

- Aerobic organisms on sheep blood agar:
  - *E. coli*: circular, dull gray, smooth, convex
  - *Klebsiella* species: grayish-white, translucent to opaque, mucoid, circular, dome shaped
  - *P. mirabilis*: pale white, with swarming growth in waves forming concentric circles
  - *P. aeruginosa*: grayish-white, translucent to opaque, circular with irregular edges
  - *S. pyogenes* (group A strep): grayish-white, transparent to translucent, matte or glossy, large zone of hemolysis
  - *S. agalactiae* (group B strep): larger than group A colonies, translucent to opaque, flat, glossy, narrow zone of beta-hemolysis; some strains are nonhemolytic
  - *S. aureus*: soft, opaque or pale gold, and circular
  - *Salmonella* species*: opaque or translucent, smooth, 2–4 mm in diameter
- Facultative anaerobic organisms:
  - *B. fragilis*: gray or white, smooth, shiny, circular on sheep blood agar
  - *Prevotella* species: gray, shiny, circular, turning brown to black after a week of growth on laked blood agar with kanamycin and vancomycin

*Causes osteomyelitis in sickle cell patients. Not a common pathogen in other hosts.

Major Skin, Soft-Tissue, and Bone Infection Pathogens

Many major pathogens of the skin, soft tissues, and bone are also considered parts of the skin's normal flora. However, other pyogenic, or pus-producing, organisms can also cause infections of these tissues. A cut or break in the skin allows bacteria to enter into deeper layers of the skin causing opportunistic infections. Pyogenic organisms release toxic leucocidins that kill host neutrophils and produce pus as a result of accumulating cells and bacteria. *S. aureus* is the most common pathogen causing skin and tissue infections. Infections of the skin and soft tissue are listed below, defined by their site of and cause of infection:

- **Impetigo:** infection affecting healthy superficial skin
- **Cellulitis:** infection of the deeper layers of the skin and soft tissues, occurs on any part of the body
- **Erysipelas**: *S. pyogenes* infection of superficial cutaneous skin on the face or legs only
- **Folliculitis:** localized infection of one hair follicle
- **Boil, furuncle**: painful, hardened, and red bump associated with deep hair follicle infection
- **Carbuncle:** red, swollen, and painful cluster of furuncles under the skin
- **Abscess:** acute or chronic inflammation with a localized collection of pus
- **Osteomyelitis** is a bacterial infection of the bone tissue. Bacteria reach the bone through the bloodstream, introduction of skin flora by recent surgery or open fracture, intravenous drug use, or as an extension of a local injury from the following sources: soft tissues, urogenital tract, or upper and lower respiratory tract.

Genital Tract

Genital Cultures

Commercial collection kits contain the supplies required for specimen collection and transport including a sterile swab with a plastic shaft and a Dacron or rayon tip and a sterile transport tube with the appropriate media to sustain organism viability. Stuart media and Amies charcoal media are often used for the preservation of organisms detected in genital tract samples. Genital tract specimens are collected with the following methods:

- **Urethral** collection is best when preformed more than 1 hour after urination. After discharge is removed from the opening of the urethra, a sterile swab is inserted 2–4 cm into the urethra, rotated for 2–3 seconds to ensure adequate sampling, and then the swab is removed.
- **Vaginal** collection requires excess discharge to be wiped from the opening of the vaginal canal before a swab is inserted. Once inserted into the vaginal canal, the swab is rotated to collect secretions from the mucosal membranes.
- **Cervical** and **endocervical** collection uses a speculum to view the cervical canal; however, lubrication cannot be used when inserting the device because it can be harmful to organisms for culture. Mucus and vaginal material are removed with a swab that is then discarded. A second sterile swab is inserted into the cervix, and the canal is swabbed in a firm but gentle manner. Endocervical samples for chlamydia require more vigorous swabbing to collect epithelial cells.

Indigenous Organisms of Genital Tract

In healthy individuals, most of the internal organs of the genitourinary tract, the kidneys, bladder, ureters, testes, and ovaries, are sterile environments. However, the lower portion of the male and female urethra are inhabited by common normal skin flora, and the female vagina has indigenous species of its own. The following are organisms that comprise the urogenital tract normal flora, along with their corresponding Gram stain and colony morphologies on sheep blood agar:

- Male and female urethra:
  - Gram-positive cocci
    - *S. epidermidis*: opaque, gray, smooth, raised, nonhemolytic
    - *Enterococcus faecalis*: small, smooth, gray nonhemolytic
  - Gram-positive bacilli
    - *Corynebacterium* species: small to medium, gray, white, or yellow, nonhemolytic
  - Gram-negative diplococci
    - *Neisseria* species: small, white to gray-brown, smooth, butter-like, translucent with a green hue on agar underneath
- Vagina:
  - Gram-positive cocci
    - *Staphylococcus* species: opaque, white to yellow, smooth, circular
    - *Micrococcus* species: opaque, white to bright yellow, smooth, raised
    - *Viridans streptococci*: gray, translucent, umbonate center, alpha-hemolytic
    - *Enterococcus* species: small, gray, circular
  - Gram-positive bacilli
    - *Lactobacillus* species: small to medium, gray, alpha-hemolytic
    - *Corynebacterium* species: see description above
  - Gram-negative bacilli
    - *Escherichia coli*: circular, dull gray, smooth, convex.

Methods for Detection of Pathogens Associated with Vaginitis

Detection of Trichomonas

Trichomonas vaginalis can be detected in fresh-void urine from males and females, prostatic secretions, and the vaginal canal. The most common detection of *Trichomonas* is through direct observation on a **wet mount** or in urine sediment. A small amount of sample and a drop of saline are added to a glass slide, and a coverslip is placed on the slide. Microscopic detection of *Trichomonas* reveals a pear-shaped trophozoite similar in size to a neutrophil, moving by its flagella in jerky, undulating movements. If microscopic analysis cannot immediately be observed, *Trichomonas* is still detectable, but it may not be motile and will take on a more spherical shape making it more difficult to differentiate from a WBC. **Immunochromatographic dipsticks** that detect *T.* vaginalis antigens are available, and they eliminate the need for live organisms and immediate testing.

Detection of Candida

Candida species can be detected under microscopic examination using a variety of methods and stains. Yeast can be observed directly with a light microscope in wet mount or urine sediment samples. The use of **KOH** reagent will lyse cells and clear excess debris from samples, aiding in the visualization of yeast and fungal elements. **Calcofluor-white** stain is used to detect yeast species under a UV microscope by fluorescing fungal elements as a bright-white color that is easily visualized. Easily distinguishable from bacteria, *Candida* presents on a Gram stain as Gram-positive buds, pseudohyphae, or true hyphae. A culture and biochemical testing of urine and vaginal samples containing *Candida* organisms can be used to determine the specific species of yeast responsible for the infection.

Detection of Bacterial Vaginosis

Bacterial vaginosis (BV) is most commonly associated with an overgrowth of *Gardnerella vaginalis*, but it can be caused by up to 35 unique species of aerobic and anaerobic bacteria. The presence of **clue cells** in urine sediment or on a wet mount are indicative of a BV infection. Clue cells are vaginal squamous epithelial cells that are covered in bacteria, giving the cytoplasm a lacy appearance. Wet-prep samples will exhibit clusters of sloughed-off clue cells covered in Gram-variable bacilli and coccobacilli. A Gram stain of a vaginal swab positive for BV will show mixed flora with a decrease in the normal vaginal flora, *Lactobacillus* species. Although more advanced methods are available, the mix of flora shown on a Gram stain can be enumerated and a diagnosis of BV may be made. Molecular PCR methods are also available for detecting species of bacteria known to cause BV.

Culture Detection

Detection of Neisseria Gonorrhoeae and Chlamydia Trachomatis

N. gonorrhoeae is a fastidious organism with specific storage and growth requirements for culture. Specimens collected for *N. gonorrhoeae* culture should be set up as soon as possible for the best viability of the organism. If inoculating the medium is delayed, samples suspected for a gonorrheal infection must stay at room temperature because refrigeration destroys viable organism. This organism may take up to 48 hours to grow, requires the enrichment of chocolate and Thayer–Martin agars, and must be incubated in a 5–10% CO_2 environment.

C. trachomatis is an incredibly fastidious organism that requires complex and extensive nutrients for cultivation and growth. Due to its intracellular obligations, *C. trachomatis* requires a host cell, such as McCoy cells, to properly grow in a culture setting. Cells are inoculated with sample, incubated in 5–10% CO_2 for 48–72 hours, and observed for brown intracellular growth. Samples suspected of chlamydial infections should be submitted to the lab immediately or frozen at –70 °C for organisms to remain viable.

Detection of Streptococcus Agalactiae

Women in the third trimester of pregnancy are screened for *Streptococcus agalactiae*, or group B strep, colonization in their vaginal canal and rectum. Infants are able to contract a group B strep infection during delivery that can cause sepsis if not treated promptly and properly. Samples for culture of group B strep are inoculated onto sheep blood agar with vertical stabs made in the agar to promote hemolysis, and they are incubated overnight in 5–10% CO_2. *S. agalactiae* is indicated by colony growth with a narrow zone of beta-hemolysis underneath each colony. A CAMP test can be performed on sheep blood agar to distinguish group B strep from other beta-hemolytic streptococcus species. Diffusible extracellular CAMP proteins produced by *S. agalactiae* react with beta-lysin produced by *S. aureus* to create an arrowhead-shaped zone of hemolysis at the intersection of an *S. agalactiae* streak made perpendicular to a streak of *S. aureus.*

Molecular Detection of N. Gonorrhoeae, C. Trachomatis, and S. Agalactiae

Molecular methods for the detection of *N. gonorrhoeae, C. trachomatis,* and *S. agalactiae* are advantageous because they do not rely on organisms' viability and are more specific and time efficient than culture methods. Probe technologies use hybridization and amplification of the bacterial genetic material to detect its presence in samples. **Hybridization** detects bacterial ribosomal RNA with the use of chemiluminescent DNA probes or an RNA/DNA hybrid using antibody-mediated recognition. Some hybridization techniques allow for the detection of *N. gonorrhoeae* and *C. trachomatis* to be determined from a single sample. **Amplification** methods are more sensitive by employing the detection and amplification of nucleic acids in organism-specific genes. **PCR** methods are able to detect small amounts of DNA or RNA in a sample and replicate, or amplify, a target nucleic acid sequence for the detection of specific organisms.

Common Genitourinary Tract Pathogens

Infections of the genitourinary tract are commonly caused by opportunistic pathogens and manifest into urethritis, vaginitis, and cervicitis. Bacterial vaginitis is a polymicrobial infection that occurs when the balance of normal vaginal flora is disrupted. Vaginitis can also develop from the sexual transmission of the parasite *Trichomonas vaginalis*. Opportunistic fungal infections caused by *Candida albicans* arise when normal flora are inhibited by the use of antibiotics, and these infections often lead to itching, irritation, thick discharge, and burning while urinating. Sexual transmission of *N. gonorrhoeae* and *C. trachomatis* will also lead to genitourinary tract infections and are causative agents in pelvic inflammatory disease that may induce infertility in women. Other common symptoms of gonorrheal and chlamydial infections include lower abdominal pain, discharge from the penis in males, vaginal discharge in females, and painful urination. Herpes simplex virus type 1 (HSV-1) and herpes simplex virus type 2 (HSV-2) are spread by sexual contact causing itching, bumps, rashes, or sores near the genitals, as well as painful urination. Syphilis infections caused by the sexual transmission of *Treponema pallidum* begin with enlarged lymph nodes near the groin and painless sores on the body and genitals. If not treated, syphilis infections can progress into its secondary, latent, and tertiary stages that lead to irreversible systemic damage.

Urine

Urine Samples

Random samples may be collected at any time, with no additional preparation or cleansing. Samples of this nature may be used for urine chemistry testing (creatinine, total protein, electrolytes, microalbumin), but they are to be avoided for routine urinalysis or culture testing due to the possibility of erroneous results and an increased chance of contamination.

Midstream clean catch collection comprises cleansing the skin near and around the urethra. Following cleansing, the patient will void first into the toilet and then collect the remaining urine (or an adequate amount) into a collection cup. This method is ideal for urinalysis, bacterial culture, and sensitivity testing.

Catheterized specimens are collected by passing a hollow tube, or catheter, through the urethra and into the bladder. This technique is most commonly used for bacterial culture testing, but it may be used for other routine tests as well.

Suprapubic samples are collected in a sterile environment when a needle is placed through the abdomen and into the bladder. Aspirated urine provides a sterile sample that is free of outside contamination and is ideal for bacterial cultures and cytologic examination.

Nephrostomy tubes are catheters placed through the skin and directly into the kidney. They are used to drain or collect urine when output through the ureters in not possible. Samples may be used for routine urinalysis testing or bacterial culture.

Colony Counts in Urine Cultures

Colony counts are extremely important to the process of evaluating urine cultures. Following inoculation and incubation, media are observed for the growth of bacterial colonies, colonies are enumerated, and they are reported as follows:

Observation	Report*
No colony growth	<1,000 colonies
<10	1,000
10	10,000
100	100,000
>100	>100,000

*The colony count is in colony forming units per mL = (number of colonies) × 100.

No growth observed on media after 48 hours of incubation is expected in normal clean-catch, catheterized, suprapubic aspirate and in surgically obtained urine samples. **Fewer than 10 colonies** observed is not considered a significant finding in clean-catch or catheterized specimens, and no further workup is needed. However, any bacterial growth of urine collected from sterile sources is significant and requires further investigation. Cultures with **colony counts between 10 and 100** may be tested further if a patient is having symptoms indicative of a urinary tract infection (UTI). Correlation with other laboratory findings and the patient's clinical signs will influence the decision to test further or not. Growth of **>100 colonies of mixed organisms** exhibiting one predominant organism is a significant finding, and the predominant bacteria will be tested further. Cultures containing three or more organisms with no predominant one indicates a contaminated specimen, no further testing is done, and the collection of a new sample is suggested. A colony count **>100 of a pure, single organism** is indicative of a UTI, and further workup is required to properly identify the organism and perform antibiotic sensitivity testing for guide treatment options.

Correlation Between Urinalysis Results and Urine Culture Evaluation

Microscopic and macroscopic urinalysis findings are evaluated and correlated with urine culture findings in the determination of UTIs. Nitrite, pH, and leukocyte esterase chemical reactions on a urine dipstick indicate the presence or absence of bacteria in a sample. Common UTI-causing bacteria, including *E. coli, Klebsiella*, *Proteus*, *Pseudomonas*, and *Enterobacter* species, will reduce nitrate to nitrite, creating a **positive nitrite** dipstick result. Leukocyte esterase is an enzyme found in neutrophils, and a **positive leukocyte esterase** result indicates a UTI because WBCs are commonly found in areas of infection. An **alkaline pH** may indicate the presence of infection-causing bacteria in urine because some bacteria hydrolyze urea into the alkaline substance ammonia. Macroscopic observations of **WBCs** and **bacteria** in urine sediment are also correlated with urine culture results in the determination of a UTI. The noted urinalysis results alone are only indications of an infection and provide guidance in culture evaluation. Following urinalysis results, urine culture growth, quantification, and organism identification are used to confirm or deny the presence of a UTI.

Identification Methods (Theory, Interpretation, and Application)

Colony Morphology on Microbiology Cultures

A bacterial colony is a visible mass of identical organisms that grows from a single bacterial cell. Different genera, species, and strains of bacteria present with distinct visual appearances that are used as the first step in isolating and identifying infectious agents. Evaluating colony morphology also aids in determining the purity of a culture by more easily recognizing contamination of other organisms. Within 18–24 hours after being inoculated with sample, organisms growing on microbiology media are visually observed. A hand lens or magnifying glass can be used to aid in identifying key characteristics. Colony morphology is evaluated by the following characteristics:

- Colony size
- Form and margins
- Elevation
- Surface features, texture, and consistency
- Color, transparency, and iridescence.

Categorization and Interpretation of Colony Morphology Characteristics

Colony morphology is categorized by size, form, margins, and elevation characteristics in the following ways:

- **Colony size** is categorized by diameter:
  - Pinpoint or punctiform < 1 mm
  - Small 1–2 mm
  - Medium 3–4 mm
  - Large > 5 mm

The form, margins, and elevation of a colony give it a distinctive shape:

- **Forms** are categorized as
  - Circular, symmetrical circle
  - Irregular, lacking symmetry
  - Filamentous, exhibiting threadlike branching
  - Rhizoid, exhibiting a branching, rootlike shape

- The **margins**, or edges, of a colony are most commonly evaluated as
    - Entire, meaning smooth
    - Undulate, meaning wavy
    - Lobular, fingerlike growth spreading outward
    - Scalloped, rounded projections resembling a scallop shell
    - Filiform, thin and wavy layers spreading outward.
- The **elevation** of bacterial colonies refers to its cross-sectional shape. Colony elevations are categorized by the following shapes:
    - Flat
    - Raised
    - Convex, curved or rounded upward
    - Crateriform, sunken in the middle
    - Umbonate, with the middle protruding upward.

Surface texture and consistency are described as having the following characteristics:

- **Textures** are described with the following terms:
    - Smooth,
    - Wrinkled, shriveled
    - Rough, granular
    - Dull, no shine
    - Glistening, shining
- The **consistency** of colonies is described as the following:
    - Moist
    - Dry
    - Viscid, thick and sticky
    - Mucoid, moist and sticky
    - Butyrous, butter-like

Colonies can exhibit a variety of transparencies and pigmentations:

- Colony **transparency** is categorized as
    - Transparent, clear, see-through
    - Translucent, semiclear, frosted-glass appearance
    - Opaque, unable to see through
    - Iridescent, color changing in reflective light
- Sheep blood and chocolate agars often yield the following **colony colors**:
    - White
    - Cream
    - Yellow
- Differential and selective medias can produce many colors based on the organism's biochemical properties such as:
    - Pink
    - Green
    - Blue
    - Black

Rapid Tests Used for Presumptive Identification

Catalase and Coagulase Tests

The following rapid tests are used for presumptive identification of organisms:

- **Catalase:** This test is used to determine the presence of the catalase enzyme in an organism and differentiate catalase-positive staphylococci from catalase-negative streptococci organisms. An organism colony is placed on a glass slide, followed by a drop of 3% hydrogen peroxide. If catalase is present, the enzyme will break down hydrogen peroxide into O_2 and water.
    - **Catalase positive**: bubbling produced
    - **Catalase negative**: no visible bubbling
- **Coagulase:** This test is used to differentiate coagulase-positive *S. aureus* from other *Staphylococcus* species. Commercial kits are available to detect bound coagulase, or clumping factor, by adding reagent rabbit plasma to an organism colony on a glass slide. If present, bound coagulase and protein A on the cell wall agglutinates with reagent for a positive reaction.
    - **Coagulase positive**: visible clumping on the slide.
    - **Coagulase negative**: no visible clumping or agglutination. Free or unbound coagulase can be detected in a tube with gel containing rabbit plasma. The presence of free coagulase will form a visible fibrin clot after 4 hours of incubation at 35 °C. If no clot is observed at 4 hours, incubation is extended to 24 hours.

Oxidase and Indole Tests

The following rapid tests are used for the presumptive identification of organisms:

- **Oxidase:** This test is used for a presumptive identification of *Neisseria* species and *P. aeruginosa.* A colony of organism is added to filter paper impregnated with Kovac's oxidase reagent (tetramethyl-*p*-phenylenediamine), and a color change, or lack of, is observed. Organisms producing the cytochrome oxidase enzyme will oxidize the reagent indicating a positive test result, whereas organisms that do not produce the enzyme will be oxidase negative.
    - **Oxidase positive:** development of a dark-purple color within 10 seconds
    - **Oxidase negative:** colorless, or remains the original color of the colony
- **Indole**: This test is used for a presumptive identification of *E. coli* and differentiation of swarming *Proteus* species. Organisms that produce the enzyme tryptophanase break down tryptophan amino acids, yielding indole. Filter paper is saturated with indole reagent, and a colony of organism is rubbed onto the filter paper. Indole-positive organisms are determined by indole's ability to combine with indicator aldehydes to form a color compound.
    - **Indole positive**: rapid development of a blue or green-blue color
    - **Indole negative**: no color change.

PYR and Urease Tests

The following rapid tests are used for presumptive identification of organisms:

- **PYR**: This test is used to identify *Enterococcus* species and group A beta-hemolytic streptococci through the presence of the enzyme pyrrolidonyl. Filter paper is impregnated with the substrate PYR that is acted on by pyrrolidonyl. The paper is inoculated with the organism being tested, the color developing reagent N,N-dimethylaminocinnamaldehyde is added, and the results are interpreted after 5 minutes.
    - **PYR positive:** development of a bright-red color
    - **PYR negative:** no color change, or a yellow-orange color
- **Urease:** This test is used to detect *C. neoformans* in sputum samples and differentiate pathogenic *Shigella* and *Salmonella* species from nonpathogenic *Proteus* species in stool cultures. Urease-producing organisms hydrolyze urea-releasing ammonia that changes the alkalinity of a sample placed on pH paper. The production of ammonia reacts with the phenol red indicator and causes a color change in urease-positive organisms.
    - **Urease positive:** color change to magenta
    - **Urease negative**: no color change, pH paper remains yellow.

Conventional Biochemical Identification

Triple Sugar Iron (TSI) Agar

A triple sugar iron (**TSI**) agar slant is used for presumptive identification of many Gram-negative bacilli, most commonly the enteric pathogens in the *Enterobacteriaceae* family. This method is based on an organism's ability or inability to produce gas and H_2S and to ferment certain sugars. TSI agar contains the following:

- Sugars — glucose, lactose, and sucrose
- Nutrient source — peptone
- Sulfur source — sodium thiosulfate
- Indicator — ferric ammonium citrate
- pH indicator — phenol red.

TSI is inoculated using a needle carrying a pure colony of the organism to be identified. The needle is stabbed through the middle of the agar and into the bottom, or **butt**, of the agar. The **slant** is also inoculated by streaking the organism along its surface while removing the needle. TSI is interpreted after 18–24 hours of incubation at 35 °C.

The following characteristics and changes observed in TSI are as follows:

Notation	Color Change	Metabolic Change
K/K	Slant, red; butt, red	No sugars fermented, no reaction
K/A	Slant, red; butt, yellow	Glucose fermented; lactose and sucrose not fermented
A/A	Slant, yellow; butt, yellow	Glucose fermented; lactose, sucrose, or both fermented
G	Bubbles/splitting in the butt of the agar	Gas production
H_2S	Black precipitate	H_2S production

Decarboxylase Testing

Decarboxylase testing, also called Moeller's method, measures an organism's ability to hydrolyze an amino acid to form an amine and often aids in the identification of organisms of the *Enterobacteriaceae* family. Hydrolysis of the carboxyl portion of an amino acid to form an alkaline-reacting amine produces a change in color in the test tubes.

For testing, a very heavy suspension is prepared by combining brain heart infusion broth with a young colony of organism that has been grown on 5% sheep blood agar for 18–24 hours. Three decarboxylase broths containing arginine, lysine, and ornithine and a control broth with no amino acid added are then inoculated with the suspension. Glucose-nonfermenting organisms will be inoculated with four drops of organism suspension, and glucose-fermenting organisms will be inoculated with one drop. Cover the medium with a 4 mm layer of sterile mineral oil, incubate at 35–37 °C, and examine at 24, 48, 72, and 96 hours of incubation.

- **Decarboxylase positive**: purple color change compared to orange in the control tube
- **Decarboxylase negative**: No color change, or yellow color in the test and control tubes.

Carbohydrate Utilization Testing

Carbohydrate utilization testing is performed to definitively identify yeast species in clinical specimens. Yeasts and yeast-like fungi can be identified by a carbohydrate utilization profile because they each use specific carbohydrate substrates. To perform carbohydrate utilization testing, a yeast is combined with saline or distilled water to create a 4.0 McFarland standard suspension. The suspension is then used to cover the surface of a yeast nitrogen base agar plate containing bromocresol purple and is allowed to dry. Sterile forceps are used to place selected carbohydrate disks about 30 mm apart on the surface of the agar. After 24–48 hours of incubation at 30 °C, the plate is observed for carbohydrate utilization by the presence of a color change or growth around a disk. The results obtained by carbohydrate utilization tests create a profile for the organism tested that is compared to profiles established in mycology laboratory manuals for organism identification.

- **Carbohydrate utilization positive**: color change or growth around the disk
- **Carbohydrate utilization negative**: no color change or growth around the disk.

Motility Testing

Motility testing is done to determine if an organism is motile or not, allowing for further differentiation among organisms. There are two methods for determining motility, the hanging drop method and the semisolid agar method. Each method's procedure and interpretation are as follows:

- Hanging drop:
    - Use a 25 °C, actively growing, 6- to 24-hour-old broth culture.
    - Place one drop of culture into the center of a coverslip.
    - Place one drop of immersion oil on each corner of the coverslip.
    - Place a depression slide on top of the coverslip, allowing the corners to seal, and invert the slide with the coverslip on top and the sample in the convex portion of the slide.
    - Examine with the 40× objective.
- **Positive:** true motility — organisms change position in respect to one another, commonly darting across the field.
- **Negative:** organisms appear active, but they remain in the same position relative to other organisms and debris,

- Semisolid agar:
  - Using a straight needle, touch an 18- to 24-hour old colony growing on agar medium.
  - Stab a needle 1/3 to 1/2 of the depth of the agar in the middle of the tube.
  - Incubate 35–37 °C, and examine daily for up to 7 days.
- **Positive:** from the site of inoculation, organisms will spread out into the medium.
- **Negative:** organisms will remain at the site of inoculation.

X and V Factors

X and V factor testing is done to aid in the identification and differentiation of *Haemophilus* species based on the organisms' use of the growth factors. X factor consists of hemin, whereas V factor is composed of NAD. *H. influenzae* is the most important organism identified by this test because it can cause meningitis and pneumonia.

This test begins with a light suspension of organism in saline. A sterile swab is dipped into the suspension and rolled across the surface of a trypticase soy agar plate. X, V, and XV factor disks are placed 4–5 cm apart on the agar's surface. The agar is incubated at 35 °C, and organism growth is observed and evaluated the next day:

- **Positive**:
  - X and V: growth around the XV disk only
  - V factor: growth around the V disk, light growth around the XV disk, and no growth around the X disk
  - X factor: growth around the X disk, light growth around the XV disk, and no growth around the V disk
- **Negative:** growth over the entire surface of the agar

Commercial Kits Used in Microbiology Testing

Commercial test kits are used for the rapid detection of various microbiologic pathogens. The following methodologies are commonly used:

- **Latex agglutination** kits allow for qualitative and semiquantitative evaluation of virulent organisms such as meningitis-causing *Cryptococcus*. Reagent latex beads are coated in organism-specific antibodies and are then combined with the patient sample. Agglutination between reagent antibodies and organism surface antigens represents the presence of the organism in question.
- **Monoclonal antibody** test kits are also used in microbiology testing for antigens produced by *H. pylori* or toxins given off by toxigenic *C. difficile.* If the target organism or toxin is present in a sample, it will attach to reagent antibodies imbedded in the test cartridge. The antigen–antibody complex formed will migrate to the test window and produce a colored line.

Automated Testing Methods Used in Microbiology Labs

Automated systems are used in microbiology for blood culture monitoring, organism identification, and antibiotic susceptibility testing. Incubated systems continuously monitor blood culture bottles for chemical reactions that indicate bacterial growth. Carbon dioxide (CO_2) generation is indicative of bacterial growth in blood culture bottles, and automated systems will alert of a positive blood culture when a specific CO_2 threshold is passed. Organism identification and antibiotic susceptibility testing are achieved with instrumentation comprised of the following components: incubator, automated reader, data terminal, printer, and the ability to be connected to the LIS.

Panels used for these systems are plastic trays with microwells coated in biochemical or antibiotic-specific reagents that are inoculated with a suspension of bacteria. Panels are available based on organism Gram stains and growth requirements to optimize the identification of an isolate. Turbidity, colorimetry, and fluorescent or matrix-assisted laser desorption ionization time-of-flight mass spectrometry (MALDI-TOF MS) methods are used to determine biochemical reactions that are compared to those of known isolates in the instrument's computerized database. Automated systems allow for rapid and confident identification of pathogens.

Automated specimen processing and total automation systems have been developed for the microbiology laboratory, with conveyors, streaking mechanisms, and incubators, among other technologies. However, automated systems rely on classic time-consuming culture techniques and require extensive knowledge for handling the various types of microbiological specimens.

Matrix-Assisted Laser Desorption Ionization Time-of-Flight Mass Spectrometry

Matrix-assisted laser desorption ionization time-of-flight mass spectrometry (MALDI-TOF MS) provides microbial identification and characterization in a fast, precise, and cost-effective manner. MALDI-TOF MS allows for organism identification even in a mixed colony culture, but it does not provide antibiotic susceptibility information.

This method is divided into two phases: ionization and time of flight. Ionization consists of a sample being fixed to a crystalline matrix and bombarded by a laser. The laser vaporizes molecules into a vacuum and ionizes without decomposing or fragmenting them. The TOF MS phase of the process separates ions based on their mass-to-charge ratio and determines the time that each molecule takes to reach a detector. Molecular patterns are profiled and compared to profiles of known microbes to identify and characterize an organism.

Multiplex Molecular Methods

Multiplex molecular methods allow for testing of multiple pathogens at the same time aiding in detecting infections that may otherwise go undiagnosed. PCR molecular methodology is used with the presence of multiple primer pairs specific to various bacteria, viruses, and parasites. A primer for each pathogen in a multiplex system is 18–22 base pairs in size, establishes specificity for the pathogen, and requires primers of similar melting points for the best results. The detection and amplification of multiple targets in one test cycle are advantageous for microbiology testing by requiring a smaller sample and less time to diagnose a patient and begin appropriate care. Most commonly, multiplex systems are used in the detection of respiratory or gastrointestinal pathogens that are highly contagious and are difficult to differentiate from one another based on their clinical signs and symptoms.

Antimicrobial Susceptibility Testing and Antibiotic Resistance

Antimicrobial Susceptibility and Resistance Testing

Antimicrobial susceptibility and antibiotic resistance testing is required to find the correct agent and the appropriate concentration to eliminate a bacterial infection. The most commonly used testing methods are dilutions and disk diffusion, but automated methods are also widely available and used. If automated methods are unclear or raise questions, traditional diffusion and dilution methods are used to clarify any discrepancies. **Broth dilution** methods require multiple tubes containing varying concentrations of antibiotics with a suspension of the test isolate added. Organism growth in each dilution is observed for the determination of minimum inhibitory concentration (MIC) and minimum bactericidal concentration. The **MIC** is the lowest concentration of drug necessary to inhibit organism growth and multiplication. The lowest concentration of a drug that will result in the death of a bacterial population is known as the **minimum bactericidal concentration. Disk diffusion** methods determine antibiotic resistance or susceptibility by observing the zone of bacterial growth inhibition surrounding antibiotic-impregnated disks on culture media. A result of no bacterial growth, or **susceptible**, indicates that the organism will most likely will respond to treatment with the agent. **Intermediate** growth indicates that a high dose of agent may be necessary for successful treatment, whereas no zone of inhibition indicates antibiotic **resistance** and that treatment with an agent will most likely fail. Antimicrobial susceptibility and antibiotic resistance testing is an important step in the process of treating patient infections, and the tests in vivo are an estimate of the effectiveness that the agent will have against an organism in vivo.

Phenotypic Detection of Resistance

Beta-Lactamase

The **beta-lactamase**, or **nitrocefin, test** is a rapid method that detects the presence of beta-lactamase enzyme production in strains of *S. aureus, N. gonorrhoeae, Moraxella. catarrhalis,* and *H. influenzae.* Beta-lactamase enzymes hydrolyze the beta-lactam rings of penicillin and cephalosporin antibiotics, rendering them inactive. This method uses paper disks impregnated with nitrocefin, a chromogenic cephalosporin that changes color when the amide bond in the beta-lactam ring is hydrolyzed by the enzyme. The procedure and interpretation of beta-lactamase phenotype testing are described below:

- Procedure
  - Using sterile forceps, place a nitrocefin disk on an empty petri dish or microscope slide.
  - Allow the disk to come to room temperature.
  - Moisten the disk with one drop of sterile deionized water.
  - Use a sterilized loop of applicator stick to remove an isolated colony and spread it on the surface of the disk.
  - Observe the disk for the development of color.
- Interpretation
  - **Positive**, penicillin and cephalosporin resistance: red-orange color
  - **Negative**, penicillin and cephalosporin susceptible: yellow color.

Extended-Spectrum Beta-Lactamases (ESBLs)

Extended spectrum beta-lactamase (ESBL)-producing strains of *Escherichia* and *Klebsiella* organisms are detected by the **double-disk synergy method**. Organisms possessing the ESBL enzyme are able to hydrolyze the oxyimino side chain of extended-spectrum cephalosporins, rendering them inactive. Therefore, antibiotic options for the treatment of infections caused by these organisms are extremely limited, with carbapenems being the antimicrobial of choice. The procedure and interpretation of double-disk synergy testing for ESBL detection are described below:

- Procedure:
  - Prepare a 0.5 McFarland standard suspension with an ESBL-suspected isolate.
  - Inoculate the entire surface of a Mueller–Hinton agar plate with the suspension.
  - Place a disk impregnated with the third-generation cephalosporin cefotaxime in the middle of the plate.
  - Place an amoxicillin/clavulanate-impregnated disk on the agar roughly 20 mm from the cefotaxime disk.
  - Incubate for 16–18 hours at 37 °C.

- Interpretation:
  - **Positive, extended-spectrum cephalosporin-resistant**: zone of inhibition around the ceftazidime disk expanded by and in the direction of the clavulanate disk
  - **Negative, extended-spectrum cephalosporin-susceptible**: no expanded zone of inhibition

Inducible Clindamycin Resistance

The **inducible clindamycin resistance test**, or **D test**, is used to detect inducible clindamycin resistance in strains of *S. aureus* that were clindamycin sensitive and erythromycin resistant. These strains possess enzymes that have the capability to induce resistance during antimicrobial therapy. Routine antibiotic susceptibility testing is unable to detect these strains and may cause a failure in the clinical treatment of MRSA infections. The D test is a disk diffusion method that is able to detect inducible resistance prior to beginning antimicrobial therapy. The D test procedure and interpretation of results are described below:

- Procedure:
  - Prepare a 0.5 McFarland standard suspension with erythromycin-resistant *S. aureus* isolates.
  - Inoculate the entire surface of a Mueller–Hinton agar plate with the suspension.
  - Place a clindamycin disk and an erythromycin disk 15–20 mm apart in the center of the plate.
  - Incubate for 16–18 hours at 37 °C.
- Interpretation:
  - **D phenotype (D+):** a blunt, D-shaped zone of inhibition around the clindamycin disk
  - **Noninduction phenotypes (negative):** a clear, circular zone of inhibition around the clindamycin disk.

Carbapenamases

The **modified Hodge test** detects pathogens possessing the beta-lactamase enzyme, carbapenemase, that inactivates carbapenem and all other beta-lactam antibiotics. Infections caused by carbapenem-resistant *Enterobacteriaceae* (CRE) bacteria are extremely dangerous, and detection is necessary for effective treatment. The principle of this test is based on a carbapenemase-producing test isolate's ability to enable the carbapenem susceptible indictor organism to expand its growth along the test isolate inoculum steak. The modified Hodge test procedure and interpretation of results are described below:

- Procedure:
  - Prepare a 0.5 McFarland standard suspension of the following:
    - Known, indicator organism, *E. coli*
    - Suspected CRE test isolate
    - CRE-positive quality control organism
    - CRE-negative quality control organism
  - With sterile saline, make a 1:10 dilution of the indicator organism.
  - Inoculate the entire surface of a Mueller–Hinton agar plate with the diluted indicator suspension and allow it to dry for 3–5 minutes.
  - Place a 10 µg meropenem- or ertapenem-impregnated disk in the center of the agar.
  - Streak the test isolate suspension in a straight line from the edge of the disk to the edge of the plate. Repeat this step with each quality-control organism.
  - Incubate for 16–24 hours at 37 °C.

- Interpretation:
  - **Positive, carbapenem resistant**: *E. coli* growth presents with a clover leaf-like indentation at the intersection of the test isolate and *E. coli* in the disk zone of inhibition.
  - **Negative, carbapenem susceptible:** no *E. coli* growth along the test organism streak in the disk diffusion zone.

Detection Methods for Genetic Determinants of Antimicrobial Resistance

Detecting genes with known antibiotic resistant properties is most commonly accomplished with PCR testing, but other molecular methods may be used as well. Genetic determination for drug resistance must be coupled with phenotypic assays to determine the level or extent of resistance present. Below are the test methods used for the genetic detection of drug resistance in pathogenic organisms:

- **mecA** — MRSA
  - **PCR** with gene-specific primers and probes
  - **Enzymatic detection PCR**: enzyme-labeled PCR gene probes are detected by immunosorbent assays
- **vanA** — resistance to high levels of vancomycin
  - **PCR** with gene-specific primers and probes
  - **Pulse-field gel electrophoresis:** separates organism DNA, pattern produced in gel determines the presence or absence of a gene
  - **Multilocus enzyme electrophoresis**: specific proteins are separated in gel, and a probe detects the presence of absence of the proteins
- **blaKPC** — beta-lactamase gene from *K. pneumoniae*
  - **Real-time PCR with fluorescent-labeled probe**: PCR amplification with forward and reverse primers, hybridization of gene DNA, if present, fluorescent probe allows for detection by real-time PCR.

Patterns of Intrinsic Antibiotic Resistance Exhibited by Common Pathogens

Intrinsic resistance to an antibiotic or family of antibiotics occurs naturally in certain organisms without the need for genetic mutation or the acquisition of genes. Naturally occurring mechanisms that induce antibiotic resistance include reduced outer membrane permeability by porins, efflux pumps actively pumping antibiotics out of the bacterial cell, and enzymes inactivating the drug. **Porins** act as pores in the cell wall membrane, allowing molecules in and out of the cell. The size and number of porins present in bacterial cell walls can exclude the entrance of certain sized antibiotic molecules. The structural difference between Gram-positive and Gram-negative organisms' cell walls acts as an intrinsic resistance to penicillin and glycoprotein activity in Gram-negative bacteria because larger molecules cannot pass through the cell wall. Gram-negative bacteria also have **efflux pumps** inside the cell that actively pump out antibiotics that have entered the cell. Through actively removing drugs from the cell, agents are not able to reach the appropriate bactericidal concentration, rendering them ineffective. Gram-negative bacteria use a combination of these mechanisms to cause resistance to different antibiotics.

Examples of common pathogens exhibiting patterns of intrinsic resistance are listed below:

- *E. coli*
  - AcrAB-TolC:
    - active efflux and inactivation of beta-lactams by beta-lactamase
    - active efflux and limited uptake of tetracyclines and chloramphenicol
    - active efflux, modified target, and limited uptake of fluoroquinolones
- *P. aeruginosa*
  - mexAB, mexXY: multidrug-resisting efflux pumps
- *K. pneumoniae*
  - inactivation of beta-lactams by beta-lactamase and plasmids

MRSA/MSSA, VRE, ESBL/CRE Screening

Specimen Sources

Screening for the colonization of antibiotic-resistant bacteria is common for patients in healthcare facilities. Colonization occurs when the potential pathogen resides in the body with no present signs or symptoms of infection. Patients colonized with these bacteria are at increased risk for severe antibiotic-resistant infections. Resistant bacteria also have the potential to spread from patient to patient in healthcare facilities on the hands of healthcare workers and visitors, body fluids, or contaminated objects and surfaces. Appropriate specimens for the screening of common multidrug-resistant bacteria colonization are described below:

- **Swab of the left and right nares** because staphylococcus bacteria often colonize in the mucous membranes of the nose
  - Methicillin-resistant *S. aureus* **(MRSA)** and methicillin-sensitive *S. aureus* **(MSSA)**
- **Rectal swab** because these bacteria survive and colonize in the gastrointestinal tract
  - Vancomycin-resistant *Enterococci* **(VRE)**
  - Extended-spectrum beta-lactamases **(ESBLs)**
  - Carbapenem-resistant *Enterobacteriaceae* **(CRE)**

Culture Methods

Culture methods available for the screening and detection of antibiotic-resistant organisms use a combination of selective media and antibiotic-impregnated agar or disks. **Chromogenic agar** is a selective media containing nutrients and inhibitors specific to the cultivation of the target organism. If present, target organism colonies can easily be recognized by their color. Culture methods for common antibiotic-resistant organisms are described below:

- MRSA/MSSA
  - **Oxacillin disk on Mueller–Hinton agar**: MRSA exhibits a zone of inhibition ≤10 mm from the disk.
  - Chromogenic agar

- VRE
  - **Bile esculin azide agar with 6µg/mL of vancomycin and confirmatory MIC:** growth of *Enterococci* colonies indicates vancomycin resistance. Colonies appear black on the agar and require MIC testing to confirm resistance.
  - **Brain heart infusion agar with 6 µg/mL of vancomycin:** requires suspension of pure isolate colonies, no bacterial growth after 24 hours of incubation detects vancomycin susceptibility, any bacterial growth confirms resistance.
- ESBL
  - **Third-generation cephalosporin and clavulanic acid disks on Mueller–Hinton agar**: in the presence of clavulanic acid, ESBL organisms will present an increased zone of inhibition on agar.
- CRE
  - Chromogenic agar

Antibiotic Resistant Bacteria

Antibiotic-resistant bacterial infections can be acquired in the community or in a hospital setting. Hospital-acquired infections are linked to a variety of sources and modes of transmission including the following:

- Surgical or invasive device implantation site
- Central line-associated bloodstream infections
- Catheter-associated UTIs
- Ventilator-associated pneumonia
- Contact with healthcare workers' or visitors' contaminated hands.

These bacteria inhabit parts of the body as normal flora and become pathogens when they are introduced to parts of the body where they don't normally reside. MRSA and MSSA organisms are normally found as commensal organisms on the surface of the skin and mucous membranes, whereas VRE, ESBL, and CRE can colonize in the gastrointestinal tract without causing infection. These bacteria possess all of the virulence factors associated with their antibiotic susceptible strains, as well as genetic mutations and enzymes that resist commonly used antibiotic therapy. Resistance to antibiotics is a growing concern as treating such infections becomes increasingly more difficult.

Biosafety Level 3 Pathogens and Select Agents (Bioterrorism)

Specimen Sources of Biosafety Level 3 Pathogens and Agents of Bioterrorism

Biosafety level 3 pathogens are agents that have the potential to cause serious or fatal disease when aerosols are inhaled into the body. Specimens suspected of being biosafety level 3 pathogens require handling under a biological safety cabinet with engineering features to control air movement. Common biosafety level 3 pathogens include tuberculosis and the mold stages of systemic fungi. Specimen sources include sputum and blood.

Specimens suspected of containing agents of bioterrorism must be handled with extreme care and following strict protocols to ensure public safety. Agents of bioterrorism can be recovered in the following clinical specimens:

- Fluid and tissue from cutaneous lesions
- Stool
- Blood
- Sputum

Bacillus Anthracis

Bacillus anthracis react and present in the following ways:

- **Biochemical reactions:**

Catalase	+
Oxidase	–
Urease	–
TSI	K/K
H_2S	–
Motility	–
Indole	+
Nitrate reduction	+

- **Gram stain:** Gram-positive spore-forming bacilli in a long chain, resembling bamboo shoots
- **Growth requirements:** aerobic, and facultative anaerobe, grow best at 35–37 °C
- **Colony morphology:** nonhemolytic, dry, ground glass surface, with irregular edges, and comma protrusions called "Medusa head" on sheep blood agar
- **Rapid test**: RedLine Alert Test — FDA-approved immunochromatographic kit test for presumptive *B. anthracis* identification from suspicious bacterial colonies grown on sheep blood agar.

Yersinia Pestis

Yersinia pestis react and present in the following ways:

- **Biochemical reactions:**

Oxidase	–
Urease	–
Catalase	+
Indole	–
TSI	K/A

- **Gram stain**: Gram-negative bacilli with bipolar staining, resembling a safety pin.
- **Growth requirements**: aerobic and facultative anaerobe, grow best at 25–30 °C.
- **Colony morphology**: pinpoint growth at 24 hours, and rough, cauliflower appearance at 48 hours on sheep blood agar. Colonies are colorless to peach on MacConkey, salmon colored on Hektoen agar, and colorless to yellow on XLD agar.
- **Rapid test**: Presumptive identification of *Y. pestis* can be determined with ELISA or immunochromatographic methodologies that detect a capsular antigen specific to the organism.

Brucella Species

Brucella species react and present in the following ways:

- **Biochemical reactions:**

Oxidase	+
Urease	+
Nitrate	+
Motility	−

- **Gram stain**: Gram-negative coccobacilli, resembling grains of sand.
- **Growth requirements**: aerobic, facultative intracellular parasite, grow best at 37 °C in 5–10% CO_2. Cultures must be incubated for 21–30 days to confirm negative.
- **Colony morphology**: small, smooth, convex, translucent to opaque, nonhemolytic on sheep blood agar. Colonies appear yellow, but they may turn brown as they age.
- **Rapid test**: a particle agglutination test with a positive *Brucella* antibody titer of 1:160 or greater is used as a presumptive identification.

Francisella Tularensis

Francisella tularensis react and present in the following ways:

- **Biochemical reactions:**

Oxidase	−
Urease	−
Catalase	weak +
Beta-lactamase	+
H_2S with lead acetate	+

- **Gram stain**: faint staining, Gram-negative pleomorphic coccobacilli
- **Growth requirements**: strict aerobe, requires cysteine for optimal growth at 35–37 °C
- **Colony morphology**: tiny, gray-white on chocolate agar and small, green-blue colonies on cysteine heart agar after 48 hours of growth
- **Rapid test**: fluorescent antibody stains, immunohistological stains, and antibody agglutination tests are available for the identification of *F. tularensis.*

Roles of Laboratory Response Network and Regional Laboratories Regarding Agents of Bioterrorism

Established by the Centers for Disease Control and Prevention, the **Laboratory Response Network** is a group of laboratories capable of properly responding to biological and chemical threats and other public health emergencies. The Laboratory Response Network is composed of labs from the following sectors: federal, state and local public health, military, food testing, veterinary, environmental, and international. This network allows for the best preparedness and response to biological and chemical terrorism.

Samples suspected of containing biological toxins or microbiological agents that threaten public health are most commonly found or recognized at sentinel laboratories. A **sentinel laboratory** is the foundation of the Laboratory Response Network and is defined as any laboratory capable of detecting and referring chemical or microbial agents. The most common sentinel laboratories include critical access and larger hospital, environmental, food testing, and veterinary labs. Once a threatening agent is recognized and all other organisms have been ruled out, samples are referred to state or local public reference laboratories for confirmation testing. Upon confirmation, regional and public health laboratories are responsible for reporting and referring confirmed bioterrorism agents to the CDC for sample characterization and further investigation.

Analytic Procedures—Mycology, Mycobacteriology, Parasitology, and Virology

Mycobacterium and *Nocardia* Species Testing

Mycobacterium and *Nocardia* species of bacteria are capable of causing a variety of disease states including pulmonary infections and infections of the subcutaneous tissue. The most common specimen collected for pulmonary infections due to these bacteria is **sputum**. First morning sputum samples collected on three consecutive days are ideal for detecting infections caused by these bacteria. **Bronchial** or **gastric washings**, **urine**, and **tissue** samples are also acceptable for *Mycobacterium* and *Nocardia* species recovery. All specimens suspected of such infections should be collected aseptically into sterile, tight-capped containers and transported to the lab as soon as possible. Urine and gastric samples may be refrigerated prior to testing, if needed, to neutralize their acidity.

Acid-Fast Reaction, Growth Patterns, and Colony Morphology for Mycobacterium and Nocardia Species Testing

Listed below are the acid-fast reaction, growth patterns, and colony morphology characteristics of *Mycobacterium* and *Nocardia* species on Löwenstein–Jensen culture media:

- *M. tuberculosis*
  - **Acid-fast:** positive, bright red
  - **Growth pattern:** obligate aerobe, enhanced growth in 5–10% CO_2, visible growth after 3–6 weeks of incubation
  - **Colony morphology:** off white to buff, dry, rough, raised, and wrinkled
- *M. leprae*
  - **Acid-fast:** positive, bright red
  - Growth pattern and colony morphology: cannot be cultivated in vitro
- *M. avium*
  - **Acid-fast:** positive, bright red
  - **Growth pattern:** aerobe, enhanced growth in 5–10% CO_2, visible growth after 3–6 weeks of incubation
  - Colony morphology: buff and smooth
- *Nocardia* species
  - **Acid-fast:** partial, pink, filamentous morphology with branching
  - **Growth pattern:** aerobe, enhanced growth in 5–10% CO_2, visible growth after 3–10 days of incubation
  - **Colony morphology:** yellow to orange, waxy, bumpy, or velvety, with downy aerial hyphae.

Mycobacterium and Nocardia Pathogens

Mycobacteria and *Nocardia* infections occur in immunocompromised patients. These bacteria are opportunistic pathogens that occur naturally in soil, water, and the following sources: ***M. tuberculosis,*** dust, carpets, clothes, unpasteurized milk; ***M. leprae,*** human peripheral nerves; ***M.***

avium, food; and ***Nocardia***, normal human oral flora. The pathogen transmission, clinical presentation, and epidemiology are described below:

- ***M. tuberculosis*** infects approximately one-third of the world's population via respiratory droplet inhalation. Although many patients remain asymptomatic, immunocompromised patients with active tuberculosis exhibit the following symptoms: fever, weight loss, night sweats, weakness, chest pains, and a cough producing sputum and blood. Infections present in three stages: **primary**, active inflammation and granuloma formation that resolves; **latent**, residual bacteria exist in the body; and **postprimary**, dormant bacteria reactivate in the upper lobes of the lungs.
- ***M. leprae*** causes Hansen's disease, or leprosy, to the skin, mucous membranes, and nerves of those infected. Leprosy is transmittable via inhalation of bacteria or contact with exudates of lesions. Although *M. leprae* has low pathogenicity, clinical manifestations of the disease may become severe and appear after 6 months to more than 40 years of incubation.
- ***M. avium*** is transmittable through inhalation or consumption of contaminants and is not infectious to most. In severely immunocompromised hosts, *M. avium* causes lymphadenitis or pulmonary and disseminated disease.
- ***Nocardia asteroides*** and ***N. brasiliensis*** cause nocardiosis. Infections to healthy hosts occur as skin abscesses, cellulitis, or lymphocutaneous via traumatic inoculation of subcutaneous tissues. Bacterial inhalation causes progressive pneumonia and disseminated disease in immunocompromised patients.

Detection of Mycobacterium and Nocardia Species

Direct detection methods of *Mycobacterium* and *Nocardia* organisms include microscopic examination with specialized stains and molecular methodologies. Acid-fast stains for clinical specimens colorize bacteria based on the presence or absence of mycolic acid in the bacterial cell wall. **Ziehl–Neelsen** and **Kinyoun** stains are used to observe acid-fast bacteria using a light microscope, whereas **auramine-rhodamine** stain requires a fluorescent microscope. Samples containing mycobacteria will show bright-red bacilli using Ziehl–Neelsen and Kinyoun stains and will fluoresce a yellow to orange color when stained with auramine-rhodamine. The microscopic observation of acid-fast bacilli in any number is considered significant and requires further workup. **Nucleic acid probe** methods can be used to detect the presence of *M. tuberculosis* and *M. avium* genetic material in bacterial colonies grown on culture media. Molecular detection of *M. tuberculosis* directly from clinical specimens can be achieved by using **nucleic acid amplification testing** methods.

Virology Testing

Virology samples should be collected as soon as possible after a patient begins to exhibit signs and symptoms of an infection due to a viral agent. Specimens from various sources and in a variety of transport or preservation media can be submitted for testing. Acceptable specimen sources and special requirements that allow for viral testing are described below:

- Respiratory specimens:
    - **Nasopharyngeal and throat swabs**: easily accessible, acceptable but often contaminated with normal oral flora organisms
    - **Nasopharyngeal aspirates:** improved recovery of viruses versus nasopharyngeal and throat swabs
    - **Bronchial lavages and washings:** ideal for detection of lower respiratory tract viruses.

- **Stool or rectal swabs**: detection of enteric viruses including rotavirus and adenovirus, stool preferred over swabs.
- **Urine**: low numbers of certain viruses are detectable; requires three separate first-morning-void, clean-catch specimens up to 10 mL each. Centrifugation and pH neutralization of urine are recommended prior to testing to avoid bacterial and pH contamination.
- **Sterile body fluids and tissues:** sent to the laboratory in sterile containers with a secure lid.
- **Fluid or cells from skin or cervical lesions collected on a swab:** require transport media to maintain viral integrity. Transport media contain antibiotics to avoid bacterial growth and contamination, and they contain fetal calf serum or albumin as a source of nutrients.

Parasitology

Specimens and Preservation Methods for Parasitology Testing

Stool is the most common parasite specimen collected. Samples must be collected into a clean, dry container with a secure lid, and they must not be contaminated by urine, water, or enemas. Contamination from urine has the ability to destroy motile organisms, water may contain free living organisms, and protozoa may not be detectable for 5–10 days following the administration of barium enemas. Recovery of parasites may be hindered up to 2 weeks after the cessation of certain antibiotics. The most concentrated, early morning and first-void **sputum** and **urine** specimens are collected into dry, sterile containers with a secure lid. **Genital swabs** submitted for parasitic detection require saline to keep them moist for optimal organism recovery. **Skin** and **tissue** samples are best submitted to the laboratory in dry, sterile containers with a secure lid. Fresh **blood** from a fingerstick is the preferred sample for thick and thin blood smear preparations; however, blood collection via venipuncture into an EDTA tube is also acceptable.

Methods of sample storage and preservation based on the type of parasite suspected are as follows:

- **Refrigeration:** eggs, larvae, and amoebic cysts. If amoebic trophozoites are suspected, do not refrigerate.
- 10% formalin and merthiolate-iodine-formalin: eggs, larvae, and amoebic cysts.
- **Polyvinyl alcohol (PVA):** amoebic trophozoites; stained specimen slides can be permanently preserved using this method.
- **Sodium acetate-acetic acid-formalin:** amoebic trophozoites; an environmentally safer alternative to PVA.
- **Schaudinn's fluid:** trophs and cysts, fixative for fresh stool samples.

Pathogenic Helminths

Parasitic worms occur naturally in soil. The route of transmission, epidemiology, and disease states associated with helminths are described below:

- **Large intestinal roundworm**, *Ascaris lumbricoides*
  - **Transmission:** fecal–oral route
  - **Epidemiology:** tropical climate and poor sanitation
  - Life cycle:
    - Eggs hatch in the duodenum and penetrate the intestinal wall.
    - Adults live and reproduce in the small intestine.
    - Eggs are passed in feces remain active in soil for 2–6 weeks.
  - **Disease:** intestinal obstruction and pneumonitis caused by larvae migration to lungs

- **Pinworm,** Enterobius vermicularis
  - **Transmission:** fecal–oral route
  - **Epidemiology:** school-age children
  - Life cycle:
    - Adult female matures in the small intestine, incubating for 1–2 months.
    - Migrates to colon, lays eggs around the anus at night.
    - Reinfection and infecting others are possible by contact as long as eggs are laid.
  - **Disease:** itchy anal region and associated secondary bacterial infection
- **Whipworm,** Trichuris trichiura
  - **Transmission:** fecal–oral route
  - **Epidemiology:** tropical climate and poor sanitation
  - Life cycle:
    - Eggs hatch in the small intestine.
    - Adult worms live and reproduce in the large intestine for 3 months after ingestion.
  - **Disease:** bloody, mucous diarrhea and prolapsed rectum in heavy infection
- **New World hookworm,** *Necator americanus,* and **Old World hookworm,** *Ancylostoma duodenale*
  - **Transmission:** skin penetration
  - **Epidemiology:** worldwide distribution
  - Life cycle:
    - Larvae move to the lungs via the venous system; they are coughed up and swallowed.
    - Adult worms live and reproduce attached to the small intestinal wall.
  - **Disease:** life cycle-associated
    - Cutaneous — allergic reactions or "ground itch"
    - Pulmonary — pneumonitis
    - Intestinal — anemia and protein deficiency from blood loss at the attachment site.

Blood and Tissue Microfilariae and Nematode Pathogens

The etiology, epidemiology, transmission, and diseases of blood and tissue nematodes and microfilariae are described below:

- **Pork worm,** Trichinella spiralis
  - **Transmission:** Ingesting larvae in undercooked pork.
  - **Etiology and epidemiology:** Worldwide, rural areas, survival requires a host: rodents, domestic pigs, wild boars, other mammals.
  - Life cycle:
    - Encysted larvae are ingested, and they mature over several weeks in the small intestine.
    - Adults produce larvae that migrate through tissues and muscle.
  - **Disease:** resembles food poisoning, muscle cell destruction, eosinophilia, possible myocardial involvement.
  - **Microfilariae,** early life stage nematodes — an arthropod intermediate host is required. Vectors introduce third-stage filarial larvae that penetrate into human skin via bite wounds during blood feedings.

- *Wuchereria bancrofti*
  - **Vector:** Anopheles, *Culex* mosquitoes
  - Epidemiology: Worldwide
  - Life cycle:
    - ❖ Adults live and reproduce in the lymphatic system.
    - ❖ Microfilariae migrate through lymph and blood channels.
  - **Disease:** elephantiasis — permanent lymphatic blockage, genitalia and lower extremities
- **Eye worm**, *Loa Loa*
  - **Vector:** Chrysops (deer) fly
  - **Epidemiology:** West and Central Africa
  - Life cycle:
    - ❖ Adults live and reproduce in subcutaneous tissues.
    - ❖ Microfilariae in peripheral blood during the day and the lungs at night.
  - **Disease:** "caliber swelling" — localized swelling, with itching on arms, legs, and near joints; blindness
- *Onchocerca volvulus*
  - **Vector:** Simulium (black) fly
  - **Epidemiology:** "river blindness" leading cause of blindness in Africa
  - Life cycle:
    - ❖ Adults live and reproduce in subcutaneous connective tissue for 10–15 years.
    - ❖ Microfilariae in the skin and connective tissues lymphatics.
  - **Disease:** severe dermatitis, blindness, onchocercoma — nodule containing an encapsulated adult.

Cestode Parasitic Pathogens

The etiology, epidemiology, transmission, and diseases of tapeworms are described below:

- **Beef tapeworm**, *Taenia saginata*
  - **Transmission:** ingestion of larvae in undercooked beef
  - **Etiology and epidemiology:** common in Eastern Europe, Russia, Eastern Africa, and Latin America; poor sanitation; free-ranging cattle
  - Life cycle:
    - ❖ Eggs enter the environment by infected human feces.
    - ❖ Livestock eat vegetation with eggs that migrate to striated muscle and become cysticerci, where they can be ingested by humans in undercooked meat.
    - ❖ Cysticerci attach to the small intestine.
  - **Disease:** taeniasis — abdominal pain, loss of appetite, weight loss
- **Pork tapeworm**, *Taenia solium*
  - **Transmission:** ingestion of larvae in undercooked pork
  - **Etiology and epidemiology:** highest infection rates are in Latin America, Asia, and Africa; poor sanitation; free-ranging pigs
  - **Life cycle:** the same as *T. saginata*
  - **Disease:** cysticercosis — rare, larval cysts in the brain and muscles, causing seizures

- **Dwarf tapeworm,** *Hymenolepis nana*
  - **Transmission**: ingestion of eggs
  - **Etiology and epidemiology:** the most common tapeworm in the US
  - Life cycle:
    - Eggs passed in human feces survive for 10 days in the environment.
    - Eggs are ingested by a beetle or flea intermediate host and develop into cysticercoids that are ingested by humans or rodents.
    - Adults mature, reside, and reproduce in the small intestine.
  - **Disease:** most asymptomatic, heavy infections are due to autoinfection — weakness, headache, abdominal pain, diarrhea, anorexia.

Trematode and Protozoa Parasitic Pathogens

Pathogenic parasite etiology, epidemiology, transmission, and diseases are described below:

- ***Schistosomes***, blood flukes
  - **Transmission:** free-swimming cercariae are released from the snail into the water and penetrate the skin
  - **Etiology and epidemiology:** found in the Western Hemisphere, not the US — snail host not present
  - Disease:
    - "Swimmer's itch" — dermatitis
    - Eosinophilia, bloody urine and diarrhea
    - Progressive chronic inflammatory disease involving the liver, intestines, and bladder
- ***Entamoeba histolytica***
  - **Transmission:** fecal–oral, ingestion of contaminated food or water
  - **Etiology and epidemiology:** most common in tropical climates and poor sanitation
  - **Disease:** amebiasis — intestinal tract ulcers, liver and lung abscesses
- ***Giardia lamblia***
  - **Transmission:** fecal–oral; ingestion of contaminated drinking or recreational water is the most common mode of transmission
  - **Etiology and epidemiology:** distributed worldwide in water, soil food, or on surfaces; common in daycare centers and in acquired immunodeficiency syndrome (AIDS) patients
  - **Disease:** giardiasis-diarrhea, duodenitis, malabsorption of fats
- ***Plasmodium* species**
  - **Transmission:** bloodstream inoculated via bite of female *Anopheles* mosquito
  - **Etiology and epidemiology:** most associated with low altitude, tropical and subtropical climates. *P. falciparum* — predominant species worldwide
  - **Disease:** nonspecific symptoms — fever, chills, headache, myalgia, weakness, vomiting, diarrhea, splenomegaly, anemia, hypoglycemia, pulmonary or renal dysfunction, neurologic changes
    - ***P. vivax*** — benign tertian
    - ***P. ovale*** — tertian malaria
    - ***P. falciparum*** — malignant tertian malaria, blackwater fever
    - ***P. malariae*** — quartan malaria.

- ***Babesia microti***
  - **Transmission:** bloodstream inoculated via deer tick bite or transmitted during blood transfusions
  - **Etiology and epidemiology:** most common in the Northeastern and Upper Midwestern US; no geographical limit on transmission via blood transfusion
  - **Disease:** babesiosis — fever, fatigue, myalgia, GI symptoms, dark urine, mild splenomegaly or hepatomegaly, jaundice.

Protozoa Parasitic Pathogens

The etiology, epidemiology, transmission, and diseases of protozoa are described below:

- ***Trypanosoma cruzi***
  - **Transmission**: feces of an infected "kissing bug" is scratched or rubbed into its bite wound on humans, also transmittable by blood transfusion
  - **Etiology and epidemiology:** North and South America, mainly rural Latin America
  - **Disease:** Chagas' disease
    - ❖ **Acute** — asymptomatic or mild fever and swelling around the inoculation site
    - ❖ **Chronic** — arrhythmias, poorly pumping heart, dilated esophagus or colon causing issues eating or passing stool
- ***Leishmania***
  - **Transmission:** released into human via bite of infected sandfly
  - **Etiology and epidemiology:** New World disease found in Asia, the Middle East, Africa, and Southern Europe. Old World disease found in Mexico and Central and South America. It does not occur in Australia, the Pacific Islands, Chile, or Uruguay.
  - **Disease:** cutaneous leishmaniasis
    - ❖ ***Leishmania donovani*** — visceral leishmaniasis (kala-azar), fever, weight loss, hepatosplenomegaly
    - ❖ ***L. tropica*** — Old World cutaneous leishmaniasis, also known as Oriental sore, skin sores
    - ❖ ***L. braziliensis*** — New World cutaneous or mucocutaneous; sores in the nose, mouth, or throat
- ***Cryptosporidium parvum***
  - **Transmission:** fecal–oral, ingestion of contaminated drinking or recreational water is the most common mode of transmission
  - **Etiology and epidemiology:** most common cause of waterborne disease in the US
  - **Disease:** Cryptosporidiosis
    - ❖ **Immunocompetent host** — asymptomatic or self-limiting, watery diarrhea, vomiting, abdominal cramps
    - ❖ **Immunocompromised host** — symptoms listed above, severe diarrhea, can also affect other parts of the GI tract or the respiratory tract.

Microscopic Observation and Identification of Parasites

Ova and parasites are identified microscopically by key characteristics using a variety of stains and slide preparations. Fresh samples can be observed as a **wet mount**, mixed with saline to observe motility and iodine to kill trophozoites and enhance nuclear material. Fresh and preserved specimens can be permanently stained for the detection, identification, quantification, and permanent recording of parasites. The **trichrome** stain is the most common stain used for identifying intestinal parasites. It is rapid and simple, and it yields uniformly stained parasites, yeast, human cells, and artifacts. Cysts, trophozoites, and small protozoa undetected on wet mount can be identified with trichrome stains. The **modified trichrome** stain is diagnostic for detecting unicellular, intracellular microsporidian parasites. Blood smears stained with **Wright** and **Giemsa** stains provide rapid detection of malarial parasite rings in RBCs. **Acid-fast** staining identifies coccidian oocysts that are difficult to detect with other stains, and it is diagnostic for *Cryptosporidium, Isospora*, and *Cyclospora* species. Intestinal parasites can be quantified and their microfilarial sheath can be observed by staining with **iron hematoxylin**.

Key microscopic characteristics evaluated for helminth eggs and other parasite identification include:

- **Shape**: oval, round, ellipse, symmetrical, elongated, lightbulb or barrel shaped
- **Size**: measured in microns
- **Color:** colorless, yellow, brown
- **Texture, outer shell appearance:** operculated, smooth, scalloped edge, lateral or terminal spine, polar or bipolar filaments.

If recovered, adult worms can be observed for key identifying features including flat or round body shape, pointed or notched tails, the shape and number of teeth, sheath, and the presence and arrangement of nuclei on the tail.

Direct and Molecular Techniques to Detect Parasitic Infections

Microscopy examination of permanently stained specimen slides is the most common and most widely used direct technique for detecting parasites. Large parasites or adult worms can be recovered and visually inspected for identification. Pinworm infections can be detected by using a paddle for collecting a sample from the perianal region. The sticky portion of the paddle is gently pressed against the skin surrounding the rectum three to four times. Samples are collected first thing in the morning because adult female pinworms lay eggs in this area each night. The **pinworm prep** paddle is visually observed for the presence of pinworm eggs, which would diagnose an infection.

Other methods for the detection of parasites have been developed for the determination of parasitic infections. Rapid tests kits use **enzyme immunoassay** and **immunofluorescent assay** methodologies to detect antigens produced as a result of parasites in the body. Enzyme immunoassay methods detect parasitic antigens with parasite-specific monoclonal antibodies, and immunofluorescent assay tests use the same methodology with the addition of fluorescent dyes to represent the antigen–antibody complexes formed. **Real-time PCR** and **multiplex PCR** methods are used to detect molecular material of ova and parasites in specimens. Multiplex assays allow for the detection of many different parasites at the same time and use a single sample. Molecular multiplex methods use a variety of molecular primers to target gene sequences of multiple organisms.

Mycology

Specimens for Mycology Testing

Cultures for fungal organisms can be set up from samples of any tissue or body fluid including hair, skin, nails, tissue, sputum, urine, blood, bone marrow, CSF, and other normally sterile body fluids. Samples must be collected in screw-cap tubes or tape plates to avoid accidental opening, spilling, and drying of specimens in transport. Swabbed samples are acceptable for culture but are the least desirable transport system due to the increased drying and contamination potential. All mycology samples should be transported to the lab as soon as possible for the best chance of recovering organisms. Specimens remain the most viable when held at room temperature and should be saved for at least 6 weeks because fungi grow slowly.

Mycology Pathogens

Found worldwide, fungi are naturally occurring organisms that are able to cause infection when they enter the lungs by inhalation or when they enter the tissues by trauma. Some species of fungi are part of the human normal flora that cause opportunistic infections in immunocompromised hosts. Hosts most susceptible to fungal infections include premature babies and neonates, HIV/AIDS patients, and those taking an immunosuppressant drug.

Candida normally live as commensal organisms on the skin and in the mouth, throat, GI tract, and vagina. ***C. albicans***, the most common species to cause infection, causes thrush infections in the throat or mouth and yeast infections of the skin, genitals, and blood. ***C. auris*** is associated with hospital outbreaks and is considered a rising pathogen due to its multidrug-resistant nature.

Cryptococcus neoformans is found in soil and in pigeon and other bird feces. Inhalation of fungi from the environment causes a pneumonia-like illness, with meningitis and encephalitis occurring in severely immunocompromised patients.

Aspergillus spores inhaled from the air cause aspergillosis, which presents as allergic reactions and lung, cutaneous, or invasive infections. ***A. fumigatus*** is the most common pathogenic species, followed by ***A. flavus***, which often affects agriculturists with farmer's lung.

Histoplasma capsulatum occurs in soil and in bird and bat feces and causes histoplasmosis when inhaled. Symptoms range from mild: fever, head and muscle aches, dry cough, and fatigue; to chronic: mimics tuberculosis symptoms; to disseminated: fatal if left untreated.

Pneumocystis jiroveci causes atypical interstitial plasma-cell pneumonia when respiratory droplets of an infected human or other mammal are inhaled.

Yeast Identifications

The results of **biochemical reactions** of yeast isolates are used to differentiate major pathogens from one another. *Candida albicans*, the most common pathogenic yeast, and *Cryptococcus neoformans*, a potentially fatal pathogen, can be differentiated from one another based on their urease test reactions, with *C. albicans* presenting as urease negative and *C. neoformans* reacting as urease positive.

Automated methods for the identification of pathogenic yeast species aid in providing rapid and confident determination of major pathogens. These methods use a panel or test card loaded with chemicals with the specific purpose of differentiating yeast species from one another. Biochemical reactions obtained from a specimen or culture isolate are compared to an information database within automated systems. The database compares biochemical patterns and potential pattern variations of known yeast species to those obtained from the unknown isolate to determine its identification. Automated methods can obtain an organism identification in as little as 4 hours, allowing for the rapid diagnosis and treatment of yeast infections.

MALDI-TOF MS allows for early identification and disease diagnosis of fungal infections in a fast and precise manner. Yeast species can be identified by MALDI-TOF MS even in a mixed-colony culture by matching unique specimen reactions to computer database records of known yeast species.

Fungal Pathogens

Most fungal species are often first identified by Gram stain procedures or microscopic examination of urine sediment. In a **Gram stain**, yeast will appear as budding cells or pseudohyphae pigmented purple or a blue-black color. Preparing hair, skin, or nail samples with **potassium hydroxide (KOH)** on a slide with a coverslip allows for nonfungal cells and debris to be cleared and makes fungal elements more easily visible. KOH-prepared slides can be stained with **Calcofluor-white** stain and viewed under a fluorescent microscope. Fungal elements are detected by fluorescing on a black background in a blue-white or bright-green color, depending on the microscope filters used. **India ink** is added to centrifuged sediment of CSF samples for the rapid detection of *C. neoformans.* If present, encapsulated *C. neoformans* buds will appear on a black background with a large clear area around them. Filamentous and branching *Nocardia* species can be differentiated from other actinomycetes with the **acid-fast** stain. **Gömöri's methenamine silver** stain aids in the detection of *P. jiroveci* by staining carbohydrates in the organisms' cell walls black to brown colors.

Key characteristics of detecting and identifying fungal pathogens microscopically include:

- Intracellular or extracellular
- Shape: budding, pseudohyphae, hyphae, filamentous
- Encapsulated or no capsule present

Examples of microscopic morphology of pathogens are as follows:

- ***Candida* species:** yeast with pseudohyphae
    - ***C. albicans*:** small, extracellular yeast buds and pseudohyphae
- ***C. neoformans*:** encapsulated yeast, no pseudohyphae
- ***Histoplasma capsulatum*:** very small, intracellular yeast in tissue samples.

Selective Culture Media and Germ Tube Test to Identify Mycological Pathogens

Many fungal species are fastidious organisms that require certain nutrients to grow. Fungi are also slow growing on culture media and require bactericidal antibiotics to avoid bacterial overgrowth and increase fungal recovery. The following culture media are used in identifying fungal pathogens:

- **Sabouraud agar:** for the recovery of dermatophytes from cutaneous samples and yeast from vaginal cultures
- **Sabouraud heart infusion agar:** for the primary recovery and isolation of fastidious saprophytic and dimorphic fungi
- **Sabouraud dextrose agar:** subculture recovered fungi to enhance sporulation and provides more characteristic colony morphology for identification
- **Mycobiotic agar:** comprised of Sabouraud dextrose agar with added antibiotics for the primary recovery of dermatophytes
    - Cycloheximide: inhibits saprophytic and nonpathogenic fungi
    - Chloramphenicol: inhibits bacterial growth added
- **Czapek's agar**: to subculture *Aspergillus* fungi for species differentiation
- **Niger seed agar**: for *C. neoformans* identification.

The **germ tube test** is a simple, rapid test for *C. albicans* identification. The procedure is based on the species' ability to produce germ tubes from their yeast cells. An amount of 0.5 mL of sheep or rabbit serum and a yeast colony are added to a test tube and incubated for 2–3 hours at 35–37 °C.

Following incubation, a drop of the serum suspension is added to a microscope slide with a coverslip and observed microscopically under low power. The presence of germ tubes extending from yeast cells indicate *C. albicans*. Germ tubes are hypha-like extensions of yeast cells with no constrictions at the point where the extension originates.

Post-Analytic Procedures

Proper Documentation Practices in Laboratories

Good laboratory practices include proper documentation of laboratory operations. Patient results, quality control and calibration values, competency testing, and documentation of troubleshooting are important for monitoring a laboratory's performance and following a continuous quality improvement plan. Accuracy in documenting patient laboratory results is necessary for providing appropriate patient care. Printed or electronic reports allow for physicians to follow up on and review results and are more accurate with less chance of clerical errors than verbal results. Computer interfaces between the analyzers and the LIS provide the documentation of correct patient results in a more efficient manner, with delta checks, or internal warnings of change between an individual patient's previous and current results. Delta checks alert staff to manually review patient results for accuracy and rule out any preanalytical or analytical mishaps. Comprehensive documentation of quality control and calibration results allows for the evaluation of analyzers' functionality and establish trends in analyte analysis.

Reporting Urgent or Critical Values

Critical or panic values are defined as possibly life-threatening laboratory results that must be acknowledged and communicated to the patient's physician as soon as possible. An automated LIS will flag critical values to alert staff of the need to review and communicate results. Required information while reporting critical values varies among individual labs, but commonly the following information must be documented along with panic laboratory results: the date and time the results were given to the physician; the name of the physician or qualified healthcare professional that the results were relayed to; and the name of the laboratory staff member who reviewed, relayed, and verified the result. Other pertinent information regarding the sample may also be documented, including noting that the sample was inspected for preanalytical or analytical errors or that the testing was repeated to verify the legitimacy of the results.

Reviewing Laboratory Results and the Result Autoverification Process

All laboratory results must be reviewed and approved by staff before they are released to providers. Reviewing the results is necessary for ensuring that laboratory procedures are being followed, the instrumentation is working properly, and that the results reflect the true state of a patient's health status. Providing accurate test results is imperative to the physician's decision-making process for providing appropriate care to patients.

Computer-based algorithms are able to automatically review and verify laboratory results without manual intervention. Laboratories are able to design, customize, implement, and validate autoverification rules based on the needs of their individual patient populations. Autoverification rules and limits are established by rule-based, neural network, or pattern-recognition computer algorithms. Although normal results with minimal variation from pervious results will automatically be released by the system, abnormal results will display flags and will require manual review. Flags for manual review are developed for the following circumstances: critical values, values outside of analyzer limitations, and results failing the checks and balances set up within the system.

Issuing Corrected Reports

The process of detecting and correcting inaccurate results that have been mistakenly verified is necessary to assuring appropriate patient diagnosis and care. Once an error is detected, the ordering provider must be promptly notified of the inaccurate result, the error must be corrected, and an accurate result must be provided to the ordering physician. The Clinical Laboratory Improvement Amendments of 1988 (CLIA '88) regulations mandate that all corrected reports issued are accompanied by a written report of the circumstances leading to the erroneous result, the actions taken to correct the issue, and a proposed plan to address changes in operations that will prevent similar mistakes in the future.

Reporting Results to Infection Control and Public Health Departments

Laboratory results indicating and confirming certain infectious diseases are required to be reported to infection control and public health departments. Results reported to hospital infection control departments are often used in the evaluation of care quality and monitoring hospital versus community-acquired infections. Disease states such as pneumonia or *C. difficile* infections are closely followed by infection prevention departments to ensure that hospital standard operating procedures allow for the optimal environment for patient care. Local and state health departments require the reporting of communicable diseases and pathogens with the potential to cause an outbreak or public health hazard to reduce the morbidity and mortality of diseases. Positive results for sexually transmitted and hepatitis, or *E. coli* 0157 infections, and potential agents of bioterrorism are examples of laboratory tests submitted to public health departments. Patient demographics and contact information are also provided to these departments for their use in evaluating and studying the state of public health and detection of certain outbreaks in the area.

Laboratory Operations

Quality Assessment and Troubleshooting

Quality Assurance

Quality assurance is a set of policies, procedures, and practices derived from the consideration of any and all factors that may affect patient care. Laboratory quality assurance programs are necessary for producing reliable test results. These functions are divided into three categories, determined by when they occur in the analysis process.

Preanalytical functions are actions taken before a sample has begun being tested that can affect the patient care process. Examples of preanalytical functions are specimen collection, labeling, transport, and preservation prior to analysis. Quality assurance policies ensure that preanalytical processes allow for proper testing to be performed on correct patient samples.

Analytical functions take place during the testing process itself. Instrument and assay validation, quality control data, and result verification belong to the analytical category of quality assurance. Comprehensive education and training of testing personnel also belong to quality assurance programs. Following quality assurance policies and standards allows for accurate results to be obtained and reported by laboratory professionals.

Postanalytical functions of a quality assurance program occur after the analysis of a specimen. Included in this category is providing proper documentation for a clinical specimen, ensuring that the correct result is being reported to clinical staff, and revealing any actions taken regarding the interpretation of results.

Calibration and Quality Control Checks of Instruments

Generally, all instruments used to generate, measure, and assess data should be routinely calibrated and tested, based on standards and standard operating procedures. The frequency may vary, but some require daily **calibration** while others need calibration every few months. Equipment should also be calibrated if mechanical or other problems have occurred. Calibration may be done manually or semi- or completely automatically, and procedures may vary, but usually include:

- Testing calibrators, solutions, or samples with known values, to determine accuracy of measurement.
- Carefully preparing calibrators, including correct volumes.
- Following directions exactly (according to manufacturer's guidelines), maintaining the proper conditions (light, heat, ventilation), and using calibrators in the correct order and manner.
- Noting the need for adjustments to the equipment or process.

Calibration is part of quality control, but those instruments, supplies, or equipment that are not involved in directly generating, measuring, or assessing data generally do not require calibration but are maintained as part of general quality control.

Point-of-Care Testing (POCT)

Point-of-care testing (**POCT**) is described as diagnostic laboratory testing performed near the patient in settings such as at the patient bedside or in physician offices. The complexity of POCT is determined by assessing the knowledge, training, reagent and material preparation, technique for operation, quality control characteristics, maintenance, troubleshooting, and interpretation required for each method.

Categories of POCT:

- **Waived**: Simple testing procedure with little chance of negative patient outcome IF performed inaccurately, little judgment is required. Any over-the-counter test approved by the FDA. Examples include influenza and rapid strep tests.
- **Moderate complexity**: Typically automated, more complex than waived tests, most laboratory tests are in this category. Examples include blood counts and routine chemistries.
- **High complexity**: Nonautomated assays requiring highly trained personnel and considerable use of judgment. Examples include microbiology procedures and blood bank crossmatches.
- **Provider-performed microscopy**: Subcategory of moderate complexity testing, in-office slide examination of body fluid performed by the physician or provider, e.g., wet mount.

CLIA '88 Standards for POCT Facilities and Advantages of POCT

POCT testing is regulated, and facilities must be licensed under the Clinical Laboratory Improvement Amendments of 1988 (**CLIA '88**). Federal guidelines require POCT sites to adhere to good laboratory practice standards, comprised of training of personnel, competency evaluations, and quality control performance. State and city governments may enact more strict or specific regulations as they see fit.

POCT is more accessible than traditional laboratory testing methods, requires a smaller sample volume, and has a quicker turnaround time. This increases patient convenience, while acting to reduce lengths of hospital stays and improve care management. The cost of providing POCT and the associated training, competency, and quality standards must be taken into consideration to maintain the provision of appropriate patient care.

Compliance

Laboratory compliance encompasses policies, practices, and procedures that must be followed to ensure accurate results and good patient care. Regulatory agencies set standards to establish good laboratory practices and provide guidance for clinical laboratories. Compliance with these practices is instrumental in the success of laboratories and the facilities that support them. Failure to follow these practices, or other standards set by governing bodies, can result in events that adversely affect patient outcomes. Noncompliance can be detected through inspections, whistleblower complaints, or unsatisfactory patient events. Recognition and resolution of laboratory noncompliance must be acknowledged and submitted to governing bodies in order for a laboratory to remain in good standing and prove that efforts are being made to support good laboratory practices.

Voluntary Accrediting and Mandatory Regulatory Agencies and Acts for Laboratory Operations

Mandatory regulatory agencies:

- **Department of Health and Human Services** (DHHS) — oversees the following:
    - **Food and Drug Administration** (FDA) — regulates medical devices and blood products; approves new tests, technology, and instruments for laboratories
    - **Centers for Medicare and Medicaid Services** (CMS) — agency responsible for CLIA '88, Medicare and Medicaid Services
    - **Office of the Inspector General** (OIG) — part of CMS, laboratories can participate in a voluntary compliance program to prevent fraud and abuse
    - **Centers for Disease Control and Prevention** (CDC) — develops disease prevention guidelines and standards
- **Department of Transportation** (DOT) — Hazardous Materials Standard requires specific training and procedures for shipping biohazardous materials
- **United States Postal Service** (USPS) — directions for properly packaging biological specimens for shipping
- **Occupational Safety and Health Administration** (OSHA) — employee safety regulations
- **Equal Employment Opportunity Commission** (EEOC) — prohibits job discrimination
- **Health Insurance Portability and Accountability Act** (HIPAA) — protects confidentiality of patients' healthcare information
- **Clinical Laboratory Improvement Act of 1988** (CLIA '88) — standards for laboratory practice and quality to ensure the accuracy of testing

Voluntary Accrediting Agencies: all in accordance with CLIA '88 standards:

- **The Joint Commission** (TJC) — inspects and accredits hospitals and healthcare facilities
- **College of American Pathologists** (CAP) — clinical laboratories
- **Commission for Office Laboratory Accreditation** (COLA) — community hospital and physician office laboratories.

Inspections, Proficiency Testing, and Competency Assessment Programs in Laboratories

Under CLIA '88, all laboratories must be certified every 2 years to continue to prove that they are operating under the appropriate standards for testing. Although the extent of the regulations enforced is determined by the complexity of testing done in a facility, all laboratory testing sites must take part in the following activities:

- Quality assurance and quality control
- Proficiency testing
- Performance improvement
- Personnel qualifications
- Patient test management

Proficiency testing is part of the laboratory's quality assurance program. Unknown test samples are sent to a group of participating labs for testing, and their results are compared to one another. Proficiency testing allows for laboratories to evaluate the accuracy of their procedures, assays, instruments, and personnel.

A **competency assessment** program comprises periodic evaluations of staff and testing personnel. Supervisory staff must review each shift's work for any errors and omissions. Competency assessment provides laboratories with a way to ensure that testing personnel are properly trained and that they are following policies and procedures, and it acknowledges any improvements that can be made for patient and employee safety.

Hardware

Computer hardware consists of all of the physical parts of a computer. All machinery and equipment that makes up the computer and its related components are considered hardware. This includes computer disks, cables, the CPU (central processing unit), printers, keyboard, modem, and any other physical parts of the computer. A computer's hardware is what indicates what a computer is capable of doing.

Software

Computer software, on the other hand, is all of the programs that tell a computer how to operate. Software can be divided into application software, which are programs that manipulate and process data, and system software, which control the computer and other programs. Software is written in various programming languages, and the software is responsible for controlling what the hardware does and how the hardware operates.

Benefits of Computerized Data Automation in the Laboratory

Computerized automation of laboratory data has several advantages. For one, with the computer taking care of recording and storing data, laboratory technicians have more time to do other clinical tasks, such as performing laboratory tests. This increases laboratory productivity. Data stored on a computer, instead of paper laboratory reports, requires less storage space and can be encrypted for confidentiality. Another reason that computer automation is beneficial is that with data stored in a computer system, doctors and nurses can access such data much faster than if paper reports had to be mailed or faxed to them. In some cases, doctors can log onto a hospital computer system to see test results right away. And, using a computer to record data leads to fewer filing and billing errors on the part of the laboratory technicians.

Maintaining the Security of Computers and Databases

Security of laboratory computers and databases is a very important issue in the medical laboratory. Patient confidentiality must be kept at all times, and patients' data must not get into the wrong hands or be viewed by the wrong set of eyes. Because of this, there are various methods that laboratories can use to keep their computers and databases safe. Using passwords and identification numbers or names for each laboratory technician or doctor is a widely used method for security. Also, limiting the access to the computers can help as well. Using voice recognition technologies or keys that must be inserted into locks on the computers can keep computers and data safe. Various software programs, such as anti-virus, anti-spyware, and encryption software can enhance security. It must be noted, however, that security measures should not greatly impact the ease of using the computers.

Review Video: Ethics and Confidentiality in Counseling
Visit mometrix.com/academy and enter code: 250384

Safety

Laboratory's Responsibility in Preventing Infections Due to Bloodborne Pathogens

OSHA requires laboratories to operate following **universal** or **standard precautions**. Such precautions are defined as treating every bodily fluid as potentially infectious or containing bloodborne pathogens. Common bloodborne pathogens are HIV and hepatitis B and C. To protect employees in the event of an accidental exposure, employers must provide hepatitis B vaccinations at no cost to employees in positions with moderate to high risk of exposure.

Laboratories must provide staff with the proper **personal protective equipment**, PPE, for them to perform their jobs safely. PPE minimizes the risk of exposure to potentially infectious samples by providing an extra barrier between samples and the staff's skin or mucous membranes. Additionally, engineered equipment is used to provide protection for laboratory staff from potentially infectious materials.

Common PPE:

- Gloves
- Lab coats
- Safety goggles

Engineered safety equipment:

- Work shields — protection from splashes
- Needle safety devices — protect against needlestick injuries
- Biohazard safety hoods — protection from aerosol-inducing samples.

OSHA

OSHA's acts and standards make up a federally created system put in place to ensure workplace safety. OSHA standards include requirements for warning labels, alerts for potential hazards, appropriate PPE, exposure procedures, and the implementation of proper training and employee education. Laboratories must create, educate, and follow a formal safety program, provide specifically mandated plans for chemical and biohazardous exposure, as well as hygiene standards, and identify various hazards in the workplace.

Safety Data Sheets (SDS) for Chemicals and Reagents

Safety data sheets (SDS) exist as the core of OHSA's safety standards. An SDS is required for every chemical present in the laboratory, to provide information regarding its physical and chemical properties, safe handling, proper storage and disposal, and the potential hazards associated. SDS information is provided by chemical manufacturers and suppliers and must accompany each chemical upon shipment.

Information on SDS:

- Trade name
- Chemical name and synonyms
- Chemical family
- Manufacturer's name and address
- Emergency phone number for more info related to the chemical
- Hazardous ingredients

- Physical data
- Fire and explosion data
- Health hazard and protection information
    - Effects of overexposure/exceeding threshold of allowable exposure
    - PPE and equipment requirements
    - First aid practices
    - Spill information and directions
    - Procedures for proper disposal.

OSHA-Mandated Regulations for Occupational Exposure to Bloodborne Pathogens

The OSHA-mandated "Occupational Exposure to Bloodborne Pathogens" standard requires laboratories to create, implement, and comply with plans to ensure laboratory staff safety from potential infectious pathogens. Employees must be educated at least annually on their laboratory's chemical and biohazard waste management and emergency exposure procedures. In the event of an exposure, policies and procedures involving such emergencies must always be available to laboratory staff to safely and properly handle all injuries, materials, and waste products.

Training and Proper Procedures for Packaging and Transporting Category A and Category B Biological Specimens

All laboratory personnel who take part in the packaging and shipment of biohazardous materials must complete a comprehensive training course within 90 days of hire and once every 2 years after that. Proper education and training are pertinent for limiting exposure during transport and providing information on a package's contents if exposure occurs.

Category A: a specimen that is capable of causing a permanent disability or a life-threatening or fatal disease to a healthy individual upon exposure

Category B: a specimen that is not in a form capable of causing a permanent disability or a life-threatening or fatal disease to a healthy individual upon exposure

"Exempt specimen": used only by USPS and the International Air Transport Association, defined as a specimen unlikely to cause disease in humans or animals and with a minimal likelihood of a pathogen being present.

Packaging guidelines for shipping:

- Primary packaging that is leakproof
- Absorbent material if the specimen is not a solid
- Secondary packaging that is also leakproof
- Itemized list of the package contents
- A third, rigid outer layer that is able to withstand a 4-foot drop test without breaking/opening
- Biohazard labeling on the outside of the packaging:
    - Category A — UN2814 Infectious substance, affecting humans
    - Category B — UN3373 Biological substance

Laboratory Mathematics

Significant Figures

Significant figures enable scientists to determine which measurements are very precise and which measurements are not as precise. Every measurement has uncertainty. When recording data, the use of the correct number of significant figures indicates the precision of the equipment being used to measure the data. In general, measurements are recorded only to the first uncertain digit. This means that the final recorded digit is considered to be uncertain. Every calculated value using collected data has uncertainty. Significant figures determine where to round when doing calculations with data. Also, significant figures prevent the answers to calculations from being stated with higher precision than the data used in the calculation would actually support.

When using significant figures in calculations, there are two sets of rules: one for addition and subtraction, and one for multiplication and division. For addition and subtraction calculations, answers should be rounded to the leftmost uncertain digit. For example, when adding measurements of 2.3 g and 10.81 g, the correct answer would be 13.1 g. The first term's uncertain digit is in the tenths place, while the second term's uncertain digit is in the hundredths place. Thus, the answer is rounded to the tenths place. In multiplication and division calculations, answers should be rounded to the exact number of significant figures in the factor that has the smallest number of significant figures. For example, when multiplying 3.2 by 4.001, the correct answer may only have 2 significant figures because 3.2 only has 2 significant figures. Therefore, the correct answer is 13. If the first factor were instead 3.20 or 3.200 (indicating that this value was known with greater precision), the answer would be 12.8 or 12.80, respectively.

Data Errors and Error Analysis

No measurements are ever 100% accurate. There is always some amount of error regardless of how careful the observer or how good his equipment. The important thing for the scientist to know is how much error is present in a given measurement. Two commonly misunderstood terms regarding error are accuracy and precision. Accuracy is a measure of how close a measurement is to the true value. Precision is a measure of how close repeated measurements are to one another. Error is usually quantified using a confidence interval and an uncertainty value. For instance, if the quantity is measured as 100 ± 2 on a 95% confidence interval, this means that there is a 95% chance that the actual value falls between 98 and 102.

Data Analysis

The **measure of central tendency** is a statistical value that gives a general tendency for the center of a group of data. There are several different ways of describing the measure of central tendency. Each one has a unique way it is calculated, and each one gives a slightly different perspective on the data set. Whenever you give a measure of central tendency, always make sure the units are the same. If the data has different units, such as hours, minutes, and seconds, convert all the data to the same unit, and use the same unit in the measure of central tendency. If no units are given in the data, do not give units for the measure of central tendency.

Mean

The statistical **mean** of a group of data is the same as the arithmetic average of that group. To find the mean of a set of data, first convert each value to the same units, if necessary. Then find the sum of all the values, and count the total number of data values, making sure you take into consideration each individual value. If a value appears more than once, count it more than once. Divide the sum of the values by the total number of values and apply the units, if any. Note that the mean does not have to be one of the data values in the set, and may not divide evenly.

$$\text{mean} = \frac{\text{sum of the data values}}{\text{quantity of data values}}$$

While the mean is relatively easy to calculate and averages are understood by most people, the mean can be very misleading if it is used as the sole measure of central tendency. If the data set has outliers (data values that are unusually high or unusually low compared to the rest of the data values), the mean can be very distorted, especially if the data set has a small number of values. If unusually high values are countered with unusually low values, the mean is not affected as much. For example, if five of twenty students in a class get a 100 on a test, but the other 15 students have an average of 60 on the same test, the class average would appear as 70. Whenever the mean is skewed by outliers, it is always a good idea to include the median as an alternate measure of central tendency.

MEDIAN

The statistical **median** is the value in the middle of the set of data. To find the median, list all data values in order from smallest to largest or from largest to smallest. Any value that is repeated in the set must be listed the number of times it appears. If there are an odd number of data values, the median is the value in the middle of the list. If there is an even number of data values, the median is the arithmetic mean of the two middle values.

The big disadvantage of using the median as a measure of central tendency is that is relies solely on a value's relative size as compared to the other values in the set. When the individual values in a set of data are evenly dispersed, the median can be an accurate tool. However, if there is a group of rather large values or a group of rather small values that are not offset by a different group of values, the information that can be inferred from the median may not be accurate because the distribution of values is skewed.

MODE

The statistical **mode** is the data value that occurs the most frequently in the data set. It is possible to have exactly one mode, more than one mode, or no mode. To find the mode of a set of data, arrange the data like you do to find the median (all values in order, listing all multiples of data values). Count the number of times each value appears in the data set. If all values appear an equal number of times, there is no mode. If one value appears more than any other value, that value is the mode. If two or more values appear the same number of times, but there are other values that appear fewer times and no values that appear more times, all of those values are the modes.

The main disadvantage of the mode is that the values of the other data in the set have no bearing on the mode. The mode may be the largest value, the smallest value, or a value anywhere in between in the set. The mode only tells which value or values, if any, occurred the greatest number of times. It does not give any suggestions about the remaining values in the set.

Beer's Law

Beer's law is defined as $A = abc$, where A is the absorbance, a is the absorptivity, b is the path of light in centimeters (cm), and c is the concentration of the absorbing compound. Consider the following example:

For a certain spectrophotometric procedure, the absorbance of a standard solution (concentration is 25 mg/dL) is 0.75 (in a 1 cm cell). The absorbance of the sample solution is 0.35 (in a 1 cm cell). Calculate the concentration of the sample solution.

Both b (the path of light in centimeters) and a (the absorptivity) are constant. So, using Beer's law, the equation for the relationship is: $\frac{c_{sample}}{c_{standard}} = \frac{A_{sample}}{A_{standard}}$. All of the values in that equation are known except for the concentration of the sample:

$$c_{sample} = \frac{A_{sample} \times c_{standard}}{A_{standard}}$$

$$= \frac{0.35 \times 25}{0.75} \frac{\text{mg}}{\text{dL}}$$

$$= 11.7 \text{ mg/dL}$$

Molarity and Molality of a Solution

Molarity and molality are measures of the concentration of a solution. Molarity (M) is the amount of solute in moles per the amount of solution in liters. A 1.0 M solution consists of 1.0 mole of solute for each 1.0 L of solution. Molality (m) is the amount of solute in moles per the amount of solvent in kilograms. A 1.0 m solution consists of 1.0 mole of solute for each 1.0 kg of solvent. Often, when performing these calculations, the amount of solute is given in grams. To convert from grams of solute to moles of solute, multiply the grams of solute by the molar mass of the solute:

$$Molarity\ (\text{M}) = \frac{moles\ of\ solute\ (\text{mol})}{liters\ of\ solution\ (\text{L})}$$

$$Molality\ (\text{m}) = \frac{moles\ of\ solute\ (\text{mol})}{kilograms\ of\ solvent\ (\text{kg})}$$

Molarity of a Solution Example

Determine the molarity of a solution that contains 20.0 grams of NaCl in 500 mL of solution.

The molarity of a solution is equal to moles per liter. In this example, we need to calculate what one mole (gram molecular weight) is of NaCl first. A mole of a compound is equal to the sum of the atomic weights of the elements in that compound. So, for NaCl, one mole is equal to the atomic weight of sodium plus the atomic weight of chlorine, $23.0\frac{\text{g}}{\text{mol}} + 35.5\frac{\text{g}}{\text{mol}} = 58.5\frac{\text{g}}{\text{mol}}$. Next, it is best to determine the concentration of the solution in terms of grams per liter. So, in our example, the solution is $\frac{20.0\text{ g}}{500\text{ mL}}$. This is equivalent to $\frac{20.0\text{ g}}{0.5\text{ L}} = 40\frac{\text{g}}{\text{L}}$. Next, the number of moles of NaCl present in the solution must be calculated. Take the grams of NaCl present in 1 liter of solution and divide it by the weight of one mole of NaCl:

$\frac{40\text{ g}}{58.5\frac{\text{g}}{\text{mol}}} = 0.68$ mol. Since molarity is equal to moles per liter, the molarity of this solution is therefore $0.68\frac{\text{mol}}{\text{L}}$, or the solution is a 0.68 M NaCl solution.

Osmolality

Osmolality is defined as the moles per 1 kilogram (kg) of solvent multiplied by the number of particles into which the molecules of solute dissociate. For instance, consider calculating the osmolality of 54 g glucose and 11.7 g NaCl in 2 kg of water.

To calculate the osmolality, first we need to calculate how many moles of solute (both glucose and NaCl) are present.

For glucose, $54\text{ g} = \frac{54\text{ g}}{180\frac{\text{g}}{\text{mol}}} = 0.3$ mol. For NaCl, $11.7\text{ g} = \frac{11.7\text{ g}}{58.5\frac{\text{g}}{\text{mol}}} = 0.2$ mol.

Then, we need to look at how each solute dissociates. Glucose does not dissociate. However, 0.2 mol NaCl will dissociate into two particles, 0.2 mol Na^+ and 0.2 mol Cl^-. So, to calculate the number of osmoles (Osm) present, we would add 0.3 Osm glucose to 0.2 Osm Na^+ and 0.2 Osm Cl^-. This totals 0.7 Osm present. Because we are dealing with 2 kg of water, however, and osmolality is noted as moles per kilogram, we need to divide 0.7 Osm by 2 kg of water, to give an osmolality of 0.35.

Preparing a Solution Example

Determine how many grams of KCl are required to prepare 250 mL of a 3 M solution.

A 1 M solution is equal to 1 mole of solute divided by 1 liter of solution. To begin, the molecular weight of 1 mole of KCl must be calculated: 39.1 g + 35.5 g = 74.6 g. Therefore, 1 liter of a 1 M solution of KCl contains 74.6 g. However, since we are interested in a 3 M solution, the number of grams contained in a 1 M solution must be multiplied by 3. Therefore, a 3 M solution contains $3 \times 74.6\frac{\text{g}}{\text{L}} = 223.8\frac{\text{g}}{\text{L}}$. In this case, though, only 250 mL or 0.250 L of the 3 M solution are needed. So, the 3 M solution needs to be multiplied by the volume needed. This equation then becomes: $223.8\frac{\text{g}}{\text{L}} \times 0.250\text{ L} = 56.0$ g KCl. Therefore, in order to prepare 250 mL of a 3 M solution of KCl, 56.0 g of KCl are needed.

Preparing a Dilute Solution from a Stock Solution

In order to prepare a dilute solution from a stock solution, the molarity and the needed volume of the diluted solution as well as the molarity of the stock solution must be known. The volume of the stock solution to be diluted can be calculated using the formula $V_{\text{stock}}M_{\text{stock}} = V_{\text{dilute}}M_{\text{dilute}}$, where V_{stock} is the unknown variable, M_{stock} is the molarity of the stock solution, V_{dilute} is the needed volume of the dilute solution, and M_{dilute} is the needed molarity of the dilute solution. Solving this formula for V_{stock} yields $V_{\text{stock}} = \frac{V_{\text{dilute}}M_{\text{dilute}}}{M_{\text{stock}}}$. Then, dilute the calculated amount of stock solution (V_{stock}) to the total volume required of the diluted solution.

Determining Final Concentrations of Solutions Examples

When calculating a final concentration of a solution after multiple dilutions, the initial concentration of the solution is multiplied by each of the dilutions as a fraction. Consider the following examples:

A 2 M solution diluted 2:5 and then diluted 1:4

To calculate the final concentration of this 2 M solution after being diluted 2: 5 and 1: 4, the equation used would be $(2\text{ M}) \times \frac{2}{5} \times \frac{1}{4}$. The final concentration would then be 0.2 M.

A 5 M solution diluted 1:2, then diluted 2:3, and then diluted 3:5

In this situation, the equation used to calculate the final concentration of the solution after undergoing multiple dilutions as stated would be $(5\text{ M}) \times \frac{1}{2} \times \frac{2}{3} \times \frac{3}{5}$. The final concentration of this solution is then calculated to be 1 M.

A 4 M solution diluted 3:7, then diluted 6:13, and then diluted 1:2

In this particular situation, the equation used to calculate the final concentration of the solution after undergoing three separate dilutions as stated in the problem would be $(4\text{ M}) \times \frac{3}{7} \times \frac{6}{13} \times \frac{1}{2}$. Using this equation, the final concentration of the solution can be calculated to be approximately 0.4 M.

Calculating Concentration in Milliequivalents Per Liter

To calculate a concentration in milliequivalents per liter when given concentration in milligrams per deciliter, the following equation needs to be used:

$$\frac{\frac{\text{mg}}{\text{dL}} \times \frac{10\text{ dL}}{\text{L}} \times valence}{atomic\ mass} = \text{mEq/L}$$

Calculate the concentration in milliequivalents per liter $(\frac{\text{mEq}}{\text{L}})$ of a serum potassium level of $22.3\,\frac{\text{mg}}{\text{dL}}$.

For potassium, the valence is 1, and the atomic mass is 39. These values can be obtained by using a periodic table. Therefore, the equation then becomes:

$$\frac{\left(22.3\,\frac{\text{mg}}{\text{dL}}\right) \times \left(\frac{10\text{ dL}}{\text{L}}\right) \times 1}{39\,\frac{\text{g}}{\text{mol}}} = 5.7\text{ mEq/L}$$

Calculate the concentration in milliequivalents per liter of a serum calcium level of $9.0\,\frac{\text{mg}}{\text{dL}}$.

For calcium, the valence is 2, and the atomic mass is 40. Therefore:

$$\frac{\left(9.0\,\frac{\text{mg}}{\text{dL}}\right) \times \left(\frac{10\text{ dL}}{\text{L}}\right) \times 2}{40\,\frac{\text{g}}{\text{mol}}} = 4.5\text{ mEq/L}$$

Sensitivity, Specificity, and Predictive Value

Getting answers with a high probability of being accurate is the best that can be hoped for in a medical test. A test can produce two kinds of errors: a false positive result (meaning that the presence of disease is detected when there is, in fact, no disease) or a false negative result indicating no disease is present when it actually is.

- Test **sensitivity**: Measures a screening test's ability to correctly identify the presence of a disease, it is the ratio of tests with positive outcomes to the total number of affected (true positive) patients tested.
- Test **specificity**: Measures a screening test's ability to correctly identify the absence of disease.

A test with both high sensitivity and high specificity can be expected to have high **predictive value**.

- True-positive (TP): the test is positive, and the patient has acquired a disease.
- False-positive (FP): the test is positive but the patient does not have the disease.
- True-negative (TN): the test is negative, but the patient does not have a disease.
- False-negative (FN): the test is negative; the patient does have the disease.
- Level of sensitivity in testing: probability of a positive test result when a patient has the disease, as indicated by the ratio, TP/(TP + FN).
- Degree of specificity: the probability that a negative test truly indicates a disease-free patient, represented by the ratio, TN/(TN + FP).
- Positive predictive value: the probability that a test will produce positive results for patients who have the disease, indicated in the ratio, TP/(TP + FP).
- Negative predictive value: denotes the probability that no disease exists in patients testing negative, stated in the ratio: TN/(TN + FN).

Manual and Automated Methodology and Instrumentation

Setting Up, Balancing, and Operating a Centrifuge

Centrifuges spin solutions to separate out solid materials by forcing them away from the center to form a pellet. Centrifuges come in various sizes and may be free floating/horizontal or angle-head (45-degree angle). Different specimens require different G-forces or **relative centrifugal force** (RCF) and different durations. The RCF is the spinning force relative to Earth's gravitation and depends on the revolutions per minute (RPM) and the radius of revolution (RR) measured in mm from the center to the end of the test tube (It can also be found using a nomogram chart.):

$$RCF = 1.12 \times RR \times \left(\frac{RPM}{1000}\right)^2$$

Procedure:

1. Use equal numbers of tubes in the buckets on opposite sites. Weigh tubes to ensure the load is balanced and use a tube filled with water if testing an odd number.
2. Close and lock centrifuge, turn it on, and follow instructions for settings.
3. Spin for necessary duration (such as 15 to 20 minutes). If excessive vibration (from imbalance) or sound of cracking vial occurs, turn off machine.
4. When completed, remove buckets carefully to avoid jarring the pellets.
5. Open buckets and remove tubes, checking for sediments.

Microscopes

The microscope most commonly used is the **light microscope** (either monocular or binocular). This microscope uses external light or light from an internal filament that allows the light to pass upward through the specimen so that the specimen appears dark against the lighter background, although the light may be inverted, illuminating from the top, for such things as a culture in a liquid medium. **Phase contrast microscopes** that do not require staining of the specimen are used to assess cell growth, especially for organisms that are transparent with standard light microscope. The **dark field microscope** uses a special dark-field condenser that makes the specimen appear light against a dark background, useful for observing spirochetes. The **fluorescent microscope** utilizes an ultraviolet light for illumination. This microscope is used when fluorescent dye is attached to a specimen because the dye glows when exposed to ultraviolet light, useful for fluorescent antibody testing.

Ocular Micrometer

The ocular micrometer is a glass disk that fits into the microscope eyepiece and provides an engraved ruler for measurement within the ocular lens. The **ocular micrometer calibration** procedure is as follows:

1. Remove eyepiece and unscrew the ocular eye lens and position the ocular micrometer with the engraved ruler with 100 divisions face down, replace the lens, and place the ocular with the micrometer into the ocular tube and microscope with 10× objective.
2. Place a stage micrometer slide with an engraved scale that closely matches in the ocular micrometer length and number of divisions on the microscope stage and focus on the parallel sets of rulers so that the 0-mm lines on the ocular micrometer and stage micrometer align.
3. Locate another set of lines that align at the furthest distance from the 0-mm lines.
4. Count the number of lines between the 0-mm alignment and the distant alignment on both the ocular micrometer scale and the stage micrometer scale.
5. Use formulas to determine the proportion of a mm measured by 1 ocular unit:
6. Stage micrometer reading × 1000 micrometers/ocular micrometer reading × 1 mm = ocular units.
7. For 40× objective: 0.1 mm × 1000 micrometer/50 units × 1 mm.

Manual Instrumentation

Borosilicate glassware is heat and chemical resistant; soda lime glassware, less expensive and less resistant; and plastic ware, less expensive and less breakable but not heat resistant and cannot be used with some reagents and chemicals. Commonly used manual laboratory instrumentation includes:

- **Test tubes**: Used to heat and hold reagents to assess chemical reactions. Vary in size and usually rimless. Held in plastic or metal test tube racks. Centrifuge tubes (15 mL) are similar but have tapered ends to hold pellet. Cuvettes are rectangular test tubes to hold solutions for photometry, placed only in plastic racks to avoid scratching.
- **Funnels (plain and separating)**: Supported in ring stand and used for filtration or to separate immiscible liquids.
- **General purpose and volumetric glassware**: Includes graduated cylinders, volumetric flasks, pipettes, and burettes and used for measuring volumes. Pipettes or eyedroppers are used to transfer liquids. Mouth pipettes should never be used. Reagent bottles hold reagents. Beakers are used to heat liquids.

Cleaning and maintenance of manual instrumentation: All glassware and plastic ware should be rinsed immediately after use in hot tap water to prevent substances from drying. The rinsed ware is soaked in low suds detergent solution (2%) for at least an hour. The ware is then scrubbed with appropriately-sized brushes inside and out. Chromic acid may be used to remove coagulated organic material. Each item is washed 5 times under running tap water to remove all detergent followed by 3 rinses with distilled or deionized water. After the washing and rinsing are completed, the equipment is dried in an oven at 140 °C if heat resistant or placed in a drying rack overnight. Prior to first use of newly purchased glassware, items made of borosilicate glass should be cleaned with detergent, washed under tap water, and rinsed with distilled/deionized water. Items made of soda lime glass should be soaked overnight in 5% hydrochloric acid, diluted 6 times to 30% to neutralize free alkali before washing under tap water, and rinsed with distilled/deionized water.

Advantages and Disadvantages of Automated Laboratory Instrumentation

Automated laboratory instrumentation is becoming the norm, and a laboratory may have total laboratory automation or system-based automation. Automated laboratory instrumentation has a number of advantages over manual procedures:

- Test results can be obtained faster and are often more accurate because they are not dependent on varying techniques and subjective judgment.
- Test results are more reliable and consistent, and can be easily reproduced.
- Data can be more easily stored, transferred, manipulated, and reported.
- Fewer laboratory personnel are needed because the automated systems can do the work of many technicians.
- Errors are minimized.
- Workflow is more efficient.

However, there are also some disadvantages: If a machine breaks down, there may be considerable delay in manually producing lab reports because of inadequate staffing or equipment. Additionally, staff members must be trained in trouble shooting and maintenance of equipment and service technicians must be available. The automation equipment may be prohibitively expensive, especially for a small laboratory.

MLT Practice Test

Want to take this practice test in an online interactive format?
Check out the bonus page, which includes interactive practice questions and much more: **https://www.mometrix.com/bonus948/mlt**

1. What is the minimum hemoglobin concentration for a male allogeneic donor required by the FDA?

a. 125 g/L
b. 11 g/dL
c. 12.5 g/dL
d. 13.0 g/dL

2. Platelets can be stored at 20–24 °C for five days, except in cases where an FDA-approved protocol is used to extend the storage period. How many days can the storage period be extended to in these cases?

a. 10 days
b. 7 days
c. 42 days
d. 21 days

3. Which of the following is an antibody to a high-incidence antigen?

a. Anti-Lu^a
b. Anti-Lu^b
c. Anti-Js^a
d. Anti-Kp^a

4. Which of the following tests is appropriate for detecting red blood cells coated with antibodies in vivo?

a. Direct antiglobulin
b. Indirect antiglobulin
c. Antibody detection
d. Indirect Coombs

5. Your medical facility has established that patients 3 months of age or older shall not have more than 2.5% of their total blood volume collected in a 24-hour period. You have orders for labs for an 8-month-old baby girl who weighs 11.5 kg with an estimated total blood volume of 750 mL. You notice that the baby girl has already had two blood draws today that total 13 ml. What is the greatest volume of blood you can safely collect without going over the maximum allowable daily limit?

a. 8.0 mL
b. 6.5 mL
c. 5.0 mL
d. 7.5 mL

6. Which of the following antibodies represents a clinically insignificant antibody if it is NOT reactive at 37 °C?

a. Anti-Le^b
b. Anti-k
c. Anti-Jk^b
d. Anti-C

7. Which of the following strategies would be appropriate to include as part of a hospital system's blood management program?

a. Intraoperative administration of epoetin alfa
b. Acute normovolemic hemodilution with sodium ferric gluconate
c. Laboratory evaluation 30 days prior to surgery
d. Post-surgical administration of tranexamic acid

8. A patient is experiencing low back pain, and you receive a urine specimen for urinalysis. The pH for the urine is acidic, and upon microscopic examination you observe lemon-shaped crystals like those in the image. What is the identification of the crystals observed?

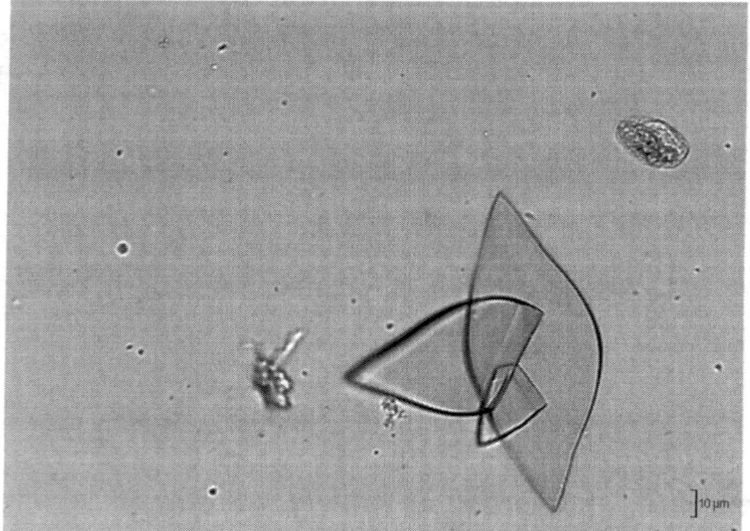

a. Triple phosphate
b. Calcium phosphate
c. Cholesterol
d. Uric acid

9. A 22-year-old male presents to the emergency department with a chief complaint of painful scrotal swelling. Which of the following would be the most likely finding in a urinalysis?

a. *Schistosoma haematobium*
b. *Trichomonas vaginalis*
c. *Neisseria gonorrhoeae*
d. *Chlamydia trachomatis*

10. A total of four tubes of cerebrospinal fluid (CSF) are collected during a lumbar puncture. Which collection tube should be utilized for cell counts?

a. The first tube
b. The second tube
c. The third tube
d. The fourth tube

11. You are working in the chemistry department when you receive a STAT order for a CSF from a patient with suspected bacterial meningitis. Which results would you expect to see?

a. Decreased glucose, decreased protein, decreased lactate
b. Decreased glucose, decreased protein, increased lactate
c. Decreased glucose, increased protein, increased lactate
d. Decreased glucose, increased protein, decreased lactate

12. A 30-year-old male comes to your laboratory for a 2-hour oral glucose tolerance test. His fasting serum glucose is 108 mg/dL and his 2-hour postprandial glucose is 145 mg/dL. What is the best interpretation of these results?

a. Impaired glucose tolerance, indicating diabetes
b. Normal glucose tolerance, indicating normal glucose metabolism
c. Impaired glucose tolerance, indicating prediabetes
d. Impaired glucose tolerance, indicating hypoglycemia

13. An increased level of which type of lipoprotein would be expected in a non-fasting serum specimen?

a. Cholesterol
b. Triglycerides
c. Low-density lipoprotein
d. High-density lipoprotein

14. The following results from a hepatic function panel come across the LIS for you to review. Based on these values, what disease process could this patient have?

TEST	PATIENT	REF RANGE
ALP	460	40–120 U/L
ALT	45	5–40 U/L
AST	52	9–40 U/L
TP	7.2	6.3–8.2 g/dL
ALB	4.5	3.5–5 g/dL
TB	2.2	0.1–1.2 mg/dL
DB	1.4	0.0–0.3 mg/dL

a. Acute viral hepatitis
b. Cholestasis
c. Sickle cell anemia
d. Hepatocellular carcinoma

15. Which component is the primary contributor to the osmotic pressure of blood?

a. Alpha globulin
b. Immunoglobulin G
c. Fibrinogen
d. Albumin

16. Which protein is considered to be the iron storage protein?

a. Ferritin
b. Transferrin
c. C-reactive protein
d. Gamma globulins

17. Which acid-base disorder is represented by the blood gas values shown?

pH	7.31
pCO_2	38
HCO_3	20

a. Respiratory acidosis
b. Metabolic acidosis
c. Compensated metabolic acidosis
d. Compensated respiratory acidosis

18. Which of the following acid-base imbalances can be caused by hyperventilation?

a. Metabolic alkalosis
b. Respiratory acidosis
c. Respiratory alkalosis
d. Compensated metabolic alkalosis

19. You're reviewing results from the immunoassay analyzer and discover a quantitative hCG result that is outside of the analytic measurement range (AMR). You will need to perform a dilution and repeat the test. If the AMR is 25,000 mIU/mL and the test results showed 85,000 mIU/mL, which dilution factor should bring the result into the reportable range?

a. 1:1
b. 1:2
c. 1:3
d. 1:5

20. Which hormone is released as a result of low calcium levels in the blood?

a. ACTH
b. PTH
c. Biotin
d. IGF-1

21. A deficiency of which of the following causes decreased prothrombin levels and abnormal bleeding time?

a. Vitamin C
b. Riboflavin
c. Choline
d. Vitamin K

22. The removal of aging erythrocytes from circulation by macrophages releases iron. What then recycles the iron and transports it back to the bone marrow?

a. Transferrin
b. Hepcidin
c. Haptoglobin
d. Ferritin

23. Which hormone is produced by the kidneys in response to hypoxemia?

a. ADH
b. Aldosterone
c. IGF-1
d. EPO

24. Common myeloid progenitor cells in the bone marrow give rise to many different cells. Which of the following cells is NOT a product of the differentiation of the common myeloid progenitor cell?

a. Megakaryocyte
b. NK cell
c. Erythrocyte
d. Promonocyte

25. Therapeutic phlebotomy treatment of polycythemia vera can cause what type of anemia?

a. Sideroblastic anemia
b. Iron deficiency anemia
c. Megaloblastic anemia
d. Pernicious anemia

26. Schistocytes are a key morphological finding associated with what condition?

a. Thrombotic thrombocytopenic purpura
b. Sickle cell anemia
c. G6PD deficiency
d. Hereditary spherocytosis

27. A patient with suspected iron deficiency has iron studies performed. Which pattern of results would be expected?

a. Low iron, low TIBC, low iron saturation, and normal or high ferritin
b. High iron, low TIBC, high iron saturation, and high ferritin
c. Normal or high iron, normal or low TIBC, normal or high iron saturation, normal or high ferritin
d. Low iron, high TIBC, low iron saturation, low ferritin

28. You are performing a manual differential and you observe a large cell with abundant, deep blue cytoplasm, an irregular-shaped nucleus with fine chromatin, and cytoplasmic extensions that appear to hug the surrounding erythrocytes. What is the correct identification of this cell?

a. Monocyte
b. Large lymphocyte
c. Reactive lymphocyte
d. Plasma cell

29. What could be a possible cause of a spuriously low MCHC with a high MCV?

a. Electrolyte abnormality
b. Lipemia
c. Severe leukocytosis
d. RBC agglutination

30. Which term refers to the hematologic method of counting cells by measuring changes in electrical conductance?

a. Hydrodynamic focusing
b. The Coulter Principle
c. Fluorescence
d. Absorption spectrophotometry

31. A sodium citrate tube that is not filled adequately will cause what?

a. Prolonged prothrombin time
b. Shortened prothrombin time
c. Clotting of the specimen
d. Decreased calcium chelation

32. Which coagulation factors would be affected by anticoagulant therapy with warfarin?

a. Factors I, III, and XII
b. Factors II, V, and IX
c. Factors IV, VIII, and vWF
d. Factors I, V, and XI

33. Immunoglobulin M primarily exists in what structural formation?

a. Dimeric
b. Quaternary
c. Pentamer
d. Monomer

34. Type I hypersensitivity anaphylaxis is mediated by which immunoglobulin?

a. IgG
b. IgE
c. IgA
d. IgD

35. Which immune system cell can target and kill tumor cells without prior activation?

a. NK cell
b. Cytotoxic T cell
c. Macrophage
d. Mast cell

36. What is the hepatitis B status of a patient with the following results?

HBsAg	+
HBsAb	–
HBc total Ab	+
HBc IgM Ab	+

a. Inconclusive; repeat testing recommended
b. Chronic HBV infection
c. Immune status post vaccination
d. Acute HBV infection

37. A physician is requesting guidance on testing a patient for Lyme disease. Which test would best screen the patient for infection with *Borrelia burgdorferi*?

a. *Borrelia* species by PCR
b. *B. burgdorferi* IgM and IgG Ab by immunoblot
c. *B. burgdorferi* IgG Ab by immunoblot
d. *B. burgdorferi* total antibodies by ELISA

38. A pregnant female begins experiencing flu-like symptoms two weeks after adopting a shelter cat. In this case, what infectious organism should be tested for?

a. *Bartonella quintana*
b. *Toxoplasma gondii*
c. *Francisella tularensis*
d. *Yersinia pestis*

39. What is the medium of choice for setting up a throat culture?

a. MacConkey agar
b. Sheep blood agar
c. Chocolate agar
d. Modified Thayer-Martin agar

40. Which organism prefers a microaerobic atmosphere and an incubation temperature of 42 °C?

a. *Mycobacterium tuberculosis*
b. *Neisseria gonorrhoeae*
c. *Campylobacter jejuni*
d. *Clostridium perfringens*

41. What is the Kirby-Bauer test used to determine?

a. Antibiotic sensitivity
b. Lactose fermentation
c. Indole production
d. Decarboxylation

42. A stool sample from a patient with bloody diarrhea was cultured with the selective medium MacConkey with sorbitol. A mixture of colorless and pink colonies grew. What is the presumptive identification of the colorless colonies?

a. *Clostridium difficile*
b. *Staphylococcus aureus*
c. *Escherichia coli* O157:H7
d. *Shigella dysenteriae* serotype 2

43. A small, Gram-negative coccobacilli is isolated from the wound of a dog bite. What would be the most likely identification of this organism?

a. *Bartonella* species
b. *Actinomyces* species
c. *Corynebacterium* species
d. *Pasteurella* species

44. A nasal lavage specimen from a patient with a possible fungal sinusitis was sent to the laboratory for culture. You observe blue-green powdery colonies on the Sabouraud dextrose agar (SDA). You prepare a lactophenol cotton blue wet mount and observe septate hyphae, smooth conidiophore, and uniseriate phialides covering the upper two-thirds of a flask-shaped vesicle. What is your presumptive identification of this mold species?

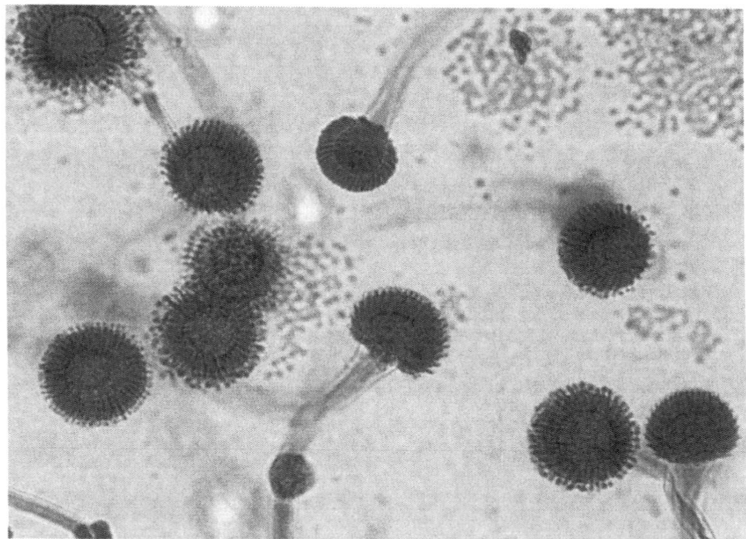

a. *Aspergillus flavus*
b. *Aspergillus fumigatus*
c. *Aspergillus terreus*
d. *Aspergillus niger*

45. A woman returns to the United States from a trip to Brazil and develops a fever, fatigue, and body aches. She visits her physician's office, where a CBC and influenza test are ordered. Upon examination of the peripheral smear, the following organism is observed. What is the identification?

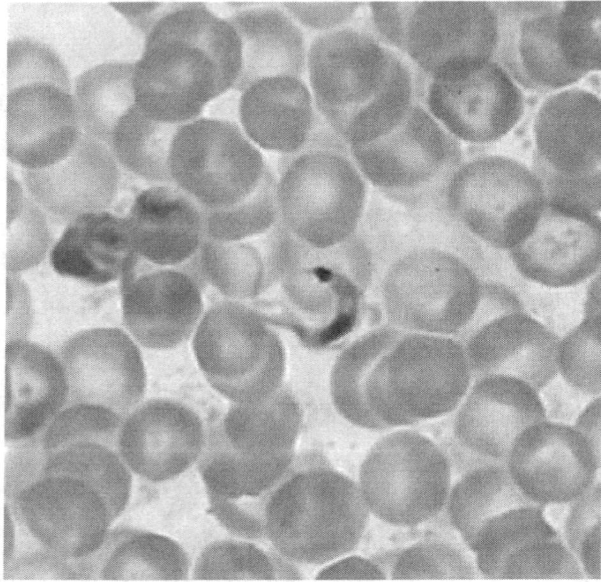

a. *Wuchereria bancrofti*
b. *Plasmodium falciparum*
c. *Trypanosoma cruzi*
d. *Leishmania braziliensis*

46. Which of the following is considered a National Notifiable Infectious Disease that must be reported to the CDC?

a. Southern tick-associated rash illness
b. Cat-scratch disease
c. Variant Creutzfeldt-Jakob disease
d. Powassan virus disease

47. Which of the following is the minimum requirement for quality control for quantitative testing under CLIA regulations?

a. Testing two levels of controls each day of patient testing
b. Testing three levels of controls each day of patient testing
c. Testing one level of control every 12 hours
d. Testing two levels of controls every 12 hours

48. What information in the safety data sheet (SDS) for any given hazardous chemical is considered nonmandatory?

a. Accidental release measures
b. Ecological information
c. Toxicological information
d. Physical properties

49. A maintenance procedure on one of your analyzers requires a clean cycle using a 5% bleach solution, but the laboratory only has an 8.5% concentrated bleach available. How much of the 8.5% bleach do you need to make 100 mL of a 5% bleach solution?

a. 87 mL
b. 59 mL
c. 55 mL
d. 50 mL

50. What can damage an objective lens on a microscope over time, rendering the lens useless?

a. 70% ethanol
b. Delicate task wipes
c. Immersion oil
d. Distilled water

Answer Key and Explanations

1. D: According to the FDA's final rule in 2015, the minimum hemoglobin concentration for a male allogeneic donor is 13.0 g/dL (130 g/L) and the minimum for a female allogeneic donor is 12.5 g/dL (125 g/L). The minimum hemoglobin concentration for an autologous donor is 11 g/dL (110 g/L).

2. B: If a laboratory is using FDA-approved storage containers, bacterial detection, and pathogen reduction devices, platelets can be stored at 20–24°C for a maximum of seven days. Platelets survive in vivo circulation for nine to ten days. Red blood cells preserved with an additive solution can be stored at 1–6°C for 42 days. Whole blood preserved with ACD/CPD/CP2D can be stored at 1–6°C for 21 days.

3. B: An antigen is considered a high-incidence antigen when it occurs in more than 99% of the population. Anti-Lu^b is an antibody to the high-incidence antigen Lu^b from the Lutheran blood group system. Anti-Lu^a is an antibody to the low-incidence antigen Lu^a from the Lutheran blood group system. Anti-Js^a is an antibody to the low-incidence antigen Js^a from the Kell blood group system. Anti-Kp^a is an antibody to the low-incidence antigen Kp^a from the Kell blood group system.

4. A: The direct antiglobulin test (DAT) is a serologic test used to detect red blood cells (RBCs) coated with antibodies (IgG) or complement (C3d) in vivo. The indirect antiglobulin test (IAT), also called indirect Coombs test, is a serologic test used to detect RBCs coated with antibodies (IgG) or complement (C3d) in vitro. The antibody screen, also called the "antibody detection test," is used to determine if unexpected antibodies that could be incompatible with donor cells are present or absent in a patient's serum.

5. C: If you collect 5 mL of blood, the 24-hour total will be 18 mL, which represents 2.4% of the total blood volume:

$$\frac{18\text{ mL}}{750\text{ mL}} \times 100\% = 0.024 \times 100\% = 2.4\%$$

This falls within the 2.5% limit. If you collect 8 mL of blood, the 24-hour total will be 21 mL, which represents 2.8% of the total blood volume, exceeding the limit. If you collect 6.5 mL of blood, the 24-hour total will be 19.5 mL, which represents 2.6% of the total blood volume, exceeding the limit. If you collect 7.5 mL of blood, the 24-hour total will be 20.5 mL, which represents 2.7% of the total blood volume, exceeding the limit.

6. A: Although the antibody anti-Le^b from the Lewis blood group system could potentially be clinically significant if it is reactive at 37 °C, it is clinically insignificant if it is not reactive at 37 °C. The other antibodies listed represent clinically significant antibodies from the Kell (anti-k), Kidd (anti-Jk^b), and Rhesus (anti-C) blood group systems.

7. C: The Society for the Advancement of Blood Management (SABM) states that at least one third of all patients scheduled for a non-emergent surgery have a treatable anemia. Laboratory evaluation of patients 30 days prior to surgery can help identify patients with treatable anemias and initiate treatment protocols to optimize hemoglobin values. The administration of epoetin alfa (Procrit®) is useful as a means of optimizing hemoglobin values for reduced transfusion need, but only when it is done in the weeks prior to surgery. Acute normovolemic hemodilution is an intraoperative procedure in which some of the patient's blood is removed, collected, and replaced with a volume expander to reduce cellular loss. Examples of volume expanders used during this procedure are Ringer's lactate, 5% albumin, 6% dextran, or 6% hetastarch. Sodium ferric gluconate is an example of an intravenous iron-replacement product and is not used as part of acute normovolemic hemodilution procedures. The administration of tranexamic acid is useful as a means of intraoperative reduction of blood loss by reducing fibrinolytic activity, but administration would be presurgical.

8. D: This image shows lemon-shaped uric acid crystals such as those that can be found in acidic urine. Uric acid crystals can also appear as barrels or needles. Triple phosphate crystals can be identified by their prism-like shape that is described as a "coffin lid" and typically occur in alkaline urine. Calcium phosphate crystals appear as needles and can be differentiated from uric acid crystals in needle form by polarization. Cholesterol crystals appear as notched rectangular shapes and can be found in both neutral and acidic urine.

9. B: *Trichomonas vaginalis* infections in males rarely cause symptoms, but when symptoms are experienced, they can include burning with urination, penile discharge, and inflammation of the prostate or epididymis. Inflammation of the epididymis can cause painful scrotal swelling. *Schistosoma haematobium* can cause testicular swelling, albeit rarely. Unless the patient has a history of travel outside of the United States, this parasite would be an unlikely culprit in this case. Epididymitis is usually caused by bacterial infections such as the sexually transmitted infections *Neisseria gonorrhoeae* and *Chlamydia trachomatis*. However, these organisms are not identified via urinalysis but instead through microbiological testing methods.

10. D: The fourth tube of CSF collected should be utilized for cell counts due to the likelihood the first three tubes have of contamination with peripheral blood during a traumatic tap. If only three tubes are collected, then the third tube will be used for cell counts first and the remainder shared for chemistry testing. The second tube is generally reserved for microbiology testing and the primary tube for non-routine testing.

11. C: Bacterial meningitis results in decreased glucose, increased protein, and increased lactate. CSF glucose metabolism can be caused by the presence of bacteria, white blood cells, or tumor cells. Decreases in CSF protein are not usually clinically significant, and increases are associated with bacterial meningitis, brain abscess, brain tumors, multiple sclerosis, Guillain-Barré syndrome, and syphilis. CSF lactate will be increased with a bacterial or fungal infection, while it will remain normal or will be only slightly elevated with a viral infection.

12. C: Impaired glucose tolerance is defined as a fasting glucose of 100–125 mg/dL and a 2-hour postprandial glucose of 140–199 mg/dL and is indicative of prediabetes. Normal glucose tolerance results are defined as a fasting glucose of <100 mg/dL and a 2-hour postprandial glucose of <140 mg/dL. Hyperglycemic (diabetic) glucose tolerance results are defined as a fasting glucose of >126 mg/dL and a 2-hour postprandial glucose of >200 mg/dL.

13. B: Postprandial triglycerides will be increased. Postprandial total cholesterol, high-density lipoprotein (HDL), and low-density lipoprotein (LDL) will be decreased.

14. B: Based on the marked elevation of alkaline phosphatase (ALP) and elevated direct bilirubin (DB), this patient could have cholestasis (decreased bile flow, such as that which occurs with a biliary obstruction). ALP levels can increase to 3–4 times normal values in the first couple days of a biliary obstruction. Cholestasis also shows an increase of direct bilirubin (DB) of >50% of the total bilirubin (TB) and normal or mildly elevated aspartate transaminase (AST) and alanine transaminase (ALT). Acute viral hepatitis will show marked elevation of AST and ALT, of >500 U/L, with normal or slight elevation of ALP. Sickle cell anemia will show marked elevation of total bilirubin due to hemolysis and usually normal levels of liver enzymes. Hepatocellular carcinoma will show mild elevation of AST and ALT, usually <300 U/L, and can have normal or elevated total bilirubin.

15. D: Albumin is the most abundant plasma protein and the primary contributor to the osmotic pressure of blood. This is in part due to the large molecular weight of albumin. The pressure created by the proteins in the blood is also referred to as the "blood colloidal osmotic pressure" (bcop). While alpha globulin and immunoglobulin G are both plasma proteins that contribute to maintaining osmotic blood pressure, they are not the primary contributor. Fibrinogen is a protein that is primarily involved in blood clotting and hemostasis.

16. A: Ferritin is referred to as the iron storage protein because it stores iron and can release it into circulation or sequester excess iron. Transferrin is a protein that binds to iron, but it primarily functions as a transport for iron, not as iron storage. C-reactive protein is an acute phase reactant and nonspecific marker for inflammation. Gamma globulins are the proteins that make up antibodies produced by plasma cells.

17. B: A low pH, normal pCO_2, and low HCO_3 indicate metabolic acidosis. Respiratory acidosis would show a low pH, elevated pCO_2, and a normal HCO_3. Compensated metabolic acidosis would show a normal pH, low pCO_2, and low HCO_3. Compensated respiratory acidosis would show a normal pH, elevated pCO_2, and elevated HCO_3.

Normal Reference Ranges:
pH: 7.35–7.45
pCO_2: 35–45 mmHg
HCO_3: 22–26 mEq/L

18. C: Hyperventilation decreases pCO_2, in turn causing an increase in the ratio of HCO_3 to pCO_2 which leads to an increase in the pH and ultimately creates a respiratory alkalosis imbalance.

	pH	**pCO_2**	**HCO_3**
Metabolic alkalosis	↓	normal	↑
Respiratory acidosis	↓	↑	normal
Respiratory alkalosis	↑	↓	normal
Compensated metabolic alkalosis	<7.4	↓	↓

19. D: The appropriate dilution factor would be 1:5 because 85,000 divided by 5 is 17,000, which is well within the AMR. The other dilution factors would not dilute the sample enough to bring the hCG into the reportable range, and the test would have to be done yet one more time.

20. B: The parathyroid glands release parathyroid hormone (PTH) in response to low calcium levels in order to maintain calcium homeostasis. PTH triggers calcium resorption from bone, the kidneys, and the intestines. Adrenocorticotropic hormone (ACTH) is produced by the anterior pituitary gland and triggers the adrenal cortex to then release cortisol and androgens. Biotin is vitamin B7 and is not involved in calcium homeostasis. Insulin-like growth factor 1 (IGF-1) is a hormone that stimulates protein synthesis and bone growth.

21. D: Vitamin K deficiency causes decreases in prothrombin as well as other clotting factors. This can cause defective clotting and prolonged bleeding. Vitamin C and riboflavin (vitamin B_2) deficiencies do not affect coagulation factors. Choline is an essential nutrient, but it does not affect coagulation factors.

22. A: Transferrin is a protein that transports iron. In the normal process of erythrocyte degradation, iron is recycled and transported back to the bone marrow by transferrin. Hepcidin is a hormone that regulates the GI tract's absorption of iron as well as the release of iron from the spleen. Haptoglobin is a protein that removes extracellular hemoglobin from circulation. Ferritin is a protein that stores iron.

23. D: EPO (erythropoietin) is produced by the kidneys in response to hypoxemia, stimulating the bone marrow's production of erythrocytes. ADH (Antidiuretic hormone) is a hormone produced by the hypothalamus that regulates water retention and excretion through the kidneys. Aldosterone is a hormone produced by the adrenal glands located on top of the kidneys. It plays a role in both blood pressure and electrolyte regulation. IGF-1(insulin-like growth factor) is a hormone produced by the liver that stimulates growth.

24. B: The NK (natural killer) cell is a product of the differentiation of the common lymphoid progenitor cell. Megakaryocytes, erythrocytes, and promonocytes are all products of the differentiation of common myeloid progenitor cells.

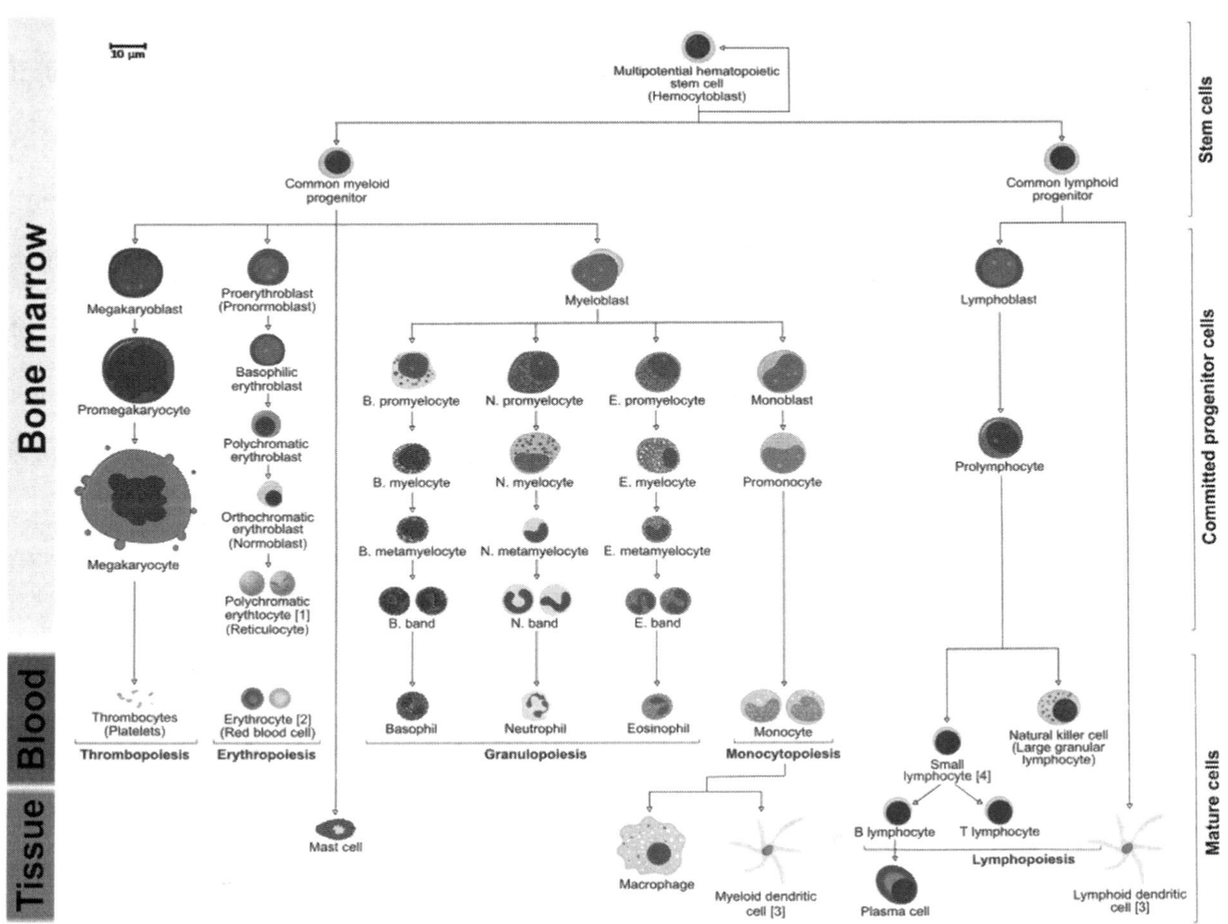

25. B: Polycythemia vera is a type of myeloproliferative neoplasm in which there is an overproduction of erythrocytes, thrombocytes, and leukocytes, or sometimes just erythrocytes. Therapeutic phlebotomy treatment to remove excess erythrocytes puts the patient at increased risk of developing iron deficiency anemia due to the increased loss of iron through phlebotomy. Sideroblastic anemia affects the body's ability to utilize iron to produce hemoglobin, resulting in iron deposits. Megaloblastic anemia is caused by impaired DNA synthesis, which can develop due to deficiencies in vitamin B_{12} or folate. Pernicious anemia is caused by a lack of vitamin B_{12} that leads to a decrease in the production of erythrocytes.

26. A: Thrombotic thrombocytopenic purpura (TTP) causes mechanical damage to erythrocytes due to the aggregation of platelets and resulting microvascular thrombi. This makes the presence of schistocytes a key finding on the peripheral slide for the diagnosis of TTP. Small numbers of schistocytes can also be present in normal samples, as well as in patients with diseases such as chronic renal failure and diabetic microangiopathy. They are also commonly found in patients with prosthetic heart valves. Sickle cell anemia's key morphological finding is, as the name suggests, sickle-shaped erythrocytes. G6PD deficiency is an RBC enzymopathy that results in a normocytic, normochromic anemia with no specific morphological findings. Hereditary spherocytosis is associated with morphological findings of spherocytes, acanthocytes, and polychromatophilic macrocytosis.

27. D: Iron deficiency will show low iron levels, high TIBC (total iron binding capacity), low iron saturation, and a low ferritin level. Anemia of chronic disease will show low iron levels, TIBC, and iron saturation and a normal or high ferritin level. Hemochromatosis will show high iron levels, low TIBC, high iron saturation, and high ferritin. Vitamin B_{12} deficiency can show all normal values, or it can possibly show high iron, low TIBC, high iron saturation, and high ferritin.

28. C: The cell described is a reactive lymphocyte. A prominent feature of the cytoplasmic projections of reactive lymphocytes is the deep blue basophilic staining seen at the edges that hug the surrounding cells. Monocytes have abundant, light blue-gray cytoplasm, sometimes with vacuoles. The nucleus may vary in shape, but it is often folded or convoluted in appearance, with loose, lacy chromatin. Large lymphocytes have abundant, pale blue cytoplasm, occasional azurophilic granules, and dense, clumped nuclear chromatin. Plasma cells are usually round to oval in shape, with a round or oval nucleus that is located eccentrically in the cytoplasm. The cytoplasm is deep blue. There is a characteristic perinuclear halo (hof) and clumped chromatin in the nucleus.

29. A: A plasma electrolyte abnormality, such as high sodium, can affect hematocrit results, which can show a spuriously low MCHC and a normal or high MCV. A possible solution to this problem would be performing a dilution of the specimen and repeating testing. Lipemia and severe leukocytosis can cause a spuriously high MCHC with a low to normal MCV. Solutions for these issues could be performing a dilution or a plasma replacement procedure. RBC agglutination can cause a spuriously high MCHC with a high MCV. Resolution of a possible cold agglutinin would involve warming the specimen to 37°C and repeating testing.

30. B: The Coulter Principle was developed by Wallace H. Coulter in the late 1940s. This technology allows for the counting and sizing of cells as measured by change in their electrical conductance. This principle is present in nearly all automated hematology cell counters. Some analyzers use hydrodynamic focusing to force cellular elements through a certain pathway. Fluorescence can be integrated into a hematology analyzer in order to detect variations in light emitted from dyed cellular components, enabling better white blood cell differentiation. Absorption spectrophotometry is a method of determining hemoglobin concentrations by measuring how much light is absorbed.

31. A: Prolonged prothrombin time will occur if a sodium citrate tube that is underfilled is used for testing. Sodium citrate chelates calcium, preventing the coagulation cascade. If the tube is less than 90% full, the concentration of sodium citrate is increased and more calcium is bound to the anticoagulant. This in turn means that less calcium is available for clot formation, ultimately prolonging the prothrombin time and the activated partial thromboplastin time.

32. B: Warfarin is an anticoagulant that inhibits the synthesis of vitamin K dependent clotting factors. Factors II, V, and IX are vitamin K dependent.

Vitamin K dependent	**NOT Vitamin K dependent**
Factor II (Prothrombin)	Factor I (Fibrinogen)
Factor V (Proaccelerin)	Factor III (Thromboplastin)
Factor VII (Proconvertin)	Factor IV (Ionized calcium)
Factor IX (Antihemophilic factor B)	Factor VIII (Antihemophilic factor A)
Factor X (Stuart-Prower factor)	Factor XI (Plasma thromboplastin antecedent)
Protein S	Factor XII (Hageman factor)
Protein C	Factor XIII (Fibrin stabilizing factor)
	vWF (von Willebrand factor)

33. C: IgM primarily exists as a pentamer—a structure composed of five monomers. This large structural formation is what gives IgM its high molecular weight. IgM can exist as a monomer but is expressed on the cell membrane of B lymphocytes. The other immunoglobulins all exist as monomers, and IgA exists in both monomer forms and dimeric forms. There are chemical quaternary polymers, but no immunoglobulin polymers exist in quaternary structure.

34. B: Type I hypersensitivity anaphylaxis is mediated by IgE. Type II hypersensitivity is mediated by IgG or IgM, as seen in blood transfusion reactions or autoimmune hemolytic anemia. IgA and IgD are not involved in any hypersensitivity reactions.

35. A: NK (natural killer) cells are able to kill tumor cells without prior activation. Cytotoxic T cells must be activated by antigen-presenting cells before they can kill tumor cells. Macrophages must be activated, such as with cytokines, in order to facilitate killing tumor cells. Mast cells are involved in the inflammatory response and are not involved in tumor immunity.

36. D: This pattern of test results indicates an acute hepatitis B virus (HBV) infection. The positive HBsAg result is a marker of a current contagious infection, and the positive HBc IgM Ab shows it is acute. Other results that can be positive during an acute HBV infection include HBcAb as well as HBV DNA and HBe Ag. Other patterns of HBV status:

	Chronic HBV	**Immune; post-vaccination**
HBsAg	+	–
HBsAb	–	+
HBc total Ab	+	–
HBc IgM Ab	–	–

37. D: The first-line screening test for infection with *Borrelia burgdorferi,* the causative agent of Lyme disease, is the *B. burgdorferi* total antibodies by ELISA (enzyme-linked immunosorbent assay). However, false positive results are possible due to other *Borrelia* species or other spirochetes. A positive or indeterminate result from ELISA testing should be followed by a confirmatory test such as a Western blot assay or immunoblot assay. If it has been ≤4 weeks since disease onset, *B. burgdorferi* IgG and IgM Ab by immunoblot would be recommended. If it has been >4 weeks, then only the IgG Ab by immunoblot needs to be tested. *Borrelia* species PCR assays can be utilized when there is a high clinical suspicion of Lyme disease but there are also negative serologic assays. PCR assays are most often used for identification of *Borrelia* species DNA in tick specimens.

38. B: *Toxoplasma gondii* is a protozoan parasite whose definitive host is the domestic cat. It is the causative agent of toxoplasmosis. Infected cats shed oocysts in their feces, which can then infect humans. Symptoms can occur within 5–23 days after infection. *Toxoplasma gondii* can be spread to the developing fetus via the placenta, which can result in miscarriage or in the fetus being born with congenital toxoplasmosis and thereby experiencing long-term health issues. *Bartonella henselae* is spread by cats with fleas and is the causative agent of cat-scratch disease, while *Bartonella quintana* is spread by body louse and is the causative agent of trench fever. *Francisella tularensis* primarily infects rabbits and rodents and can be transmitted to humans via tick or deer fly bites. It is the causative agent of tularemia. *Yersinia pestis* is spread by infected fleas from rodents and is the causative agent of the plague.

39. B: Throat cultures are primarily performed to identify group A *Streptococci*, specifically *S. pyogenes*. Sheep blood agar is the appropriate medium for culturing group A *Streptococci*, which will exhibit β-hemolytic colonies. MacConkey agar is a selective medium that favors growth of Gram-negative bacteria, so this would not be a good choice for a throat culture. Chocolate agar is made by heating and lysing sheep blood and therefore is an appropriate medium for evaluating β-hemolysis. Modified Thayer-Martin agar is a selective medium for isolating *Neisseria* species.

40. C: *Campylobacter jejuni* are Gram-negative bacilli that are microaerophilic and thermophilic. The optimum incubation conditions for recovering this organism are a temperature of 42°C and an atmosphere of 5% oxygen, 10% carbon dioxide, and 85% nitrogen. *Mycobacterium tuberculosis* and *Neisseria gonorrhoeae* are obligate aerobes. *Clostridium perfringens* is an obligate anaerobe.

41. A: The Kirby-Bauer test, also known as the disk diffusion test, is used to determine the antibiotic sensitivity of an organism. Lactose fermentation can be determined using the ONPG (ortho-nitrophenyl-β-D-galactopyranoside) test. Indole production can be determined by performing an indole test using Kovac's reagent. Decarboxylation can be determined using the arginine decarboxylase test or the lysine decarboxylase test.

42. C: Enterohemorrhagic *Escherichia coli* (EHEC) are a group of bacteria that produce shiga toxins and shiga-like toxins. EHEC are the primary cause of bloody diarrhea, with *Escherichia coli* O157:H7 being the most common. The MacConkey agar with sorbitol is a partially selective medium for the isolation of *Escherichia coli* O157:H7, which will grow in colorless colonies due to its inability to ferment sorbitol. Final identification requires serologic or molecular confirmation because this method does not differentiate between toxin-producing from non-toxin-producing strains and there are other organisms that can grow on this medium that do not ferment sorbitol. The MacConkey agar with sorbitol also includes bile salts and crystal violet, inhibiting the growth of Gram-positive organisms such as *Clostridium difficile* and *Staphylococcus aureus*. *Shigella dysenteriae* serotype 2 ferments sorbitol, so it would appear as pink colonies on this medium.

43. D: *Pasteurella* species are small, Gram-negative coccobacilli which can be transmitted via dog saliva. *Bartonella* species are Gram-negative bacilli or coccobacilli. *Bartonella henselae* can be spread via a cat scratch. *Actinomyces* species are Gram-positive bacilli that can represent normal flora of the human oral cavity. *Corynebacterium* species are Gram-positive bacilli the majority of which are nonpathogenic, but the genus also includes *C. diphtheria*, which is the causative agent of diphtheria.

44. B: *Aspergillus fumigatus* is the most likely identification of this mold species based on the macroscopic and microscopic morphological descriptions provided. *A. fumigatus* is the most common cause of fungal sinusitis, allergic aspergillosis, invasive aspergillosis, and aspergilloma ("fungus ball"). The second most common cause of invasive aspergillosis is *Aspergillus flavus*, which is sometimes mistaken for *A. fumigatus*. On SDA, *A. flavus* produces yellow-green colonies, often with white border. It can be differentiated from *A. fumigatus* on microscopic examination by its globose vesicle covered with uniseriate or biseriate phialides. Less common disease-causing *Aspergillus* species include *A. terreus* and *A. niger*. *A. terreus* can cause disseminated disease and produces beige to cinnamon brown colonies on potato dextrose agar. Its microscopic morphology includes mostly globose or dome-shaped vesicles with the upper halves covered in biseriate phialides. *A. niger* can cause aspergilloma, and it produces colonies that are white initially but then turn black due to the pigment in the conidia. On microscopic examination, *A. niger* shows a globose vesicle, biseriate phialides, and conidia with brown to black pigmentation. Confirmatory identification of mold species can be performed using matrix-assisted laser desorption ionization time-of-flight mass spectrometry (MALDI-TOF MS).

45. C: *Trypansoma cruzi* is a vector-borne parasite transmitted by the triatomine bug ("kissing bug"), causing American trypanosomiasis ("Chagas disease"). This parasite is common in Mexico and Central and South America. *T. cruzi* can be differentiated from *T. brucei gambiense* on microscopic examination by two morphological features: *T. cruzi* has a large kinetoplast and is about the size of a red blood cell while *T. brucei gambiense* has a small kinetoplast and is two times the size of a red blood cell. *T. brucei gambiense* is spread by the tsetse fly and is endemic to West and Central Africa. It is the cause of African trypanosomiasis ("African sleeping sickness"). *Wuchereria bancrofti* is a vector-borne parasite that is transmitted by mosquitoes and causes lymphatic filariasis. This parasite can be found throughout Asia, Africa, the Western Pacific, and South America. The microfilariae of *W. bancrofti* are best isolated from blood collected at night and can be observed microscopically on a smear as a large, curved body with a posterior end that is tapered to a point and an anterior end that is rounded or blunt. *Plasmodium falciparum* is one of four vector-borne parasites that cause malaria in humans. *P. falciparum* can be found throughout areas of Africa, Mexico, Central and South America, and Asia. On a peripheral blood smear, *P. falciparum* gametocytes have a crescent or banana shape, and the chromatin may be a single mass or diffuse. *Leishmania braziliensis* is a vector-borne parasite transmitted by the sand fly in areas throughout Africa, Mexico, Central and South America, and Asia. Identification of *L. braziliensis* is usually performed by skin scraping, where the amastigotes can be observed inside macrophages.

46. D: Powassan virus disease is considered a National Notifiable Infectious Disease that must be reported to the CDC. Powassan virus is a tick-borne arbovirus that can cause severe cases of encephalitis and meningitis. Southern tick-associated rash illness (STARI), cat-scratch disease, and variant Creutzfeldt-Jakob disease are all infectious diseases that are not on the CDC's list of nationally notifiable infectious diseases.

47. A: The minimum requirement set forth by CLIA for quality control for quantitative testing is two levels of control materials for each day of patient testing. More levels of controls or more frequent testing of controls may be required by the manufacturer for specific tests, and those frequency requirements would supersede the minimum CLIA requirement.

48. B: Ecological information (section 12) on an SDS is considered nonmandatory. This section provides information on environmental impacts should the chemical be released. Accidental release measures (section 6), toxicological information (section 11), and physical and chemical properties (section 9) all contain mandatory information.

49. B: The relationship between concentrations of solutions is shown by the following inverse proportion:

$$V_1 \times C_1 = V_2 \times C_2$$

V_1 = volume of starting solution
C_1 = concentration of starting solution
V_2 = volume of final solution
C_2 = concentration of final solution

Given this equation, the volume of 8.5% bleach needed to prepare 100 mL of a 5% bleach solution can be calculated by solving for V_1.

$$V_1 \times (8.5\%) = (100\text{ mL}) \times (5\%)$$

$$V_1 = \frac{(100\text{ mL}) \times (5\%)}{(8.5\%)}$$

$$V_1 = 58.8\text{ mL}$$

Since this is a cleaning procedure, 58.8 mL can be rounded to 59 mL. So, to make the solution, you need 59 mL of the 8.5% concentrated bleach diluted with water to a total volume of 100 mL in order to make a 5% solution.

50. C: If immersion oil is left on any of the objective lenses, including the 100x oil-immersion objective lens, it will eventually seep into the lens and render it useless. Oil is best absorbed by delicate task wipes rather than lens paper, which may just spread the oil around. Lenses can be cleaned with distilled water, lens cleaner, or 70% ethanol and lens paper. It is best to wipe off any oil from the objective lenses and clean the stage after each use. It is also important to protect the objective lenses from dust by using a dust cover on the microscope.

Image Credits

LICENSED UNDER CC BY-SA 3.0 (CREATIVECOMMONS.ORG/LICENSES/BY-SA/3.0/DEED.EN)

Hematopoiesis_(human)_diagram, by A. Rad,
(https://commons.wikimedia.org/wiki/File:Hematopoiesis_(human)_diagram_en.svg)

Uric acid crystals under microscope, by Doruk Salancı,
(https://commons.wikimedia.org/wiki/File:Uric_acid_crystals_(urine)_-_%C3%9Crik_asit_kristalleri_(idrar)_-_03.png)

LICENSED UNDER CC BY-SA 4.0 (CREATIVECOMMONS.ORG/LICENSES/BY-SA/4.0/)

Microscopy image of aspergillus fumigatus, by Antonio and Biagio and Cesare Arrigo,
(https://commons.wikimedia.org/wiki/File:Antonio_e_Biagio_e_Cesare_Arrigo_Aspergillus_fumigatus_01.jpg)

How to Overcome Test Anxiety

Just the thought of taking a test is enough to make most people a little nervous. A test is an important event that can have a long-term impact on your future, so it's important to take it seriously and it's natural to feel anxious about performing well. But just because anxiety is normal, that doesn't mean that it's helpful in test taking, or that you should simply accept it as part of your life. Anxiety can have a variety of effects. These effects can be mild, like making you feel slightly nervous, or severe, like blocking your ability to focus or remember even a simple detail.

If you experience test anxiety—whether severe or mild—it's important to know how to beat it. To discover this, first you need to understand what causes test anxiety.

Causes of Test Anxiety

While we often think of anxiety as an uncontrollable emotional state, it can actually be caused by simple, practical things. One of the most common causes of test anxiety is that a person does not feel adequately prepared for their test. This feeling can be the result of many different issues such as poor study habits or lack of organization, but the most common culprit is time management. Starting to study too late, failing to organize your study time to cover all of the material, or being distracted while you study will mean that you're not well prepared for the test. This may lead to cramming the night before, which will cause you to be physically and mentally exhausted for the test. Poor time management also contributes to feelings of stress, fear, and hopelessness as you realize you are not well prepared but don't know what to do about it.

Other times, test anxiety is not related to your preparation for the test but comes from unresolved fear. This may be a past failure on a test, or poor performance on tests in general. It may come from comparing yourself to others who seem to be performing better or from the stress of living up to expectations. Anxiety may be driven by fears of the future—how failure on this test would affect your educational and career goals. These fears are often completely irrational, but they can still negatively impact your test performance.

Review Video: 3 Reasons You Have Test Anxiety
Visit mometrix.com/academy and enter code: 428468

Elements of Test Anxiety

As mentioned earlier, test anxiety is considered to be an emotional state, but it has physical and mental components as well. Sometimes you may not even realize that you are suffering from test anxiety until you notice the physical symptoms. These can include trembling hands, rapid heartbeat, sweating, nausea, and tense muscles. Extreme anxiety may lead to fainting or vomiting. Obviously, any of these symptoms can have a negative impact on testing. It is important to recognize them as soon as they begin to occur so that you can address the problem before it damages your performance.

Review Video: 3 Ways to Tell You Have Test Anxiety
Visit mometrix.com/academy and enter code: 927847

The mental components of test anxiety include trouble focusing and inability to remember learned information. During a test, your mind is on high alert, which can help you recall information and stay focused for an extended period of time. However, anxiety interferes with your mind's natural processes, causing you to blank out, even on the questions you know well. The strain of testing during anxiety makes it difficult to stay focused, especially on a test that may take several hours. Extreme anxiety can take a huge mental toll, making it difficult not only to recall test information but even to understand the test questions or pull your thoughts together.

Review Video: How Test Anxiety Affects Memory
Visit mometrix.com/academy and enter code: 609003

Effects of Test Anxiety

Test anxiety is like a disease—if left untreated, it will get progressively worse. Anxiety leads to poor performance, and this reinforces the feelings of fear and failure, which in turn lead to poor performances on subsequent tests. It can grow from a mild nervousness to a crippling condition. If allowed to progress, test anxiety can have a big impact on your schooling, and consequently on your future.

Test anxiety can spread to other parts of your life. Anxiety on tests can become anxiety in any stressful situation, and blanking on a test can turn into panicking in a job situation. But fortunately, you don't have to let anxiety rule your testing and determine your grades. There are a number of relatively simple steps you can take to move past anxiety and function normally on a test and in the rest of life.

Review Video: How Test Anxiety Impacts Your Grades
Visit mometrix.com/academy and enter code: 939819

Physical Steps for Beating Test Anxiety

While test anxiety is a serious problem, the good news is that it can be overcome. It doesn't have to control your ability to think and remember information. While it may take time, you can begin taking steps today to beat anxiety.

Just as your first hint that you may be struggling with anxiety comes from the physical symptoms, the first step to treating it is also physical. Rest is crucial for having a clear, strong mind. If you are tired, it is much easier to give in to anxiety. But if you establish good sleep habits, your body and mind will be ready to perform optimally, without the strain of exhaustion. Additionally, sleeping well helps you to retain information better, so you're more likely to recall the answers when you see the test questions.

Getting good sleep means more than going to bed on time. It's important to allow your brain time to relax. Take study breaks from time to time so it doesn't get overworked, and don't study right before bed. Take time to rest your mind before trying to rest your body, or you may find it difficult to fall asleep.

Review Video: The Importance of Sleep for Your Brain
Visit mometrix.com/academy and enter code: 319338

Along with sleep, other aspects of physical health are important in preparing for a test. Good nutrition is vital for good brain function. Sugary foods and drinks may give a burst of energy but this burst is followed by a crash, both physically and emotionally. Instead, fuel your body with protein and vitamin-rich foods.

Also, drink plenty of water. Dehydration can lead to headaches and exhaustion, especially if your brain is already under stress from the rigors of the test. Particularly if your test is a long one, drink water during the breaks. And if possible, take an energy-boosting snack to eat between sections.

Review Video: How Diet Can Affect your Mood
Visit mometrix.com/academy and enter code: 624317

Along with sleep and diet, a third important part of physical health is exercise. Maintaining a steady workout schedule is helpful, but even taking 5-minute study breaks to walk can help get your blood pumping faster and clear your head. Exercise also releases endorphins, which contribute to a positive feeling and can help combat test anxiety.

When you nurture your physical health, you are also contributing to your mental health. If your body is healthy, your mind is much more likely to be healthy as well. So take time to rest, nourish your body with healthy food and water, and get moving as much as possible. Taking these physical steps will make you stronger and more able to take the mental steps necessary to overcome test anxiety.

Mental Steps for Beating Test Anxiety

Working on the mental side of test anxiety can be more challenging, but as with the physical side, there are clear steps you can take to overcome it. As mentioned earlier, test anxiety often stems from lack of preparation, so the obvious solution is to prepare for the test. Effective studying may be the most important weapon you have for beating test anxiety, but you can and should employ several other mental tools to combat fear.

First, boost your confidence by reminding yourself of past success—tests or projects that you aced. If you're putting as much effort into preparing for this test as you did for those, there's no reason you should expect to fail here. Work hard to prepare; then trust your preparation.

Second, surround yourself with encouraging people. It can be helpful to find a study group, but be sure that the people you're around will encourage a positive attitude. If you spend time with others who are anxious or cynical, this will only contribute to your own anxiety. Look for others who are motivated to study hard from a desire to succeed, not from a fear of failure.

Third, reward yourself. A test is physically and mentally tiring, even without anxiety, and it can be helpful to have something to look forward to. Plan an activity following the test, regardless of the outcome, such as going to a movie or getting ice cream.

When you are taking the test, if you find yourself beginning to feel anxious, remind yourself that you know the material. Visualize successfully completing the test. Then take a few deep, relaxing breaths and return to it. Work through the questions carefully but with confidence, knowing that you are capable of succeeding.

Developing a healthy mental approach to test taking will also aid in other areas of life. Test anxiety affects more than just the actual test—it can be damaging to your mental health and even contribute to depression. It's important to beat test anxiety before it becomes a problem for more than testing.

Review Video: Test Anxiety and Depression
Visit mometrix.com/academy and enter code: 904704

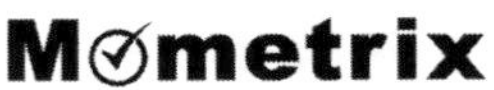

Study Strategy

Being prepared for the test is necessary to combat anxiety, but what does being prepared look like? You may study for hours on end and still not feel prepared. What you need is a strategy for test prep. The next few pages outline our recommended steps to help you plan out and conquer the challenge of preparation.

Step 1: Scope Out the Test

Learn everything you can about the format (multiple choice, essay, etc.) and what will be on the test. Gather any study materials, course outlines, or sample exams that may be available. Not only will this help you to prepare, but knowing what to expect can help to alleviate test anxiety.

Step 2: Map Out the Material

Look through the textbook or study guide and make note of how many chapters or sections it has. Then divide these over the time you have. For example, if a book has 15 chapters and you have five days to study, you need to cover three chapters each day. Even better, if you have the time, leave an extra day at the end for overall review after you have gone through the material in depth.

If time is limited, you may need to prioritize the material. Look through it and make note of which sections you think you already have a good grasp on, and which need review. While you are studying, skim quickly through the familiar sections and take more time on the challenging parts. Write out your plan so you don't get lost as you go. Having a written plan also helps you feel more in control of the study, so anxiety is less likely to arise from feeling overwhelmed at the amount to cover.

Step 3: Gather Your Tools

Decide what study method works best for you. Do you prefer to highlight in the book as you study and then go back over the highlighted portions? Or do you type out notes of the important information? Or is it helpful to make flashcards that you can carry with you? Assemble the pens, index cards, highlighters, post-it notes, and any other materials you may need so you won't be distracted by getting up to find things while you study.

If you're having a hard time retaining the information or organizing your notes, experiment with different methods. For example, try color-coding by subject with colored pens, highlighters, or post-it notes. If you learn better by hearing, try recording yourself reading your notes so you can listen while in the car, working out, or simply sitting at your desk. Ask a friend to quiz you from your flashcards, or try teaching someone the material to solidify it in your mind.

Step 4: Create Your Environment

It's important to avoid distractions while you study. This includes both the obvious distractions like visitors and the subtle distractions like an uncomfortable chair (or a too-comfortable couch that makes you want to fall asleep). Set up the best study environment possible: good lighting and a comfortable work area. If background music helps you focus, you may want to turn it on, but otherwise keep the room quiet. If you are using a computer to take notes, be sure you don't have any other windows open, especially applications like social media, games, or anything else that could distract you. Silence your phone and turn off notifications. Be sure to keep water close by so you stay hydrated while you study (but avoid unhealthy drinks and snacks).

Also, take into account the best time of day to study. Are you freshest first thing in the morning? Try to set aside some time then to work through the material. Is your mind clearer in the afternoon or evening? Schedule your study session then. Another method is to study at the same time of day that you will take the test, so that your brain gets used to working on the material at that time and will be ready to focus at test time.

Step 5: Study!

Once you have done all the study preparation, it's time to settle into the actual studying. Sit down, take a few moments to settle your mind so you can focus, and begin to follow your study plan. Don't give in to distractions or let yourself procrastinate. This is your time to prepare so you'll be ready to fearlessly approach the test. Make the most of the time and stay focused.

Of course, you don't want to burn out. If you study too long you may find that you're not retaining the information very well. Take regular study breaks. For example, taking five minutes out of every hour to walk briskly, breathing deeply and swinging your arms, can help your mind stay fresh.

As you get to the end of each chapter or section, it's a good idea to do a quick review. Remind yourself of what you learned and work on any difficult parts. When you feel that you've mastered the material, move on to the next part. At the end of your study session, briefly skim through your notes again.

But while review is helpful, cramming last minute is NOT. If at all possible, work ahead so that you won't need to fit all your study into the last day. Cramming overloads your brain with more information than it can process and retain, and your tired mind may struggle to recall even previously learned information when it is overwhelmed with last-minute study. Also, the urgent nature of cramming and the stress placed on your brain contribute to anxiety. You'll be more likely to go to the test feeling unprepared and having trouble thinking clearly.

So don't cram, and don't stay up late before the test, even just to review your notes at a leisurely pace. Your brain needs rest more than it needs to go over the information again. In fact, plan to finish your studies by noon or early afternoon the day before the test. Give your brain the rest of the day to relax or focus on other things, and get a good night's sleep. Then you will be fresh for the test and better able to recall what you've studied.

Step 6: Take a practice test

Many courses offer sample tests, either online or in the study materials. This is an excellent resource to check whether you have mastered the material, as well as to prepare for the test format and environment.

Check the test format ahead of time: the number of questions, the type (multiple choice, free response, etc.), and the time limit. Then create a plan for working through them. For example, if you have 30 minutes to take a 60-question test, your limit is 30 seconds per question. Spend less time on the questions you know well so that you can take more time on the difficult ones.

If you have time to take several practice tests, take the first one open book, with no time limit. Work through the questions at your own pace and make sure you fully understand them. Gradually work up to taking a test under test conditions: sit at a desk with all study materials put away and set a timer. Pace yourself to make sure you finish the test with time to spare and go back to check your answers if you have time.

After each test, check your answers. On the questions you missed, be sure you understand why you missed them. Did you misread the question (tests can use tricky wording)? Did you forget the information? Or was it something you hadn't learned? Go back and study any shaky areas that the practice tests reveal.

Taking these tests not only helps with your grade, but also aids in combating test anxiety. If you're already used to the test conditions, you're less likely to worry about it, and working through tests until you're scoring well gives you a confidence boost. Go through the practice tests until you feel comfortable, and then you can go into the test knowing that you're ready for it.

Test Tips

On test day, you should be confident, knowing that you've prepared well and are ready to answer the questions. But aside from preparation, there are several test day strategies you can employ to maximize your performance.

First, as stated before, get a good night's sleep the night before the test (and for several nights before that, if possible). Go into the test with a fresh, alert mind rather than staying up late to study.

Try not to change too much about your normal routine on the day of the test. It's important to eat a nutritious breakfast, but if you normally don't eat breakfast at all, consider eating just a protein bar. If you're a coffee drinker, go ahead and have your normal coffee. Just make sure you time it so that the caffeine doesn't wear off right in the middle of your test. Avoid sugary beverages, and drink enough water to stay hydrated but not so much that you need a restroom break 10 minutes into the test. If your test isn't first thing in the morning, consider going for a walk or doing a light workout before the test to get your blood flowing.

Allow yourself enough time to get ready, and leave for the test with plenty of time to spare so you won't have the anxiety of scrambling to arrive in time. Another reason to be early is to select a good seat. It's helpful to sit away from doors and windows, which can be distracting. Find a good seat, get out your supplies, and settle your mind before the test begins.

When the test begins, start by going over the instructions carefully, even if you already know what to expect. Make sure you avoid any careless mistakes by following the directions.

Then begin working through the questions, pacing yourself as you've practiced. If you're not sure on an answer, don't spend too much time on it, and don't let it shake your confidence. Either skip it and come back later, or eliminate as many wrong answers as possible and guess among the remaining ones. Don't dwell on these questions as you continue—put them out of your mind and focus on what lies ahead.

Be sure to read all of the answer choices, even if you're sure the first one is the right answer. Sometimes you'll find a better one if you keep reading. But don't second-guess yourself if you do immediately know the answer. Your gut instinct is usually right. Don't let test anxiety rob you of the information you know.

If you have time at the end of the test (and if the test format allows), go back and review your answers. Be cautious about changing any, since your first instinct tends to be correct, but make sure you didn't misread any of the questions or accidentally mark the wrong answer choice. Look over any you skipped and make an educated guess.

At the end, leave the test feeling confident. You've done your best, so don't waste time worrying about your performance or wishing you could change anything. Instead, celebrate the successful completion of this test. And finally, use this test to learn how to deal with anxiety even better next time.

Review Video: 5 Tips to Beat Test Anxiety
Visit mometrix.com/academy and enter code: 570656

Important Qualification

Not all anxiety is created equal. If your test anxiety is causing major issues in your life beyond the classroom or testing center, or if you are experiencing troubling physical symptoms related to your anxiety, it may be a sign of a serious physiological or psychological condition. If this sounds like your situation, we strongly encourage you to seek professional help.

Tell Us Your Story

We at Mometrix would like to extend our heartfelt thanks to you for letting us be a part of your journey. It is an honor to serve people from all walks of life, people like you, who are committed to building the best future they can for themselves.

We know that each person's situation is unique. But we also know that, whether you are a young student or a mother of four, you care about working to make your own life and the lives of those around you better.

That's why we want to hear your story.

We want to know why you're taking this test. We want to know about the trials you've gone through to get here. And we want to know about the successes you've experienced after taking and passing your test.

In addition to your story, which can be an inspiration both to us and to others, we value your feedback. We want to know both what you loved about our book and what you think we can improve on.

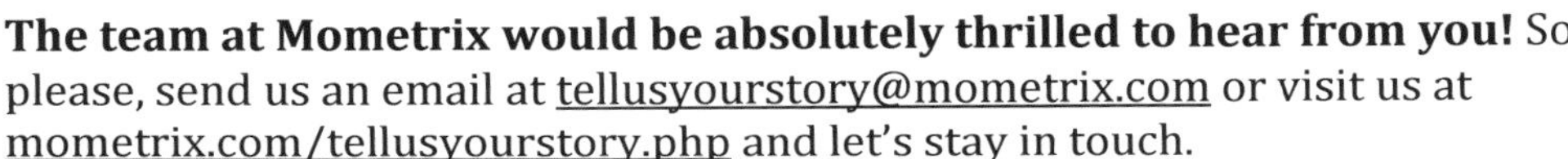

The team at Mometrix would be absolutely thrilled to hear from you! So please, send us an email at tellusyourstory@mometrix.com or visit us at mometrix.com/tellusyourstory.php and let's stay in touch.

Additional Bonus Material

Due to our efforts to try to keep this book to a manageable length, we've created a link that will give you access to all of your additional bonus material:

mometrix.com/bonus948/mlt